THE POLITICAL ECONOMY OF HEALTH CARE DEVELOPMENT AND REFORMS IN HONG KONG

To Naureen

The Political Economy of Health Care Development and Reforms in Hong Kong

VICTOR C.W. WONG
Department of Social Work
Hong Kong Baptist University

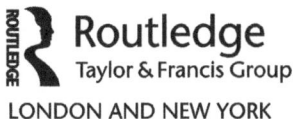

Routledge
Taylor & Francis Group

LONDON AND NEW YORK

First published 1999 by Ashgate Publishing

Reissued 2018 by Routledge
2 Park Square, Milton Park, Abingdon, Oxon, OX14 4RN
52 Vanderbilt Avenue, New York, NY 10017

Routledge is an imprint of the Taylor & Francis Group, an informa business

Publisher's Note
The publisher has gone to great lengths to ensure the quality of this reprint but points out that some imperfections in the original copies may be apparent.

Disclaimer
The publisher has made every effort to trace copyright holders and welcomes correspondence from those they have been unable to contact.

A Library of Congress record exists under LC control number: 98074643

ISBN 13: 978-1-138-33768-8 (hbk)
ISBN 13: 978-1-138-33773-2 (pbk)
ISBN 13: 978-0-429-44220-9 (ebk)

Contents

List of Tables

Acknowledgements

This book has originated from my doctoral thesis submitted to the University of Sheffield. Among many individuals who have offered invaluable help and support throughout the process of completing this book, my first and foremost gratitude goes to Professor Alan Walker. He supervised this study as my research supervisor and provided a wealth of ideas on the subjects I pursued in this book. His comments are sharp, stimulating and insightful. I am indeed very much indebted to his kindness to write for me the foreword of this book.

I would like to express my sincere thanks to David Phillips. In addition to valuable suggestions and comments on this work, he has strengthened my grasp of research issues raised in social sciences. I thank him for his valuable suggestions and support.

Thanks are due to all the persons I interviewed for their opinion on the different aspects of health care reforms in Hong Kong.

My whole-hearted thanks and gratitude must go to Sammy Chiu who encouraged me to embark on a doctoral study, and who has been my comrade in the movement for social reforms in Hong Kong since the mid-1980s.

I owe a special and lasting gratitude to my companion Naureen whose love and support enabled me to go through the whole process of the study and the preparation of this book.

Thanks are also due to May Chan for her invaluable help in word processing.

I have to acknowledge that in spite of the efforts of all the above people, all mistakes or deficiencies of this book remain my responsibility alone.

Foreword

This book is a unique account of the development and reform of health care in Hong Kong. From its origins under British colonial rule to the latest debates about the impact of demographic change, rising public expectations and advances in medical science and technology Hong Kong's health care policy and institutions are subjected to sustained critical scrutiny. It is the most comprehensive analysis available of health care policy in Hong Kong and is bound to become a standard reference work for a wide range of scholars interested in Hong Kong, China, health policy, the sociology of health care and comparative social policy.

The main focus of the book is on policy developments since 1945 and Wong shows how successive governments developed health policy in both a capitalist and Chinese context, with an emphasis initially on charity hospitals and family responsibility and, following riots in 1966/67, the growth of public provision for those who could not afford private medical care but with a strong emphasis on rationing. Thus, rather than adopting a fully public health care system Hong Kong instituted a two-tier one. The limits to the expansion and improvement of public medicine were set by the priority given by government to economic development and the maintenance of a low tax policy. The latest chapter in health financing sees the government seeking to promote private health insurance, as part of a general policy of privatisation of Hong Kong's social services, with all the predictable consequences for the exclusion of the poor and high-risk groups and increasing health inequalities.

The importance of this book lies not only in the detailed record it provides of the development of health policy and institutions in Hong Kong, it is also a major work of political economy. Wong utilises the political economy perspective to demonstrate how the state interacts with the dominant interests of capital, the public demand for health care and the power of the medical profession in the formation of health policy. The book emphasises the role of the medical profession and critically examines the nature of medical power and how it has helped to shape health care development and reform. A further important and novel contribution of this book is the consideration it gives to the role of the family and Chinese medicine alongside that of formal medicine. Wong shows how policy makers view the family as a crucial element in cost containment in minimising the hospitalisation of frail and chronically sick patients. The discourses surrounding the introduction of support for family carers focus on the family as a 'free resource'. Similarly, the use of Chinese medicine is strongly reliant on family (female) care. Both 'traditional' Chinese medicine and family care are viewed as having a major role in tackling the escalating costs of health care resulting from high-tech western medicine and demographic change.

Victor Wong is to be congratulated for producing such an informative, engaging and accessible work of scholarship. It is a major contribution to the literature on health policy and a unique account of developments in this field in Hong Kong. It is with great pleasure and pride that I endorse it.

Alan Walker
University of Sheffield

Introduction

Health care policy is certainly one of the most significant components of public policies in developed countries. On average, annual expenditure on health care accounted for 8.1 per cent of Gross Domestic Product (GDP) in twenty-four OECD countries in 1992, and public health spending as a percent of GDP reached 5.9 per cent (OECD, 1996). In Hong Kong, the public and private sectors together spent 4.7 per cent of the GDP on health care in 1995. Of this, 2.1 per cent was public spending and 2.6 per cent was private spending (Wong, 1999). However, the government of Hong Kong believes that Hong Kong's annual expenditure on health care would be about 6 per cent of the GDP if public spending on infrastructural and supporting services were included (Hong Kong Government, 1993a). One of the biggest single cost items in the public health care system is the rental value of land used for health care facilities, which is almost treated as free (Hay, 1992). If this was taken into consideration, it would no doubt increase the proportion of public health spending. Merely from the sheer size of health care spending, the importance of health care policy can be realised.

Moreover, state provision of health care has been one of the earliest and most consistent forms of public policy in western countries (Leichter, 1979). Germany pioneered public health insurance in 1883 and Austria followed suit in 1888. The UK established the National Health Insurance Scheme for general practitioner care in 1911 and the National Health Service in 1948; and the US Medicare scheme specifically targeted to the elderly commenced in 1965 (Schneider, 1982). At present, there is no state among developed capitalist countries, which fails to provide some form of public health care for its citizens. The major concern instead is the extent of state intervention in health care. In Hong Kong, state intervention in health can be traced back to the beginning of the British colonial governance. Hong Kong became a British Colony in 1843, when the Treaty of Nanking was ratified. A government medical and health service was initiated in the same year with the appointment of a colonial surgeon and the establishment of a Committee of Public Health. The colonial surgeon was at first mainly responsible for meeting the health needs of the local British army force; whilst the task of the Committee was to create and enforce a code of sanitary rules for the protection of health (Endacott, 1958). With government subsidies and donations from prominent Chinese leaders and merchants, the first Chinese hospital, named the Tung Wah Hospital, began to operate in 1870 (Sinn, 1989). This also marked an important step in state financing of health care as well as hospital medicine for the local Chinese population. What is so special about this Chinese hospital is its original practice of Chinese medicine rather than Western medicine which was not well received by the local Chinese until almost the turn of the next century.

From 1901 the government gave a grant to the Hong Kong College of Medicine for the Chinese which had been set up in 1887 with the aid of western missionaries and local doctors to encourage the Chinese to train in Western medicine (Endacott and Hinton 1962). In about 1905, the name of the College was changed to Hong Kong College of Medicine, dropping 'for the Chinese' in order to admit students of other nationalities (Choa, 1981). This College finally became part of the University of Hong Kong. State involvement in the financing of doctors' training was accompanied by the slow development of medical facilities, like specialist hospitals for the treatment of infectious diseases, and maternity hospitals. As time went by, heavily subsidised Western medicine practised in public hospitals and clinics gained much more popularity among the local Chinese population. The slow but steady expansion of medical facilities was, however, interrupted by the Second World War. In the immediate post-war years, the government concentrated upon the restoration of basic health and sanitation infrastructures and the control of infectious epidemics. At the same time, hospital care and outpatient services also began to expand. With the publication of the first medical white paper published in 1964, the policy of providing low cost or free medical and personal health services was confirmed (Hong Kong Government, 1964).

Health Care Systems and Cost Containment

The health care policies of developed countries are, however, widely diverse and based upon different systems. For example, the 'National Health Service System' of the UK is characterised by its universal coverage and general tax financing. Before the implementation of the 'internal market' reform within the NHS, the government played the dual roles of financing and providing public health care to its citizens. In countries such as Germany and Japan, health care policies are based on the 'Social Insurance System'. One of the major features of this system is its compulsory universal coverage, generally within the framework of social security. In most cases, unlike the British NHS, those countries operating social insurance systems mainly restrict state involvement to the financing of health care, while private providers are responsible for health care delivery and have their health spending reimbursed from public medical insurance bodies. The US health care system is dominated by private insurance. This 'Private Insurance Dominant System' is characterised by limited public coverage, and the dominance of employer-based or individual purchase of private health insurance run on a voluntary basis. Most hospitals and clinics belong to either profit-making or non-profit-making private bodies, with few of them owned by the state. The role of the state is restricted to helping those who are most in need, for example, old people and the poor.

Most health care systems in the world rely on both state intervention and market competition, in terms of both financing and provision. The state may either finance or provide health care in some areas, while the rest is left to the market. For example, a small private sector exists alongside the NHS in the UK (Higgins, 1988). In the case of Hong Kong, the public sector takes care of 92.1 per cent of the inpatient workload; while the private sector provides about 82 per cent of primary medical care (Hospital Authority, 1995a). Thus, as far as inpatient services are concerned, state intervention is much more significant than market competition; and it is vice versa for outpatient services. Like the British NHS, the public health care system of Hong Kong is open to all citizens and is mainly financed by general taxation.

While the health care policies and health care systems of developed countries are widely different, health care reform has generally become their watchword nowadays. Demographic changes, rising public expectations and advances in medical science and technology - whether they are the real underlying reasons or not - are most often regarded by the states in developed countries as the dominant factors triggering the cost escalation of health care. For the state, the rising cost of health care, much of it funded from public purses, has been a major factor in the drive to keep public spending under control. Cost containment has become a highly touted national priority in many developed countries. Hong Kong is no exception to this trend in western societies.

There are lots of market-oriented measures available for the purpose of cost containment, both on the demand side and the supply side. Alternative cost containment measures like socialisation of pharmaceutical products and other medical products is, however, very unlikely (Waitzkin, 1983). Then, how do we look at the context and the dynamics of the health care reform? What kind of roles and forms of intervention do the state adopt in the reform? In what way does the reform change the financing and delivery of health care? How does the reform influence people's access to public medical services? These questions are indeed worth an in-depth examination in any study of health care reform since health care policy comes to play an increasingly important role in our everyday life.

The Political Economy Perspective

The study of state intervention in health care can be approached from different perspectives. One of this is the economistic or market-oriented perspective. The focuses of this perspective are on the analysis of market success and failure in health care, and the purely economic justifications of state intervention. However, one of the major weaknesses of this perspective is its inability to explain why many health care systems were already in place before the formulation of coherent economistic arguments, mainly developed by Culyer (1971), Evans (1984) and Fuchs (1974, 1986). Moreover, this perspective has overlooked the political dimension of state intervention in health care.

Viewed in this light, the political economy perspective provides a valuable framework for understanding how the polity, economy, and society shape public policy. The central problem of the political economy perspective is the manner in which the economy and polity interact in a relationship of reciprocal causation, affecting the distribution of social goods (Walton, 1979:9). Because of the dominance of public funding for health care, this area may be more subject than others to political dealings among competing interests. In addition to this 'political' dimension, the political economy perspective also emphasises the 'economic' part, i.e. the productive and reproductive elements inherent in the policy making process (Binney and Swan, 1990:168). In the final analysis, however, a distinction between these two elements is not always easy to maintain.

In the health care field, major contributions to a political economy framework have been made in the 1970s (Lichtman, 1971; Alford, 1972; Kelman, 1971, 1975; Turshen, 1975; Navarro, 1975, 1976; Renaud, 1975, 1977; Doyal, 1979). Bearing in mind that capitalism is the dominant political form in both developed and developing countries, these authors regard it as the principal analytical context for discussing the issues of health and health care. Some of the salient characteristics of health care systems in capitalist countries are the convention of defining health care and disease in terms of the clinical or medical model; and the predominance of hospital and curative medicine and heavy reliance on drugs and medical technology. Such a context is viewed as a fundamental barrier to a more positive definition of health and a positive concerted effort in health promotion and protection (Kelman, 1975; Turshen, 1977; Renaud, 1977).

The Political Economy of Health Care: Four Essential Components

Political economy analyses of health have commonly addressed ways in which the capitalist context and the needs of capitalism affect the health needs of the population. Under this perspective, health needs are defined in political terms with particular emphasis upon access to and control and struggle over the basic material and non-material resources that sustain good health (Baer, Singer and Johnsen, 1986). Leaving medical resource distribution entirely to the market mechanism would serve to perpetuate social inequalities, the divide between the privileged and the underprivileged (Navarro, 1976). One point to be emphasised is that political economy is not a conspiracy model. The peculiarity of the capitalist context is the prominence of the process of capital accumulation. From the standpoint of profit making, minimising production costs and maximising sale and profit are the rules of the game in capitalist societies, even though these features often lead to occupational accidents and diseases and serious environmental pollution affecting in general the health of the population (McKee, 1988).

Studying the role played by the state is central to the political economy perspective since the state has relative autonomy and power to mediate between the different classes of society, and ameliorate social conditions that could threaten the capitalist order (Urry, 1981). Although there is no need to run its activities on the logic of capital accumulation, the state has to observe their impact on overall production and reproduction - the 'economic' part of the political economy. It is common for the state to allocate resources to ensure the maintenance and growth of the economy. Offe and Ronge (1982:192) are of the view that the income of the state is dependent on the economy, and thus it has a 'general interest in facilitating' the growth of the economy in order to perpetuate itself. Therefore, while the state improves social conditions, it must simultaneously help to maintain the conditions for profitable capital accumulation. In this sense, the state has to confront the difficult dual tasks of satisfying political demands for health care and keeping their overall costs as low as possible. This shed light on the reason why the reform of health care is somewhat bounded by political constraints in achieving the purpose of cost containment.

The power of the state extends beyond the distribution of resources to the reproduction of social institution, e.g. in defining and redefining the role of the family. A less-developed area of great significance in the political economy of health or health care concerns the relationship and interplay between the state and the family in health care. One of the probable reasons for this underdevelopment may be a preoccupation with the formal health care system. Substantial developments have been made towards a political economy of ageing by studying the relationship between the state and the family, and the latter's role in the care of the elderly (Qureshi and Walker, 1986, 1989). As will be discussed in detail in Chapter 1, the vast bulk of health care that people receive does not come from the formal health care system but from the informal health care system of which the family plays a dominant role. Although the focus of this book is not on the informal health care system, the reform of public health care must consider the role of the state in maintaining and reproducing the role of the family in financing and providing health care.

The study of informal or alternative medicine presents another less-developed area of research in the political economy of health care. As a Chinese society, Hong Kong is characterised by the persistence of traditional Chinese medicine consumed in the form of non-institutional medicine and within the family context, despite the continuing dominance enjoyed by Western bio-medicine. Before the 1990s, the Hong Kong government did not endorse or encourage the use of Chinese medicine which persisted or even flourished as a result of the efforts of the private sectors of the society and the Chinese people's receptiveness to the underlying philosophy and practices of Chinese medicine (Lee, 1981). In the 1990s, the Hong Kong government has, however, taken more active measures to promote Chinese medicine. An examination of the political economy of health care development in Hong Kong cannot afford to overlook the ways the state has shaped the role of Chinese medicine.

Within the political economy perspective, the medical profession is considered to be crucial in the health care system and in health care policy development. There is ample evidence that the influence of the medical profession over health care policy has been substantial (e.g. Willcocks, 1967; Harris, 1969; Freidson, 1970; Ham, 1985; Harrison, Hunter and Pollitt, 1990; Smith, 1993). The medical profession has enjoyed dominance and power over other health care providers and practitioners (including Chinese medicine practitioners in the Hong Kong context) and the patients who are placed in a subordinate or inferior position (Nettleton, 1995). Alford (1972:164) considers doctors as the professional monopolists seeking to erect barriers to protect their control over research, teaching and health care delivery. The power of the medical profession is so strong that it is not unusual for it to be in either direct or indirect conflict with the state in the shaping of health care policy.

In summary, within the political economy perspective, the four essential components in the study of health care in capitalist countries are: the capitalist context; health needs; the state; and the medical profession. All this suggests that in the formulation of health care policy, the role of the state is important, but it has to consider the needs and context of capitalism, the political demands of its citizens for health care, and the power of the medical profession.

Health Consumption

The preceding discussion shows that the political economy perspective is especially relevant in providing a framework for understanding how the polity, economy and society shape the health care system. It is certain that in any political-economic analysis of health care reform, we must eventually consider the resources available for health consumption. Conceptually, health consumption may be considered as a process of consuming use-value pertaining to the satisfaction of health needs or wants. The market, the state, the family and charities are the four important sectors providing people use-value or the means to attain use-value. In the market sector, the consumption of health care is taken in a commodity form. That is, health care is bought and sold as a commodity like any others available in the market. The guiding value underlying market transactions is exchange value with the purpose of making a profit. In the family, however, health care is normally produced solely for its use-value and is not offered for market exchange among its members. The state may provide or finance health care in order that use-value can be consumed by its citizens without them facing undesirable financial barriers in meeting their health needs. Finally, charitable organisations also play a certain role in providing or financing medical care to the underprivileged even though their role has become less significant in many developed societies today (Ellencweig, 1992).

As the state is increasingly involved in health care, state financing has constituted one of the important means for patients' consumption of use-value to meet human needs in health. The application of radical cost-containment measures will surely imply a reduced level of consumption of state-subsidised health care. In addition, the state may utilise other sectors or agents, like the family, employers, insurers and charities to provide or finance health care to meet demands or needs for health consumption.

Methodology

The public health care system is conceptualised as having three important constituent elements, namely, access, financing and delivery. Focusing on the forms of state intervention in health care rather than the entire health system allows for a more in-depth analysis of the various changes with respect to the consumption of public medicine.

To legitimate the health care reforms, the state has to back them with justifications, even though some of them may not be acceptable to some politicians and the public. Those justifications specifically made for modifying access to health care, and the financing and delivery mechanisms of the public health care system are one of the focuses of the book. In addition, reforms have to confront political constraints, both from the public and the medical profession. These constraints affect the way the justifications are made on the one hand, and influence the process of health care reforms on the other. In summary, the examination of the political economy of health care reforms includes three basic dimensions that are closely related to one another: constraints, justifications and the forms of state intervention in health care.

As to the methodology of this study, literature review, conceptualisation, documentation and interviews with politicians and policy makers are employed. Documentation covers two areas, namely, documents and opinion surveys specifically on health care reform. The sources of documents are: the government and the Hospital Authority, the Hong Kong Medical Association, and the Health Panel of the Legislative Council respectively. Opinion surveys on health care reforms were mainly collected from Legislators, newspapers and concerned organisations responsible for undertaking the surveys.

To make the analysis more strongly grounded empirically, and to obtain first-hand information from the politicians about their opinion on the current health care reforms, and especially with respect to the forms of state intervention, interviews with six politicians were conducted between August 1993 to November 1994. Politicians here refer to the members of the Legislative Council of Hong Kong, which comprised 60 members between 1991/92 and 1994/95. In order to identify a representative sample of politicians, one legislator (who was also spokesperson on health care for his political party) from each of the five most influential political parties in Hong Kong at the time of interview (namely Democratic Alliance for Betterment of Hong Kong, Hong Kong Association for Democracy and People's Livelihood, Liberal Party, Meeting Point and United Democrats of Hong Kong), and one legislator who was elected from the Medical and Health Care Functional Constituency were selected to be interviewed. As regards the viewpoints and opinion of these Legislators, secondary sources were also used for the study.

I also interviewed three other persons who were not politicians but were responsible for making, advising on or implementing health care policy in Hong Kong, and they were the ex-Secretary for Health and Welfare, a member of the Health and Medical Development Advisory Committee and the Chief Executive of the Hospital Authority. Again, secondary sources were also employed to supplement the first-hand information collected during the interviews.

Plan of the Book

The first task is to attempt an analysis of the political economy of health consumption and the forms of state intervention in health care (Chapters 1 and 2), and the power and influence of the medical profession in health care (Chapter 3). These three chapters together provide the theoretical framework for the discussion and analysis made later. The second task is to critically examine two phases of health care development in Hong Kong before the era of health care reforms began, i.e. 1945-1966 and 1966 to the mid-1980s (Chapters 4 and 5). The discussion also provides a critical review of the background for analysing the important changes taking place since the era of health care reforms started in the mid-1980s. The next important task is to examine the reforming of access, financing and delivery of the public health care system and the furthering of informal health care via the promotion of family care and Chinese medicine (Chapters 6-9). The final task is to conclude the study (Chapter 10).

1 Conceptualisation of 'Resources' for Health Consumption

Introduction

Recently, the sociology of consumption has claimed particular attention (Saunders, 1985; Burrows and Marsh, 1992). Interest has been partially stimulated by works posing a challenge either to the Marxist approaches that reduce consumption to production (Bauman, 1988); or to the economistic approaches that separate or isolate consumption from production at all, as if the former was an entity itself (Swedberg, 1986, 1987). With respect to the sociology of consumption, it is recognised that the relationship between consumption and production is sociologically problematic (Warde, 1990), and that this must be examined in relation to how consumption is socially constructed in the wider societal context (Cheal, 1990).

A significant question pertaining to consumption is the examination of the available resources enabling or facilitating individual consumption. Again, in what way the major resource for consumption is conceptualised is ultimately itself a social construction. Different theoretical perspectives have different conceptions of 'resources' for consumption. To neo-liberals, the economy or the production sphere provides the goods and services that make consumption possible; while household production activities and household consumption are defined as being outside the economy. As long as the purchase of goods is completed, consumption as an economic activity is finished irrespective of whether the household or individual has actually consumed the goods or not. Viewed as an economic transaction, personal consumption is equated with purchasing in the market, or selling of goods or services to the consumers. This emphasises the importance of money income in enabling people to get the goods or services they want. The visible economy, represented in GDP,

11

indicates the degree of abundance of resources for consumption.

Nevertheless, such a perspective has recently been seriously challenged by social theory which does not perceive production activities as being limited to the visible economy. Production activities can take place in the 'informal or hidden economy' (Portes, Castells and Benton, 1989), and in the 'household economy' (Wilk, 1989). Moreover, in addition to the market or the commercial sector, the state today occupies a structural position in providing people the means for social consumption, or even directly produces the services by itself. Neo-liberals are not unaware of the significant position of the state in facilitating consumption because it is vested with the power to tax people. They are indeed very active in formulating economistic arguments to check 'undesirable' state intervention (Mishra, 1990). The economists generally consider state (public) and market (private) consumption as two typical forms of consumption (Donaldson and Gerard, 1993). Public consumption is understood to be equivalent to state intervention; while private consumption is understood to be equivalent to market competition.

There are two major criticisms of such a simple dichotomy. First, private consumption is heavily influenced by state policy. For example, tax concessions are used to subsidise private organisations in their provision of health care benefits to their employees (Busfield, 1990). The US is perhaps the best example to illustrate this point. Therefore, this seemingly private form of consumption is yet closely related to state intervention and the foregone resources or expenditure of the state. Second, feminists have identified the household unit as being important in providing use-values to satisfy the needs of family members (Kerr and Charles, 1986; Graham, 1984, 1987). To them, the family is placed in a strategic as well as a constrained location to meet the basic needs of its members.

Concerning the study of the political economy of health care, it is therefore essential to examine what kinds of resources are available for health consumption that is not necessarily restricted to one particular source or resource. The purposes of this chapter are two-fold. First, it provides a framework to understand how the state may shape and reshape the conceptualisation of resources for health consumption, and on what basis such an exercise may be justified. Secondly, I will examine in what ways the three selected important theoretical perspectives - liberal and neo-liberal theories, the Marxist and neo-Marxist perspectives, and feminist perspectives - define the relationship between consumption and production, designate the significance of consumption, and differ in their conceptualisation of the dominant resources for health consumption. These three perspectives are selected for discussion on the basis of their typical conceptualisation of the respective roles of the private wage, the social wage and unpaid domestic labour.

In the discussion of each of these perspectives, two important points will be critically examined: the major resource for enabling or facilitating health consumption, and the role of the state in health care. This chapter argues that the political economy of health care requires an expanded conceptualisation of resources for health consumption of which the private wage, the social wage and unpaid domestic labour are the three major elements. This does not mean that they are the only resources for health consumption. For example, charities and donations are also means for consumption (Wistow et al., 1994). But these three resources provide the basis on which further analysis can be made. The state may realise the reduction or containment of the social wage via promoting employer-based private health insurance, emphasising the role and responsibilities of families in taking care of their members, encouraging voluntary work and charity and so on. As regards health care reform, state policies are essentially concerned with the remix of resources for health consumption and the legitimation of such an exercise.

Liberal and Neo-liberal Theories

The 'Economy and Society' Perspective

The liberal theory of 'economy and society' was established mainly by the work of Parsons (Parsons, 1937; Parsons and Smelser, 1956). Within this theory, Parsons drew a sharp distinction between the economy and other sub-systems of the social system as a whole, namely, polity, kinship, and cultural and community organisations. The economy is characterised by production activities for market exchange or transactions; while the household unit is portrayed as a consumption unit. The productive market economy provides the goods or services to make it possible for individual household units to consume the commodities they want. To be more exact, the households are seen as passively consuming units, as the economy provides the means (i.e. in terms of salary or wage), and the goods or services for consumption.

As regards consumption, it is considered to be an expression of value commitments or cultural meanings that are shaped through the socialisation of the personality and the institutionalisation of cultural values (Holton and Turner, 1986). So, consumption activities do not take place within a vacuum, but are closely related to other sub-systems that have played an important role in defining or shaping the value(s) of consumption. However, this overlooks the dimension of power relations or the coercive manipulation exercised by the corporate and professional power. Busfield (1992) argues that in company health schemes it is the corporation that designs the package or chooses the type of insurance for its employees, and thus corporate power is decisive in determining how employees consume health care. Further, Parsons has often been criticised for overlooking the structural power enjoyed by the medical profession which secures the compliance of patients to a bio-medical regimen (Morgan, Calnan and Manning, 1985; Turner, 1988). Besides, unlike other commodities, health care has little or no identity value (Warde, 1992) that helps to reflect the value commitments people hold. Health care, like being confined in a hospital bed, is not valued for its own sake, but for what it does towards producing health.

Since the 'economy and society' perspective was developed in the context of a laissez-faire economy in the US, individual well-being is presumed to be closely related to the private wage that is realised through one's exchange of labour for a salary. Money incomes or personal incomes earned by breadwinners are considered essential in providing individuals and their families the means of financing their market consumption. This theory, therefore, assumes that individual income would totally go into the family purse for the sake of consumption. This has in fact largely ignored the dynamics within the family, and the impact that the overall social and economic context has been placed on it. Many critics, especially feminists, have challenged such a taken-for-granted assumption (Pahl, 1988; Edwards, 1981).

An overemphasis put on the private wage has underestimated the importance of other available resources that can make consumption possible. Households may have access to health care through other means, for example, by virtue of their rights as members of companies, communities or nation-states. In the case of fringe benefits provided by companies, it is not difficult to understand them as a component of the private wage received by an employee. However, the economy and society theory has not examined why the private wage should also be extended to the family member(s) of the employee who does/do not work for a salary. Further, the private wage is not immune from state subsidies. Titmuss (1976), in his study of the division of welfare in society, has already highlighted how occupational and fiscal welfare are related to state policies. Non-working members of a specific community may benefit from the provision of subsidised health care on the basis of mutual-aid; while the citizens of a country may be entitled to health care operated on the citizenship principle. Moreover, production activities are not limited to the economy; the family may provide health care to its members through self-help. That is, both production and consumption activities can take place within the household.

After such a brief and critical discussion of the economy and society theory, three points can be summarised here. First, this perspective cannot provide a broader basis on which to conceptualise the resources for health consumption. Second, a rigid separation of production from consumption has overlooked the complexity of the processes of production and consumption. Third, as far as consumption is concerned, the private purse tends to be wrongly equated to the family purse. Although the Parsonian conception of the relationship between economy and society has been largely discarded within academic circles (e.g. Giddens, 1984), such a dual conception or dichotomy can still have important influences within policy-making circles. It seems that putting an equal sign between personal income and family income is an available excuse for the state to shift more its financing responsibility in social services back to the family - even though the consumers of public services are not the family breadwinners, or wage earners by themselves.

The Respective Role of the State and the Market

The focus of classical economic theory is certainly on the market. Adam Smith (1985), in his book, *An Inquiry into the Nature and Causes of the Wealth of Nations*, considered market exchange as being primary in the generation of wealth. Although the role of the state is somewhat secondary with respect to this purpose, the authority exercised by the state had in his view a positive contribution to make. However, the role of the state should only be limited to providing basic public works and public institutions, like roads and canals as cited by Smith. However, he did not single out health care and discuss it with reference to the market economy and the limited role of the state in this field (Reisman, 1993).

According to the laissez-faire philosophy of Smith, neo-liberals believe that market principles should be largely applied to health care if the goals of efficiency and freedom of choice are to be achieved. In their opinion, state intervention in health care should only be limited to public health measures and subsidies for the poor (Donaldson and Gerard, 1993). To better understand the standpoint of neo-liberals, we have to examine the meanings of externalities and public goods on which they 'legitimately' justify public health interventions.

Industrial pollution of the air and water are the most common problems of externalities. Such externalities or negative spillovers arise because 'economic agents take into account only the direct effect upon themselves, not the effect on others' (Atkinson and Stiglitz, 1980:7-8). Externalities are, therefore, undesirable side effects generated by the economic agents on the society as a whole. On the other hand, public goods are one of the externalities generating social side effects, whose provision or consumption is both non-rival (one's consumption does not preclude other's consumption) and non-excludable (one's consumption actually forces others' consumption) (Knapp, 1984:93). Some public health interventions, like sanitation works, disease-control programmes, health-promotion campaigns, are some examples of public goods that may help to reduce the side effects of negative externalities. 'Free-riders' of such programme benefits cannot be excluded, while the beneficiaries cannot be forced to pay. Public goods have to be provided by the state in order that the whole community can enjoy the benefits which cannot be guaranteed by the market.

Significant externalities are also associated with communicable diseases. If a person is infected with such a disease, but incapable of consuming health care, the presence of his illness will generate diswelfare to others. The free treatment of this person's illness would, therefore, be beneficial to the whole community. Since unregulated markets do not account for individual's willingness to pay for such external benefits, merely relying on the forces of market competition will lead to the generation of ill-health or externalities in the community.

The provision of certain preventive health care, like vaccination and immunisation programmes are also justified by the neo-liberals on the basis of externalities. That means an individual's consumption of public health care has direct effects on reducing the risk he or she has to face in contracting a particular disease, and on reducing the probability of others getting it as well. Neo-liberal economists are of the view that the external benefits from the type of health care provided in developed economies are relatively small nowadays. They argue that the treatment of communicable diseases is the only form of personal health care that confers external benefits, but since communicable diseases are now fairly rare, the scope of health care to be financed through competition or the market should be expanded (Green, 1986).

In addition to public health interventions, the neo-liberals' response to the criticism of the inequitable market distribution of health care is to give subsidies to the poor so as to facilitate their entry to the health care marketplace. Certainly, health consumption can be made possible by means of the provision of free public medicine by the state. However, the neo-liberals are particularly against such an arrangement. First, enhancing the market power of the poor can allow them to choose insurance plans they prefer. Free public medicine provided to the needy is supposed to restrict rather than expand their freedom. Second, competition among health insurers and providers in the market can in the long run drive down the prices of medical care and make consumers' demand heard. As will be discussed in detail in Chapter 2, there are still many other ways available for state intervention in health care.

Neo-liberals have clearly identified the state as one of the sources for providing its citizens public health, and financing those most in need to consume personal health care. Their final analysis is that market competition should play the primary role, and state intervention the secondary role in the distribution of resources. So, state resources available for health consumption should be limited to those areas where the market cannot function efficiently, and to those target groups who cannot provide for themselves. However, the economistic theories have underestimated if not overlooked the political dimension of health care. Again, like the economy and society theory, neo-liberal beliefs presume on the predominance of private wages in financing health consumption. But that can hardly be the case for those who are not eligible for public subsidies, but at the same time who are either not engaged in the labour market for a wage, or who are only engaged in a minor way. They must in some way or other depend upon resources furnished from other sources. Except in the way of explicitly identifying the relatively marginal role of the state in health care, neo-liberals share with the Parsonian society and economy theory the same restricted conception of resources for health consumption. Despite this, the arguments of neo-liberals have been used by many of the governments of developed nations to justify their attempts to emphasise personal and family responsibility in financing health consumption, and to 'effectively' contain the rising cost of health care.

Marxist and Neo-Marxist Perspectives

Marx's Framework for Understanding the Relationship between Production and Consumption

These two interrelated perspectives are the main rivals to the liberal and neo-liberal notions. Marx's model of economic processes is different from the simple dichotomy of production and consumption constructed by the 'economy and society' theory. Marx (1970) added in distribution and circulation (or exchange) between production and consumption. To him, production is the creation of commodities from raw materials. Distribution refers to the process according to which individuals receive a proportion of the commodities produced. Exchange is the process by which the buyers get the commodities they want via the generalised exchange medium of money, or by which the sellers get their profit. Consumption, then, refers to the use of goods or commodities to satisfy individual needs. In Marx's model, consumption is the final stage of a production/consumption episode. These four stages are ordered in a linear sequence of transforming natural resources to specific use values finally consumed by a particular individual. As Marx (1970:194) states, 'production represents the general, distribution and exchange the particular, and consumption the individual case'.

As regards health care or medical care, it can be provided in the form of either material products or services. For example, we can buy non-prescribed medicines or drugs over the counter. The four economic phases of a production/consumption episode do not necessarily come up with a final consumption of health care in a material form. Instead, most health care organisations and professionals are engaged in the production and provision of services rather than goods, like contact with a physician in an ambulatory care setting, and admission to the inpatient service of a hospital.

In Marx's framework, it is the mode of production, rather than the forces of production or any other economic factors, which ultimately determines the distribution and consumption of commodities, whether adequate or not. Underlying the capitalist mode of production is the relations of production between capital and the proletariat which shape the pattern of consumption. Therefore, the ultimate concern of Marx is still on production, and consumption is ultimately reduced to production even though the former is included as the final phase of a production/ consumption episode.

Within the context of the capitalist mode of production, Marx argued that individual consumption is merely for the reproduction of labour which remains an aspect of the reproduction of capital. Labour power refers to the individual's capacity to work which acts as one of the important inputs to the production process and in exchange for which the employer pays the wage. Labour is but a commodity which can be sold and bought in the market and be exploited by capital.

However, there are two major points of criticism of the reduction of (market) consumption to the reproduction of labour. First, for certain groups of population, consumption activities may be just for the sake of reproduction or maintenance of health, rather than reproduction of labour for sale in the labour market, for example, the disabled, the unemployed, older people and housewives. These groups may be willing to 'sell' their labour for a money wage, but they usually confront almost insurmountable difficulties to enter into the labour market. Second, some activities of individual consumption may even dissolve labour, for example, cigarette smoking and heavy drinking. All these activities may be useful for the purpose of the reproduction of capital as big profits can be made out of them; but they are more susceptible to reducing the productivity of labour rather than reproducing it. So, it is not fair to consider the reproduction of labour as being totally equivalent to the reproduction of capital.

Moreover, Marx's reduction of consumption to production has tended to ignore the relative autonomy of the state. Although his theory was especially critical to the classical political economy of Adam Smith, his theory shared one similar point with the latter: a minimal state and an unregulated economy, and the dominance of the private wage in the determination of the means of subsistence. All this is actually the context within which he made a savage critique against the nature of capitalism as an institution in the exploitation of labour and the proletariat. It needs to be borne in mind that Marx was writing at a time when the extent of state intervention was relatively small. It is, therefore, not surprising that Marx overlooked the role of the state in the provision or financing of welfare and health care.

Further, it is recognised that the family has played an important role in facilitating consumption, say, preparing meals and taking care of sick members. Individual consumption by non-working members of the family does not lead to any selling of labour power in the market. However, some Marxist writers are of the idea that the role of the private wage in the reproduction of labour is similar to that of the unpaid domestic work performed in the home (McIntosh, 1979; Bennholdt-Thomsen, 1981). That is, the private wage and unpaid domestic labour are considered to be functional for the reproduction of labour and then the reproduction of capital in capitalist societies. However, such an argument relies upon a form of functionalist reasoning, in which unpaid domestic work is explained by its functions for capitalism (Harris, 1983). This assumes that the boundary between the family and the state is taken for granted; but without realising the role played by the state in demarcating and shifting the boundary between the two sectors.

State-subsidised Consumption in the Eyes of Neo-Marxists

Unlike Marx, neo-Marxists have appreciated the role of the state in income redistribution, and as a financier or direct provider of social services. Castells (1973, 1978) introduced the concept of collective consumption to draw attention to the fact that some areas of consumption, like housing, education and health, were increasingly being organised by the state in advanced capitalism. Collective consumption as a form of state-subsidised consumption is the opposite to individual consumption of which the individuals are responsible for the financing of consumption. Also, the state may subsidise individual consumption in the market through tax allowances. So, with respect to collective consumption, the decisive factor is the extent of state involvement in the provision of the consumption facilities, and not at all the manner in which it is consumed. In recognition of the increasing importance of collective consumption in advanced capitalist nation-states, Castells has identified it as a new arena of conflict. One more point to be emphasised is that the conflict is no longer restricted to that between capital and labour, but also that between the state and the consumers of public services of which the latter are not necessarily the income earners.

According to Castells, another notable feature of collective consumption is that it is an important state strategy to reproduce labour on a collective basis. Under certain circumstances, there might be produced a deficiency of wages when compared with costs for consumption for the working class. In other words, despite the payment of wage, there exists a possible gap between the ability to pay and the needs of the working class (Dickinson and Russell, 1986). Castells argues that the provision of facilities for collective consumption is not amenable to provision by private markets - at least among low-income groups. The state may choose to intervene to provide these facilities to overcome the contradictions within the capitalist system that cannot sufficiently reproduce labour and ultimately capital itself (Castells, 1978; Preteceille and Terrail, 1985).

State provision of health care could indirectly facilitate the expansion of the economy in the reproduction of labour power or the provision of human capital both in terms of quantity and quality. The former refers to the number of workers provided, while the latter refers to the supply of healthy labour force. The supply of healthy labour in sufficient quantity was identified by Weisbrod et al. (1973:10) as contributing to an increase in economic output as a result of a decrease of absenteeism and a rise in efficiency. However, if everything is reduced to the reproduction of labour, it cannot explain why the state still provides collective consumption facilities in the case of widespread unemployment. Further, for prime age workers and children, the consumption of health care may be considered as being favourable for reproducing labour for the economy (George and Wilding, 1984) at present or in the future. But what of older people whom they are much marginalised in the labour market? In short, Castells has correctly pointed out that the state has occupied a structural position in the arena of collective consumption in which people come together as consumers of state services, rather than as workers receiving a private wage. However, his reduction of collective consumption to the reproduction of labour cannot sufficiently explain the scope of state intervention in social services which may not be amenable to such a purpose.

O'Connor (1973) stresses the dual functions of state expenditure (including both social consumption and social expenses) in enabling capital accumulation while at the same time legitimating the existing social order. His idea of social consumption agrees with that of collective consumption of Castells which is aimed at reproducing labour power. In contrast to social consumption, social expenses do not directly enhance capital accumulation in terms of reproducing labour, but are envisaged by him as necessary to maintain social cohesion and to legitimate the existing social order. Such an argument can explain why public health care is also provided to older people, the mentally ill, the handicapped, and the chronically ill who are deemed by capital as making no economic contribution to the market economy at all.   However, a major weakness of O'Connor's framework is that virtually anything done by the state can be nodded in on these grounds.   Gough (1979) does not see state intervention as a form of automatic response to capitalist interest and thus he avoids the problem of adopting a functionalist position and seeing the introduction of welfare provisions simply to support capital accumulation.   He also recognises that even though welfare provisions may support capital's interests or maintain social cohesion, they have also improved the welfare of the working class and are partly a result of their own struggle or claims.

The Differences between the Private Wage and the Social Wage

Neo-Marxists have clearly spelled out the important role of the state in providing resources or facilities for consumption on a collective basis. In addition to the labour wage or the private wage that can provide workers the means to consume health care, they can usually get access to health care in the form of a social wage provided by the state (Friedland and Sanders, 1986).   There are four major differences between the private wage and the social wage.

First, unlike the private wage which is manifested as the exchange value of the labour power of an individual worker and is in most cases distributed to him or her alone, the social wage is also distributed to those who do not or could not join the labour force for various reasons, for example, housewives, the retired and the handicapped. The acquisition of the social wage is therefore independent of one's selling of labour power or its commodification in the market.

Second, the private wage is individually appropriated.   Individuals are free to dispose their own income in whatever way they like.   The social wage, on the other hand, is in the first place collectively owned, and is distributed by the government to those who need it in a 'reconstituted form' (Mishra, 1984:85). The social wage may sometimes enable consumers to own their commodities. Subsidised health insurance and housing ownership are some examples.   If it is delivered in kind or in voucher, the wage is constrained for a particular purpose, say, consuming health care in the public sector, or purchasing health insurance in the market.

Third, the social relationship underlying the provision of a private wage is a commodity one as represented by the commodification of labour in the market. Whereas access to the social wage is governed by non-commodity relationships, like citizenship rights, which could be sought without being engaged in a commodity relationship with the providers.

Finally, the disposal of the private wage and the provision of the social wage are two of the major ways to realise the exchange value of goods or services. In the former case, consumers have to pay by themselves, while in the latter case, the exchange value of goods and services is realised by the government when it buys or produces them. That means from a provider's point of view that the social wage is but a form of commodity which is not free at the point of production. Whereas from a consumer's point of view, the social wage is not seen as a commodity since he or she is not required to pay the cost of production. The distinction between the private wage and the social wage can be considered as a difference in the means of realising the exchange value of commodities, whether they are human labour or market goods.

Criticisms of the Thesis of Fiscal Crisis

State expenditures cannot, however, be seen as straight-forwardly functional for capital (Pierson, 1991). The expansion of social services might generate further public demands and requests for expanding the scope of citizen's rights. Neo-Marxists, especially O'Connor (1973), see a fiscal crisis arising from tensions between the accumulation demands of capital and people's mounting needs and expectations. That is, the state will be caught in a dilemma between the contradictory functions of accumulation and legitimation as the economy further develops. However, the working class may lack consolidated strength or see no alternative to the current order. Besides, the state may also regard the promotion of an economic environment susceptible to the achievement of the accumulation purpose as a means to legitimate its rule (Mishra, 1984, 1990).

Moreover, in contrast to the neo-Marxists, Habermas (1984) accords an explicit role to the state in respect of the ideological management of welfare or service provision to overcome the 'inevitability' of fiscal crisis. The state may emphasise personal responsibility in the financing of social consumption, and re-emphasise the family as a natural unit to take care of its members. A possible shift from the state to individuals or the family, or a mix of responsibility shared between the statutory and informal sectors cannot be fully accounted without addressing the state's effort in managing ideological inputs (Hewitt, 1992).

The neo-Marxist perspective has recognised the role played by the state in the provision of a social wage that is closely associated with the resources available for individuals' consumption in advanced capitalism. Compared to the neo-liberal perspective, this perspective has no doubt well expanded the conception of resources for consumption. Nevertheless, some neo-Marxists have overestimated labour reproduction as the main reason for state intervention, and underestimated the state's capacity in manoeuvring the ideological and material context of social consumption. Irrespective of this, the concept of the social wage has effectively provided the background for an in-depth examination of state intervention in relation to health consumption.

Feminist Perspectives

Concerning the resources for consumption, the focus of the aforesaid two rival perspectives is centred around the role played by the private wage and the social wage respectively. Viewed from the liberal or neo-liberal perspective, the level of financial resources for consumption is closely related to individuals' position in and their wage gained from the labour market. Although economic activities are deemed to be atomistic or individual economic endeavours, these perspectives presume the natural sharing of individuals' private wage within the family. Feminist perspectives are especially against the neo-liberal approach in adopting the 'black-box' approach that results in treating the household as a passive consumption unit and in obscuring the role of domestic labour in the area of consumption.

The Role Played by Women in Unpaid Domestic Labour

Feminists have made efforts to identify the issues of household or domestic consumption as a major sociological problem (Kerr and Charles, 1986; Graham, 1987). Rather than simply serving as a passive consumption unit, the family plays a significant role in terms of production, in which women typically play a major role. There is no doubt that production activities can be organised on a household basis, and the goods produced can be marketed like any other commodities available in the market. However, nowadays in advanced capitalism profit-making 'economic' activities have been mostly organised on a corporate or company basis. Sociological studies of the family have shown that it is active in the production of service for self-consumption rather than for sale in the market, like home-making, food preparation, physical care of family members and so on, and that most of this work is done by women themselves (Gershuny, 1982). It is therefore women who have the major responsibility for producing and servicing goods and services for the sake of daily consumption within the family context. In this sense, family production has made consumption of services or goods possible without entirely depending on the private wage and social wage.

Domestic production and servicing not only require labour, but also the precious time of women. All this has, to some extent, deprived women the opportunity to get a full-time job remunerated with a salary in the labour market. Nevertheless, despite the considerable labour inputs of women in the family context, women's domestic work has most often gone unremunerated in the capitalist context (Walker, 1988; Cheal, 1990). For example, in the calculation of GDP, employing a maid to assist with household chores is viewed as an economic activity, while it is not so even with the same kind of work done by female kin in households. This has made women's labour and the role of the family in production less visible. Since the unpaid labour of women is of no concern to neo-liberals, the family is therefore viewed as a passive consumption unit that depends on the services and goods available from the market economy. However, feminists view the family as a unit capable of producing its own services for consumption. As discussed earlier, some Marxist functionalists explained the necessity of unpaid labour of the family as being functional for the reproduction of labour in advanced capitalism (McIntosh, 1979). However, feminists are at the forefront of criticising such a functionalist account that simply considers the family as the setting for ensuring the reproduction of labour in the market economy, even though such an approach could recognise the role of unpaid labour (Graham, 1985). Their basic argument is that the gender-biased division of labour should not be taken for granted without considering the social and economic policies of society at large.

Recent studies on family care giving have found that the female members of the family provide the bulk of care (Walker, 1981, 1982, 1991; Qureshi and Walker, 1986, 1989; Glendinning, 1992; Myles, 1991;

Renshaw et al., 1988; Wilson, 1982).   Further, the role played by the family is central to the delivery of care in the informal sector of which neighbours and volunteers just play a secondary role (Bond, 1992). Local studies in Hong Kong also agree with the point that women are ultimately central to the delivery of care provided in the family, and that family care has formed the major component of community care in Hong Kong (Chow, 1986a, 1987; Ngan, 1990). An up-dated large-scale local research project on the role of the family in community care adds more weight to this point by concluding that 'community care in Hong Kong at present effectively means family care or perhaps more appropriately care by women' (Working Group on Research for International Year of the Family, 1994:149).

Women's Role in Informal Health Care

If health care is conceptualised to be equivalent to medical care, the study of the health care system would then be focused on the formal health care system that is dominated by hospital medicine and clinic services. Within the formal health care system, health care is produced by paid and trained professionals, like doctors, nurses, dentists, physiotherapists, occupational therapists, optometrists, etc. (Frenk, 1993). Simply viewing the family as a consumption unit, neo-liberals tend to focus their attention on the examination of the formal health care system that provides the facilities for health consumption. However, adopting such a restricted conception of health care would unnecessarily undermine the importance and contribution of the informal health care system in the provision of health care 'resources'.   Unlike formal health care, informal health care is provided by unpaid carers who do not consider their activities as an occupation (Haug, 1990). In fact, informal health care is an integral part of all health care systems (Lewis and Lewis, 1977). It is even argued that the informal or lay health care system provides the bulk of health care in society (Open University, 1985a).

Then, what has the family done in the provision of health care? Feminists have developed a typology of informal health care with five areas of activity: mediating professional help, coping with crisis, providing for health, teaching about health and illness, and nursing the sick (Graham, 1984). Mothers or daughters are found to be the chief negotiators or mediators of health care bridging between the formal and informal health care systems (Abel, 1993; Haug, 1990). Coping with a health care crisis is mainly concerned with the handling of chronic conditions. Acute illness or disease may demand much energy and effort. However, if it can be cured within a short period of time, the chance of developing into a health care crisis is slim. Chronic illness lasts much longer and is characterised by recurrences and readmission into hospital whenever acute conditions take place. The management of chronic illness is indeed one of the major health care crisis for the family and the patient to cope with. Feminists believe that women usually suffer the most as a result of the inadequate supply of support services given to the chronically sick and to carers (Twigg, 1993).

Providing for health refers to the provision of a family environment that is conducive to normal health and minimises health-damaging insecurities. In this sense, household chores, like meal preparation, bed-making, washing and so on, mostly done by women, can be considered as the performance of health maintenance activities that constitute a major share of the time and energy expended in household. In Hong Kong, the making of Chinese herbal preparations for the sake of family health maintenance is a common practice. In a utilisation survey, it was found that 58 per cent of respondents who were mothers were responsible for preparing soup with Chinese medicinal materials, and 42 per cent of the same group prepared herbal tea and 38 per cent prepared herbal tonics (Working Party on Chinese Medicine, 1991). The preparation of herbal tea is easy. However, it is not so with herbal soup and herbal tonics, their preparation requires much time and effort. Taking into consideration this specific cultural factor, women's contribution to providing for health in the family should not be underestimated.

The family actively processes health information, and evaluates it concerning health problems and health care. In her study of Chinese medicine, Koo (1982) reports that it is usually women who obtain, process, and communicate health information to the young. Lee and Cheung (1989) argue that, growing up in a family context emphasising the use of traditional Chinese medicine, Chinese adolescents in Hong Kong are receptive to traditional Chinese medical ideas and methods for disease treatment and health maintenance despite the predominance of Western medicine.

With respect to nursing the sick, extra effort has to be devoted in looking after the needs of the ill than to healthy members. Local studies have also demonstrated that women in the caring of the sick shoulder the greatest burden (Chiu, Wong and Woo, 1993; Working Group on Research for International Year of the Family, 1994). As regards the treatment of diseases, Chinese medical care, and especially herbal medicine, remains quite extensively utilised by the Chinese population of Hong Kong (Lee, 1975, 1980; Wong et al., 1993a). The patients especially regard traditional Chinese medical care as an important way of treatment after initially unsuccessful attempts with Western medicine (Working Party on Chinese Medicine, 1991).   Compared to herbal soup and herbal tonics, the preparation of herbal medicine for the sick requires even longer time and effort. Like Western medicine, Chinese medicine cannot be taken just once, it has to be taken many times before the sick can be cured or relieved of their symptoms. Moreover, it may even take the (female) carers several hours to prepare each dose of herbal medicine. So the preparation of Chinese herbal medicine is both labour- and time-consuming.

Many studies have shown that illnesses attended at home greatly outnumber those attended in the formal health care system (Pratt, 1976; Brody, Poulshock and Masciocchi, 1978). The phenomenon of illnesses attended at home is especially so with the case of chronic illness (Corbin and Strauss, 1988). Informal health care work is typically made possible with the unpaid labour of women - even when it conflicts with their paying jobs, and even when there are other kins who are available to share some of the health care work (Northcott, 1983). Unlike Western medicine, Chinese medicine cannot be administered in the hospital setting in Hong Kong.   Hospital medicine is monopolised by the practice of Western medicine only. As an alternative medical practice, Chinese medicine is considered as something between formal health care and informal health care.

It can be seen that health care has not been exempt from the structural basis that has shaped and reshaped women's subordinate position within the informal health care system.   In the Hong Kong context, people's receptivity to traditional Chinese medicine and medical care has been another key factor accounting for the important role of women in health maintenance and treating the sick. The formal and informal health care systems are mutually dependent. Without the contribution of the 'free' labour of women the health care system might collapse as a whole. One of the major implications of feminist perspectives is that the unpaid caring labour contributed by women should not be taken for granted (Twigg and Atkin, 1994). Rather, the role of the family in health care has to be examined in relation to the policies of the state. If the state regards the family as the ideal context of taking care of the sick, there is a tendency for it to overlook the needs of the carers, and the medical rehabilitation needs of the patients. In this case, informal health care given within the family context may be dysfunctional, rather than functional for patients' as well as carers' health. If the contribution of the family in health care is merely taken for granted by the state, the family may have to shoulder greater responsibility in the contribution of unpaid labour which is time- and energy-consuming.

Feminist perspectives have illuminated the gender-bias in the production of informal health care on the one hand, and on how informal health care has played a significant role in sustaining the formal health care system on the other hand. This implies that the state may limit its role in certain areas, say medical rehabilitation of chronic patients. This will be examined in detail in the book later. As discussed earlier, family responsibility also includes the component of financing consumption. If the state re-emphasises family responsibility in health care, the scope is not limited to providing informal health care (as clearly identified by feminists), but also extended to financing health care - whether it is formal health care or traditional Chinese medicine. In short, by making use of the ideological and material context of the family, the state may justify the limited supply of support services to the sick and the carers, and expand the non-state financing tools and channels in financing formal and alternative health care.

Conclusion

The above analysis has provided a theoretical framework to understand how and why the conceptualisation of resources should incorporate both ideological and material dimensions. No doubt, any examination of health care reforms has to account fully for these two dimensions, as well as the role of the state. As discussed in the Introduction, health care reforms have to be undertaken through the modification of three essential components of the health care system, namely, access, finance and delivery. An examination of the forms of state intervention in health care is the task of the next chapter.

2   State Intervention in Health Care

Introduction

The dichotomy between state and market has guided many academic debates (Le Grand and Estrin, 1989; Miller, 1990). The field of health care has not been an exception to this in the public/private debate. In the real world, most health care systems in the world rely on both state intervention and market competition. Recent health care reforms undertaken in different societies of the world have been designed to blend the 'best' of state intervention and market competition on the basis of existing health policies. An interesting phenomenon is that those health care systems established on the basis of universalism are now introducing more market measures, while the typical private insurance dominant system of the US is now developing strategies to overcome market failures which prejudice universal access to basic health care (Saltman and Von Otter, 1992). As in the case of the British NHS which was founded on the principle of universalism, recent reforms are intended to introduce market principles into service delivery, such as increased competition among providers, greater managerial autonomy for hospitals, and more private-sector involvement in the public health care system (Culyer, Maynard and Posnett, 1990).

An analysis of the political economy of health consumption requires an understanding of the role of the state which is a central actor in the development of policy positions and options in health care. It also requires an examination of the important question of the public/private mix in health care. The chapter is based on a fundamental premise: To understand a health care system and its reforms, it is essential to examine the different forms of state intervention, and the variables of the health care system against which the state may modify or re-modify.

31

Typologies and Forms of State Intervention in Health Care

State Intervention and Health System Policies

Scholars in health care have developed various approaches to categorising health systems of the world (Fulcher, 1974; Field, 1989; Terris, 1978; Raffel, 1984; Roemer, 1991, 1993). In these studies, the role of the state, or the degree of state intervention in health care is recognised in some way or another. The following is a critical discussion of three different typologies of health system policies, and the major strengths and limitations of this approach in examining the role of the state in health care.

Field's Typology

Some of the typologies are developed in the way that can be applied to societies of different levels of economic resources. For example, Field (1989) offers a typology consisting of five prototypes or typical models of health care systems, namely, (1) emergent, (2) pluralistic, (3) insurance/social security, (4) national health service, and finally (5) socialised, which are different with respect to the extent of state intervention, with emergent system the lowest, and the socialised system the highest. The degree of the socialisation of health care increases as it moves from health system (1) to health system (5). On the one hand, the emergent system is characterised by mass exclusion from access to standard and basic health care service, and only a minority in a society can enjoy the privilege of basic coverage in health care. On the other hand, the socialised system is characterised by universalism in coverage or protection in health care for the whole population. Inasmuch as the nature of health care is concerned, it is considered in the emergent system as a market commodity like any others available for personal consumption or purchasing; and in the socialised system as a social good or a state-provided public service available for citizens' consumption whenever health needs arise. Within the emergent system, private wages earned by individuals and their families largely provide the funding for consuming health care. However, in the socialised system, citizens are entitled to consume health care as part of their social wage; public spending rather than the private wage or private spending predominates as the source of funding for health care. The other three types of system are different in the extent of state intervention and in the extent to which health care is regarded as a commodity.

Terris' Typology

Terris, however, distinguishes only three prototypes, namely, public assistance, national health insurance and national health service. Within Terris' framework, the prototype of public assistance corresponds to Field's health systems 1 and 2, where state intervention in health care is less significant or kept to a minimum, and market competition is predominant. The prototype of national health insurance corresponds to Field's health system 3: the state plays a significant role in making health care as an insured or guaranteed consumer good. Finally, the prototype of national health service largely corresponds to Field's health systems 4 and 5, which represents the highest degree of socialisation. Terris' categorisation serves to describe the macro picture as to what type of health system policy the nation adopts. Unlike Terris' framework, Field assumes a world-wide automatic convergence toward a socialist health system in spite of the different bases of health care system and political-economic context of the nation-states. However, the convergence theory applied to the evolution of health system has been clearly rejected by many health policy analysts (Elling, 1994). Instead, the reversal of the convergence process, or the privatisation of health care seems to carry more truth and has become today a more prominent trend in many industrialised countries.

Roemer's Typology

Perhaps the best known typology is that of Roemer (1991, 1993). Unlike other typologies, his categorisation takes into account the economic level of the nation-states (i.e., affluent, resource-rich, developing and poor). Going from the least state intervention to the most, Roemer's prototypes are: entrepreneurial, welfare-oriented, comprehensive, and socialist. As a result, 16 types of national health systems can be classified by economic level and health system policies. According to this typology, the US fits in the 'affluent entrepreneurial', the UK in the 'affluent comprehensive', Japan and Canada in the 'affluent welfare-oriented', and the former USSR in the 'affluent socialist'. Compared to Terris' and Field's frameworks, the categorisation developed by Roemer seems much more comprehensive.

Strengths and Limitations of the Categorisation of Health Systems

All these typologies of health systems, in some way or another, deal with the nature of health care and the extent of state intervention and market competition. Each particular prototype may give us a general impression as to the proportion of health costs assumed by the public sector, the extent of state control over various types of decisions, and the extent to which the state itself owns and operates health care facilities. The system policies adopted by the state also give us some ideas about the context within which health care policy is to be shaped. In addition, the typologies developed can provide a framework to compare and contrast different health systems, or to make a comparative study of different nations with respect to their health systems.

The main thrust of the typology of health system policies is the identification of criteria for the classification of each national system into different major clusters. Two major limitations characterise the typology of health system policies. First, an implicit effort seems to be made to converge the complexity of a national health care system into a rather simplistic presentation (Ellencweig, 1992). Each nation-state may not correspond exactly with a particular prototype, and nation-states of the same category may vary much in the extent of state intervention, and in the forms of state intervention taken. Second, the typologies developed may be useful in describing the basic and fundamental features of health care systems, but not so much with respect to the detailing of health care reforms taking place within a health care system. Health care reforms implemented in a nation state may have long-term effects in promoting or constraining people's access to and changing the financing and delivery of health care, but may not be as radical as to the extent of changing the health care system as a whole. Thus, there is a need to examine the possible forms of state intervention in the field of health care, which can effect significant changes within health care systems.

Forms of State Intervention in Health Care

Three Major State Functions: Regulation, Provision and Financing In general, the state is viewed as having three functions: regulation, provision/delivery, subsidy/financing (Le Grand and Robinson, 1984; Frenk, 1993). As regards regulation, it involves a large number of options. More direct regulation may be applied to the areas of health fees and health care products (e.g. ensuring the safety of drugs available in the market). Regulation may also be exercised in an indirect way. For example, the state plays an important role in regulating the inputs to health care with respect to health manpower supply and qualification (Birdsall, 1994). Moreover, the private sector may self-regulate itself in terms of ensuring the professional standard of the providers of health care and the quality of health care products. Regulation can be combined in varying degrees with the public/private mix of provision and financing. The basic point is that public financing does not have to match public provision, nor private financing to private provision. Public provision could be financed by private spending (e.g. private insurance, direct out-of-pocket payment, etc.) and private provision by public spending (e.g. publicly-funded agencies contracting services from the private sector). The state may choose to involve itself in all of these three functions, or limit its intervention to one or two of these functions with respect to certain areas of health care. Moreover, the state may either reduce or increase its role in respect of regulation, provision or financing.

Maxwell's Typology: Government Control and Government Financing
Maxwell (1974) suggested a typology of state intervention based on two dimensions: extent of government control and extent of government financing. According to this framework, government control refers to the extent of state intervention with respect to both regulation and provision; and government financing to the degree of state involvement in subsidising its citizens pertaining to the consumption of health care. Thus, such a typology can be considered to be based on the three major state functions discussed above. With a higher degree of state control and financing in health care, the degree of state intervention is higher. On the contrary, a minimal role played by the state in the control and financing of health care immediately implies a predominant private health care system. This view places the UK and the Scandinavian countries in the quadrant of high government control and financing, and the US in the quadrant of low government control and financing.

Frank and Donabedian's Typology: Control and Eligibility Frenk and Donabedian (1987) proposed another two-dimensional space formed by control and eligibility. The first dimension refers to the extent of state control over the production of health care, both in terms of ownership and financing. The second dimension reflects the basis of eligibility on which health care is distributed to the users.   Within this framework, four possibilities of state control are identified according to the axes of ownership and financing: concentrated ownership, dispersed ownership, concentrated financing, and dispersed financing.

First, the quadrant of concentrated ownership and financing implies a higher degree of state control.   Administrative arrangements are concentrated in a single state agency, and the state assumes the direct ownership of health care facilities and acts as an employer of health care providers.   In this way, control is highly vested in the hands of the state, which is characterised by a command-and-control type of regulation.

Secondly, the quadrant of dispersed ownership and financing represents the lowest degree of state control among the four quadrants. The state mainly confines its role to providing or financing some types of health care and subsidising certain segments of the population in the use of health care, with administrative arrangements widely dispersed among different responsible agencies.   The state may also actively promote the use of private providers and private spending via pro-competitive regulatory efforts.

Thirdly, a good example of the combination of dispersed ownership and concentrated financing is the case of Canada that is often portrayed as 'socialised insurance' (Evans, 1989).   Public agencies in each of the provinces of Canada serve as the health insurers for their residents.   The services are however provided primarily by private doctors or hospitals.

Finally, an example of the combination of concentrated ownership and dispersed financing is, however, not yet available in any developed economies.   Significant financing dispersion implies the prominent role of private financing.   However, dispersed financing may refer to a mixed economy of health care.   Thus, attempts made to maintain the state ownership of health care facilities and employment of the health labour force, but yet reduce the level of state subsidies, or facilitate the growth of private insurance can be seen as a trend toward such a combination.

An essential feature of this framework is the inclusion of the dimension of eligibility to state-financed or state-provided medicine.   In effect, health policies might not provide for all.   For example, designated health care benefits might only be targeted for the workers so that they can resume work as soon as possible (Light and Schuller, 1986).   Similarly, the passage of Medicare and Medicaid in the US targeted the elderly and the poor for special attention respectively (Hollinsworth et al., 1990). Numerous criteria are also available to determine the eligibility to basic health care in general, and 'favoured' health care in particular, for example, age, income, civil servant status, employment status and so on (Staples, 1989).

In their typology of state intervention, Frenk and Donabedian identified three major principles on which the state determines the population's eligibility to health care: poverty, contribution/privilege, and citizenship. Thus, the dimension of access indicates the specific relationship between the state and users of health care, that is characterised by the basis for eligibility or entitlement. Different principles of access may be applied to different areas of health care. For example, curative and preventive services may produce very different responses from the state. On the one hand, despite a great degree of state intervention, many nation-states preserve a private health care market, in which access to health care is based only on purchasing power. On the other hand, there exists no modern government in developed economies which would allow the market place to distribute all health care according to the purchasing power of consumers.

Under the principle of poverty, the state provides or finances health care as a form of public assistance to those who are least able to help themselves. Medicaid in the US is a good example. Besides, private charity generally provides health care to the needy according to this principle. The principle of contribution/privilege is based on the identification of particular groups who are deemed by the state as being important, e.g. civil servants, the army, the employed, etc. These two principles of eligibility to state services are selective in nature as they do not cover the whole population. Finally, the principle of citizenship extends eligibility to health care to the entire population, and is characterised by the principle of universalism. However, Walker's argument is that such a principle developed in the western industrialised countries is intended to guarantee certain minimum rights, rather than to create social equality (Walker, 1984a:22). So, the privileged groups, like the senior civil servants, may in actual or informal practice have earlier, convenient and effective access to better health care despite the operation of the principle of citizenship in policy terms. According to Frenk and Donabedian, the combination of four levels of state control and three principles of access defines twelve possible forms of state intervention in health care.

Forms of State Intervention: Choices Available for the State in Health Care Focusing on forms rather than health system policies enables a more in-depth analysis of the various choices available for the state in health care. For example, though mainly financed by taxation, the British NHS applies two forms of state intervention by the type of service. The state restricts its role to financing in the case of ambulatory care in which the general physicians are contracted personnel rather than the employees of the government. While in the case of hospital care, the state exercises a much more concentrated ownership even though a more dispersed ownership has now taken place following the introduction of internal market into the NHS.

The conception of the forms of state intervention has provided a valuable framework in distinguishing (i) the various principles of eligibility underpinned by different social relations with the state in which users become involved in gaining access to health care; (ii) the extent to which the state may be involved in the financing or delivery of health care, and (iii) the political choices available to the state in the shaping of health care system or health care policy. For example, the application of the citizenship principle does not necessarily imply a monopolistic role played by the state. This is possible, but should only be considered as one of the available options. Further, highlighting the principle of access allows for an assessment of people's access to health care. For instance, although the US is rich of health care resources of various sorts, it is estimated that some 50 million citizens in the US are either uninsured or seriously underinsured (Pepper Commission, 1990). This includes people who either do not qualify for Medicaid or cannot afford private insurance. The significant differential access to health care across income groups in the US is on the one hand the state's decision not to provide health care based on the citizenship principle, and on the other a feature of structural inequalities of the wider society.

Moreover, in the investigation of the forms of state intervention, four important dimensions of health care or health policy against which the state may shape or reshape have been identified: access, provision/delivery, financing/subsidy and regulation. In the real world, varying degrees of state regulation are usually exercised, whether in a direct or indirect way, or in a command-and-control or pro-competition manner. Besides, state regulation may be exercised either independently or in association with a particular public/private mix of financing and delivery in health care. Such an analysis has provided a basic and yet fundamental framework for understanding regulation as an important state function and in what way state regulation may be exercised. The next three sections will be devoted to examining the barriers to access to health care, the different aspects of delivery and finally the major sources of financing in health care.

Barriers to Access

A specific principle of access serves to identify which segment of population should be eligible to health care financed or provided by the state. In addition to the principle itself, there exist various barriers that may influence people's access to health care (Ellencweig, 1992). For example, the programme recipients of Medicare and Medicaid in the US do not receive medical care in the same manner as it is generally provided in the market place. As Medicaid pays health care providers less than Medicare, poor people experience more difficulties than their elderly counterparts in getting access to health care. It is reported that some 80 per cent of the states in the US have problems getting doctors to participate in Medicaid mainly because of the low fees (Shultz, 1991).

The state may indeed put up or allow certain barriers to access to state-subsidised medicine, or in other words, ration access to health care by various different measures in spite of its guarantee to ensure the provision or financing of health care to the entire population or certain segments of the population (Conrad and Brown, 1993; Allen, 1993). This section discusses four major types of barriers to access to health care: doctor-induced, physical, economic and social.

Doctor-induced Barriers

It is generally believed that those with means can have their health needs satisfied in the free market, through buying health insurance in advance or personal health care whenever there is a need. Purchasing power is considered to be the single criterion in governing or ensuring access to private medicine provided in the market. However, this overlooks a very important factor: availability of services (to be discussed in more detail under the heading of physical barriers). In short, if certain medical facilities or health services are not available, there is a major constraint on obtaining service even for those individuals and families who have enough income or insurance to pay for care (Fuchs, 1974).

Moreover, for medicine, unlike other consumer goods, patients are highly dependent on the professional expertise of the medical profession and most often cannot get access to the service they desire without the latter's advice or approval.   Because of the uncertainties surrounding health, disease and medical interventions, patients' power cannot easily be exercised through shopping around, or refusing to use physician services. For some analysts, it is deemed to be wholly inadequate and inappropriate to regard a patient as a consumer (Stacey, 1976).

It has been suggested that the intensive involvement of the state in health care does not necessarily imply an erosion in doctors' autonomy (Larkin, 1988).   Doctors can exercise much control over the nature of medical tasks by controlling diagnostic tests, procedures and drug prescription, and preserve the autonomy to make the decisions to treat which patients first and decisions on defining urgency.   Except for emergencies, the prioritisation of elective work or surgery mostly depends on the advice of doctors (James, 1993).   The behaviour and decisions of doctors play an important role in shaping patients' access to health care, or in other words, putting up barriers to certain patients in seeking treatment or satisfying their medical needs.

Physical Barriers

Under this heading, three different types of barriers are discussed: queues or waiting time, availability of services and finally distance and travel time.

Queues or Waiting Time   Aaron and Schwartz (1984) argue that queues or long waiting time are common measures adopted to ration access to public medicine if the criterion of need has replaced that of purchasing power. This rationing method, applied in situations where supply most often falls far short of demand, is based not on one's ability to pay, but one's ability to wait.   Unlike purchasing power, queuing is an implicit rationing means to determine who should get treatment first.   It is argued to be a necessary evil but yet the fairest measure.   However, it is difficult to ensure all those who wait are less seriously ill, or less in need.   For example, those patients with less obvious symptoms may be more amenable to therapy if they are treated quickly.   If health expenses go to curative rather than preventive measures, to maternal and child care rather than geriatric care, and privilege or priority be given to certain segments of the population and not to others, it is not simply rationing according to needs and urgency; it is rationing according to how needs and urgency are defined, or it is rationing according to desert or merit determined by the state. What is so important is that these barriers may be implemented in a very implicit way which is usually decided or shaped by the medical profession itself.

Availability of Services   Those who cannot afford to consume private medicine can only have their needs satisfied in the public sector. As discussed in Chapter 1, if the state regards the unpaid labour of the family as a resource, it may easily overlook the needs of carers, and the rehabilitation needs of the patients, and support or services might be insufficiently provided as a result. Undoubtedly, if a certain publicly-subsidised health service is made available, but is in much short supply, or is available to a particular target group only, this will still constrain access to health care.

Besides, certain services may only be provided in the private sector but not in the public sector. In this case, it really depends on the comprehensiveness or range of services provided within the public sector. Comprehensiveness has two closely interrelated aspects: range of services available and the continuity of care. The first refers to the degree of comprehensiveness of services made available in the preventive, secondary, or tertiary sectors of health care. The second refers to the continuity of care a patient receives for the prevention, treatment and rehabilitation of his or her illness. The defenders of universalism tend to define the sphere of universal coverage in comprehensive terms to embrace virtually all health care (Starr, 1993). The realisation of such a goal could help to effectively reduce some of the physical barriers to health care.

Since the formal health care system of Hong Kong is monopolised by the practice of Western medicine, patients do not have any access to publicly-subsidised Chinese medicine (Chapter 1). In May 1977, the 30th World Health Assembly urged 'interested governments to give adequate importance to the utilisation of their traditional systems of medicine' (WHO, 1985:136-7). However, up to the present moment of writing this book, there is not any intention on the part of the government to incorporate Chinese medicine into the formal health care system (see Chapter 9), which has a history of over two thousand years, and a considerable heritage of clinical experience in prevention and treatment of diseases. Thus, from a socio-cultural point of view, it can be said that the public health care system of Hong Kong does not provide comprehensive health care.

Distance and Travel Time These two factors are interrelated. That is, the longer the distance between the place of residence and the clinic or hospital, the longer the travel time will be. Long distance or travel time may also discourage patients from using free outpatient services available from public clinics and consult private practitioners instead (see Chapter 4). Perhaps the most significant aspect of geographical distance is the question of rationing: should access to quality health services depend on where one lives? (Mohan, 1995).

Economic Barriers

Fees and Charges Fees and charges are payments made to service providers where recipients of health care pay a certain percentage of the actual cost, the full cost, or even the economic cost (including an element of profit) of the service(s) used (Glennerster, 1992). As regards the use of private medicine, fees and charges in the form of direct, out-of-pocket payment or cost sharing to cover uninsured cost may serve as an explicit criterion in shaping access. Although patients are not generally required to pay an 'economic' fee for consuming public medicine, they may have to pay a fee for this purpose. It all depends on whether public medicine is fully or partially subsidised, or the extent of cost recovery the state wants to make. A fee may deter abuse. However, it may also deter the genuinely needy from using the service, even if this is not the primary intent (Judge, 1980). As doctors exercise much control in deciding whether treatment is necessary, what kind and for how long the patient shall receive it, the defenders of universalism generally do not buy the idea of charging patients.

Non-User-Fees As Le Grand (1982) and Abel-Smith (1976) have shown in their respective examination of the British NHS, even completely removing the price barrier will not be enough to equalise the use of health services by different social groups according to need because the working class has to pay a higher proportion of non-user-fees in terms of unpaid sick leave, travelling cost and other living costs, etc. Compared with the well-off population who enjoy more employers' fringe benefits, the working class have to pay a higher opportunity cost to consume health care free at the point of consumption. All these may therefore act as economic barriers by creating disincentives for utilising public or private medicine.

Social Barriers

Means Testing The employment of a means test is not limited to the practice of the principle of public assistance. Free medicine may be provided to the most needy only on the basis of their eligibility to social assistance. Without going through the means-testing process, people may only enjoy partially subsidised public medicine. However, the means test is closely associated with the undesirable effect of stigma, and this may deter many patients from getting early access to proper treatment. The eligibility requirements for free or heavily subsidised medicine may also be tightened via the imposition of a means test. Similar to the idea of means-testing, targeting is a means used to identify or select those most in need. The implication is that untargeted services are wasteful. To achieve the purpose of targeting, a means-test may be used to ration access. Bamford (1993:35) argues that targeting is in nature a rationing device, though dressed up in beautiful language.

Lower Service Quality Medical services can be sub-divided into clinical and non-clinical aspects. In most cases, patients' knowledge of the effects of medical treatments is very limited as medicine has become more highly technical and scientific. Such a difficulty about the uncertainty of the efficacy of treatment is not only limited to patients, but also to doctors as well. Even the doctors may not know about the side-effects of new medicine or mode of treatment until they have become more evident among the patients (Arrow, 1963). Because of their imperfect knowledge, it is a difficult, if not an insurmountable task for patients to judge the quality of clinical medicine. However, it is not the same case with the non-clinical aspect of health care. In contrast to the quality of clinical care, the patients can judge the quality of the non-clinical aspect of health service more easily. Lower or poorer service quality could act as an undesirable social barrier to access to public medicine, and may thus indirectly encourage people to consume private medicine instead. Poorer service quality may manifest itself in different ways: inconveniences, shorter consultation time, poor bed or hospital environment, no choice of doctors or hospitals provided to patients, etc.

Whatever the level of resources individual patients have, they inevitably face barriers to health care, though in very different ways or in different mixes. It is reasonable to believe that patients of working class background usually experience more barriers than their well-off counterparts. The well-off population usually have a louder and more articulate voice than their poorer counterparts in getting their needs heard (Klein, 1983). Moreover, whatever the level of overall resources, and whatever the system of health care, the services provided are rationed in some way or another. For example, an economic or price barrier to access is most evident to the uninsured or underinsured population in the US as a result of the absence of universal health insurance. In the UK, removing price barriers to access was one of the founding objectives of the NHS. However, patients face the physical barrier of queues or long waiting time especially with respect to non-emergency cases or selective surgeries. The point is, therefore, that different societies and different groups of people face very different sets of barriers according to widely differing criteria listed in the above discussion.

Health Care Delivery

Health care delivery has two major elements: delivery mechanism and service provision. The delivery mechanism is concerned with the organisational arrangements for delivering health care to eligible users, with varying degrees of administrative flexibility, financial incentives to providers and proneness to competition. Whereas, service provision has two aspects: service delivery approach and service differentiation. This section is devoted to examining the different aspects of these two important elements, and to providing a framework for understanding the ways the delivery of health care may be reformed via state intervention.

Delivery Mechanisms

There is a range of organisational arrangements that may realise the commitment of the state to provide a socially specified minimum standard of health care. Basically, however, there are three major kinds of delivery mechanism that the state may adopt to finance or provide health care:

public integrated model, public contract model and public reimbursement model (OECD, 1992).

Public Integrated Model This model is characterised by the integration of state functions of financing and provision, and is considered equivalent to a national health service if universal or near-universal access is ensured. That is, state-financed health care is provided to citizens in kind at the point of consumption. Before the implementation of an internal market (to be discussed under the heading of Public Contract Model) in the British NHS, it was the model used for public hospitals in the UK. This model is also characterised by the lack of user choice of doctors or hospitals and competition between medical care providers within the public sector. A centralised provision system distinguished by concentrated state ownership and financing is criticised for being too inflexible and providing too few incentives to the providers to improve efficiency and raise service quality (Lopez-Casasnovas, 1989).

While keeping the integration of financing and provision relatively intact, the state may implement measures that are more amenable to generating flexibility and incentives. For example, if the provider units, like the hospitals, are allowed to keep the difference of the budget, it would provide them an incentive to underspend. In addition, if the providers are allowed to keep extra revenue from private patients, it would provide them an incentive to attract private patients and enlarge the waiting list of public patients (Wolfe and Moran, 1993). Thus, in examining whether the health care delivery mechanism based on the integrated model is amenable to cost recovery or revenue generation, the degree of administrative flexibility and financial incentives provided to the health care providers has to be addressed.

Public Contract Model Social insurance or national health insurance implemented in Japan, Canada and many northern European countries is based on the public contract model. As one of the versions of the public contract model, social insurance has two major characteristics. First, health insurance is compulsory in the form of income-related contributions and partial or full subsidisation of contributions for the poor. If the level of premium is fixed at a certain per cent of employees' income, and if the poor are subsidised in the purchase of health insurance, it would be considered a comparatively equitable way of financing health care. Second, under the public contract model, there is normally a standard contract with doctors and hospitals concerning the method and level of payments. Negotiation over fees and charges usually takes place between insurers or sickness funds and providers' organisations under bilateral monopoly (OECD, 1992). Third, the role of the state is usually limited to financing health care, while the private sector is responsible for providing health care. In the case of Canada, providers receive payment from the central insurer and compete among one another for custom; so, the traditional differentiation between the public and private sectors is not so applicable. Compared to the integrated health care system, a social insurance system usually gives users more choices of medical care providers. As the level of payments for particular treatments or procedures has been standardised, competition between providers is over the quantity and quality of services, but not over price (Appleby, 1992).

In a different version, the internal market implemented within the British NHS may also be categorised under the public contract model, which is characterised by the separation of purchasers and providers (Øvretveit, 1995). The UK system has two variants: health authorities as purchasers, and general physicians (GPs) as budget holders. In the former case, each district health authority (DHA) serves as a budget holder (Harrison, 1991). The provider institutions have to compete for contracts with the DHAs. Competition is not just limited to public providers, but also extends to private providers. So, two types of competition can be identified: competition between provider units within the public sector, and competition between public and private providers. Primary doctor purchasing is another variant of the current health care reform taking place in the UK General physicians (GP) fundholding allow primary doctors to hold budgets to purchase drugs and a limited range of hospital test and inpatient services (Øvretveit, 1995). A major difference between GP budget holders and DHAs lies in the potential for the selection of patients. DHAs must take responsibility for all residents, while GPs may select their own patients. There may thus provide an incentive for GPs to select the potentially cheaper patients (Mullen, 1990). However, purchaser competition is also possible since patients may change their family doctors.

Public Reimbursement Model Similar to the public contract model, this model usually ensures universal or near-universal health insurance coverage. The reimbursement model is, however, characterised by the insurer's reimbursement of patients for medical care bills, in part or in whole on the one hand, and on the other by the absence or near absence of contractual relationship between insurer and provider. This model is thus distinguished by insurer's minimal interference with the transactions between doctor and patient. As providers' income is related to the quantity and price of the services provided to patients, unnecessary demands made by doctors may not be effectively restrained. Under this model, health care expenditure is thus relatively open-ended, rather than being capped in the form of global budgeting as in the case of public integrated or public contract system. In view of the paramount objective of cost-containment in present day health care reforms, European countries like Belgium and France have gradually phased out the reimbursement model and adopted the public contract model or a blend of the public contract and integrated models (OECD, 1992).

The above discussion has shown that the public/private divide is too simple a dichotomy to describe the available options for designing or reforming the organisational arrangements of a health care system. In the final analysis, the use of competition is not restricted to the private market; and the state may use a mix of intervention measures and market competition to realise health care objectives. The ideas of administrative flexibility and competition ultimately involve the selective introduction of financial incentives and market mechanisms through the exercise of state power (Saltman and von Otter, 1992). However, it is not certain that in actual practice competition and further decentralisation of the management of health care will work out desirable effects as predicted by the state. Incentives may work the other way round to realise providers' rather than users' interests. How does the delivery mechanism provide incentives within a more decentralised or competitive atmosphere, and how do these incentives shape the way health care is provided should be one of the focuses in the examination of health care reforms.

Service Provision

Service Delivery Approach This refers to the particular approach adopted in the provision of services. The medical profession plays a very important role in the production of formal health care. As Chapter 3 will show, the medical profession with its orientation and thinking much predominated by the acute care perspective tends to concentrate its attention on critical care or the acute conditions of diseases. Critics like Schwartz (1987) and Childress (1987) suggest that such an approach to formal health care assigns priority to critical care over prevention and long-term care. Confronting the prevalence of chronic illness in developed economies, the appropriateness of the acute care approach to health and disease has been subject to much criticism (Conrad, 1989). Nowadays, other health care approaches, like primary health care, community-based health care and long-term care - which all closely involve or recognise the role of the family and the community - have increasingly caught the attention of the states in the formulation of their health care strategy (Williams, 1995). As the emerging trend of the state's putting new emphasis on these non-acute-care approaches to health care has been taking place within a context giving much priority to cost containment, there is a worry that state funding may not be adequately channelled to make these approaches work effectively.

Service Differentiation   The non-clinical aspect of health services may not be delivered in a standardised way. The providers could provide different levels of services that are supposedly clinically equivalent but have different amenities or degree of convenience.   The differentiation of services provides a leverage for the providers to price the services differently.   The providers may also employ the differentiation strategy to expand 'choices' to patients.   Even more homogenous than the US health care system, the British NHS has still retained private beds (pay beds) ever since its inception in 1948, which is a demonstration of free enterprise and an important source of financial benefits to consultants within the framework of universalism (Weller and Manga, 1983).

State-financed or state-provided health care may not be delivered on the same level of service or coverage without any differentiation for the entire population.   The entire population may have basic coverage, but some may enjoy better non-clinical service and perhaps privileged access either because of their means or because of their status and position.   The health care system as a whole can be differentiated into public and private sub-systems, with the former of lower service quality and the latter of better quality.   It is also possible that a public health care system can be differentiated into two- or even multi-tiers according to the different level of amenities and non-clinical services provided.   Two points are of importance then: the degree of differentiation of services and the relative size of the upper tier(s) in relation to the lower tier.   Both the state and the health care providers can indeed play an important role in respect of service differentiation   (Chapter 7 will be devoted to discussing the implementation of B-class beds and its relationship to service differentiation within the public health care system of Hong Kong).

Health Care Financing

The mechanism by which health care is financed is another important feature. In the present day context of developed capitalist societies in the world, there are five major means available for financing health care: general tax revenues, hypothecated tax, out-of-pocket payments, employer's fringe benefits and finally private insurance (Glennerster, 1992; Holliday, 1992; Wolfe and Moran, 1993). In addition to these means, charity was another avenue for health support for many centuries before the Second World War. For example, before the establishment of the British NHS in 1948, charity substantially contributed to health care by assisting it financially and materially (Barry and Jones, 1991). Inspired by religious or mutual-help motives, charitable organisations operated hospitals or clinics and provided the major financing resource for the emerging modern health systems. However, in developed capitalist nation-states, charity as a 'third-party payer' for health care has been largely replaced by the state or private insurers (Ellencweig, 1992).

It is usual for a health care system to adopt a mixed mode of financing, though in different combinations and proportions in different societies. The key questions are therefore concerned with the actual mix of different financing tools; the state functions (in terms of regulation, financing and provision) used in adjusting the mix; and the justifications made to promote the use of a specific financing tool or a particular mix of financing in health care. This section outlines the major characteristics of the different financing means to provide a framework for analysis.

General Taxation

General tax revenues come from two major sources: direct taxation revenues from personal and profits taxes, and indirect taxation on items not directly connected with health care, e.g. duties, property, or utilities. If a health care system is predominantly financed by direct state funding out of general taxation, the government can exercise tight control over the global budget for health care, and thus in turn better achieve the cost containment objective. The use of a global budget is usually administratively easier and inexpensive since funding is directly distributed to health care agencies in a prospective way (Holliday, 1992). Another major advantage of general taxation is that the financing of health care is not over-concentrated on a single tax source (Bailey and Bruce, 1994). Besides, progressive taxation serving as a major means to finance health care is viewed as being socially just (Doorslaer, Wagstaff and Rutten, 1993).

Direct state funding out of general taxation is currently the central mechanism employed in the UK to finance health care, and the one in Hong Kong to finance hospital care. This is certainly the baseline against which all other financing options have to be judged in the Hong Kong context. As direct taxes are related to the ability to pay taxes, they are more progressive and indirect taxes regressive. If direct taxes are sufficiently progressive, the overall tax structure can be progressive. How the rates of different taxes are determined, and how much of general tax revenue is to be spent on health care are very much political economy issues. They are important questions since they influence the extent to which the state commits itself in the financing of health care on the one hand, and on the other, they help to reflect the ideological context within which the state finance or provide public services.

Hypothecated Tax

Unlike general tax revenues, an hypothecated or earmarked tax is a dedicated amount to be spent on a particular area. Hypothecated tax for health care is in nature a compulsory health tax, which is mostly collected in the form of payroll tax. Social insurance, like the hypothecation of taxes, is a way of earmarking funds for health care provision. Hypothecated taxes as a means to finance health care is commonly adopted in continental Europe.

How the rate of hypothecated taxes is determined is different from countries to countries. The same case is also applied to the relative proportion of payroll tax to be contributed by employer and employee respectively. If hypothecated tax or a health tax predominantly finances health care, it can help to reflect the level of resources that people would like to spend on in this field. However, the central control mechanism as exercised in the form of a global budget in the case of general tax revenues would also be undermined. Health çare spending might increase more rapidly if concerned debates are dominated by the medical profession in its calls for extra funding to finance expensive high-tech acute care medicine (Appleby, 1992).

Out-of-Pocket Payments

Out-of-pocket money is a usual medium to purchase commodities in the market, like food, clothes, electrical appliances, etc. As far as health care is concerned, such a financing means represents direct, full or partial payments to providers by the users themselves. The case of full, direct, out-of-pocket payments depends on patients' ability to pay since they do not receive any third-party payment or subsidy (which is paid or reimbursed by the state or private health insurers). This mode of payment may be commonly found in patients' self-initiated outpatient consultations and their purchase of over-the-counter medicines, but usually much less so with respect to expensive hospital care.

The case of partial, direct, out-of-pocket payment is considered equivalent to cost sharing. The role played by cost sharing depends on the extent to which health care consumption is publicly subsidised or reimbursed by private health insurance. That is, the greater the extent of cost sharing, the less important the role played by third-party payment and vice versa. In a health care system like the British NHS, cost sharing is realised in the form of patient fees and charges. While in social insurance or private insurance systems, cost sharing is realised via the payments of deductibles and/or co-payments. While in many other developed societies, the majority of payments are made via public funding, like social insurance contributions and general tax revenues. Given the prevalence of third-party payment for health care, out-of-pocket money is generally viewed as a source of supplementary rather than predominant funding.

Employer's Fringe Benefits

Employer's fringe benefits are provided on the basis of employment status, though the coverage may also be extended to the family members of the employees. In the field of health care, employer's fringe benefits may be taken in three different forms: employment-based insurance, employer's direct reimbursement, and employer's provision of in-kind service. In the US, the first one is the predominant one, which takes the form of a payroll deduction shared by employer and employees. The insurance premium is calculated on the basis of an actuarial estimation of the expected health risks of the group or individual covered. Besides, employers may reimburse the cost of health care paid in advance by their employees, either completely or partially; or recruit 'station-doctor(s)' to provide treatment to employees in the workplace. Since hospital care can be very expensive, employers would normally prefer the purchasing of health insurance to self-insurance. Thus, the modes of direct reimbursement and direct provision of health care in the workplace are mostly limited to outpatient medical consultations.

The extent of health care coverage and protection provided by employer's fringe benefits depends on the specific arrangements made between employers and employees either on a group or individual basis. Similar to the private wage, the package of fringe benefits reflects the social class divisions and the underlying patterns of inequality of the wider society (Titmuss, 1976; Calnan, Cant and Gabe, 1993).

Private Insurance

Voluntary employment-based insurance as discussed above is certainly a form of private insurance. Their expansion or contraction much influences the market share of private insurance in the financing of health care. But for present purposes, private insurance is separated from employer's fringe benefits. Private insurance may also be purchased on an individual rather than corporate basis. Because of the uncertainty of the incidence of illness, and the lack of information over the form, amount, and cost of future health care, private health insurance is considered by the marketeers as a feasible solution to insure against the financial costs of ill-health. However, private health insurance may be taken out because of state's provision of tax incentives or tax concessions (Chapter 1).

Private insurance is an alternative to out-of-pocket payments, publicly-subsidised medicine and social insurance, in sharing risks among the insured. At the time of consumption, the insured will be able to much lower the market price of consumption. Thus, it can give the insured a sense of security over the financial risk of health consumption (Fein, 1989). Besides, since private health insurance supplies patients with extra cash, they can jump the queue for public medicine or minimise the risk of not being treated immediately (Glaser, 1991). However, a major disadvantage of private health insurance is the actuarial calculations of risks and thus resulting in both exclusion of risky groups and variable premiums. Generally, those who are most in need of health care, like older people, the chronically ill and the disabled, would most probably be excluded from being insured as a result. Despite this major drawback, many nation-states are now implementing measures to facilitate people to take out private insurance as a means to finance health care. Such a strategy adopted not only influences how health care is financed, but may also help to promote inequalities of access to health care.

The five major financing tools discussed above can be re-categorised into two on the basis of their inclination to the centralisation or dispersion of the financing of health care, i.e. public spending and private spending. General tax revenues and hypothecated taxes are two major possible funding sources for health care if health care financing is well centralised or dominated by public spending. Out-of-pocket payments, employers' fringe benefits and private insurance become the major funding sources for health care if a health care financing system is well dispersed or dominated by private spending. In the former case, citizens are entitled to health care as part of their social wage; while in the latter case, individuals have to largely rely on their private wage to pay for their health care consumption.

To centralise the financing of health care, the state may either provide or finance health care with the use of more public funding by emphasising the role played by taxes, whether earmarked or not. To disperse the financing of health care, different sorts of state functions may be used separately or in combination to enhance the role of private spending, for example, implementing cost-sharing measures, facilitating the growth of employers' fringe benefits and private insurance.

Conclusion

It is evident that neither the simple public/private dichotomy nor simple typologies of health system are useful in analysing the complexity of current health care reforms taking place in developed societies. Rather, a mix of public/private resources, and the combination of market mechanisms and social objectives, are now deemed to be critical in reforming the health care system as a whole. A critical examination of the forms of state intervention and the major elements of a health care system can serve to conceptualise the different roles of the state in the ever changing health care system.

3   The Medical Profession and Health Care

Introduction

An important feature of health care is the significant role played by one professional group, doctors, which claims to have the scientific knowledge and expertise in health and diseases. The labelling of the doctor as a healer and a professional seems to identify him or her as being committed to patients' interest in particular, and the community at large. There is, however, another side to the coin, that the medical profession is also making the most of its expertise and professional knowledge to maximise its own political power and economic interest. As a professional group, doctors are more than healers, and may exercise as strong political power as politicians do in relation to matters related to health. Because of their significant role, and because of increasing state intervention in health care, the state has to deal with them - whether at a time of co-operation or conflict, or whether in terms of achieving health care objectives or implementing health care reforms.

This chapter is devoted to a critical examination of the nature and various dimensions of medical power, and to providing a framework for understanding the relations as well as tensions between the state and the medical profession with respect to the politics of health policy formation and shaping.

Clinical Perspective of Western Medicine

Characteristics of the Clinical Perspective of Western Medicine

Viewing through the 'Clinical Gaze'   Foucault (1973) argues that the clinical approach of Western medicine or biomedicine provides what heterms a 'clinical gaze' in viewing diseases and the human body. The gaze implies 'a way of seeing', and it is through the clinical gaze that the bodily structures and their malfunctioning become visible to doctors. The clinical status of disease is acquired through the identification of specific physiological or biochemical malfunctioning of organs or tissues. Along with disease, health acquires a clinical status, which is represented as the absence of clinical symptoms or disease (Illich, 1975:114). Thus, sickness rather than health is placed in the centre of biomedicine, and no positive concept of health is advanced from the clinical perspective (Kelman, 1975). Viewed from a clinical perspective, the paramount tasks of doctors are firstly to make the right diagnosis and then treat the symptoms and disease with appropriate medical measures accordingly.

The clinic or hospital provided an ideal setting for the development of the clinical gaze for it was the place where plenty of patients were housed, diseases were identified, medical training was undertaken, and a census of disease was kept. Historically speaking, the concept of clinic or hospital is a relatively new one. Before clinics and hospitals became much more commonplace as they are now, the home setting was the place where treatment of patients was undertaken (Open University, 1985a). Stepping into the 19th century, medical perception of human bodies and the treatment of disease became more and more clinic- or hospital-based. Precisely, the hospital as an ideal organisation within which medical examination and medical care are rendered, provides the doctors with a more 'controlled' environment for the application of clinical and biological principles, and the development of medical knowledge and clinical medicine (Waddington, 1973).

Mechanical Conception of Human Bodies The clinical gaze, emphasising the clinical examinations of the body, has reduced the human body more or less to the status of a machine whose various parts could be examined, regulated and repaired discretely (McKeown, 1971; Turshen, 1989). Based on this conception, doctors act like engineers to mend the 'wares' of human body. With further advances in anatomy and medical technology, different parts of the body, from organs, tissues to cells, can be investigated in greater detail, and clinically intervened and treated. As a consequence of the adoption of the mechanical metaphor in inspecting 'signs' and 'symptoms' of diseases, and in describing and investigating 'malfunctionings' and 'abnormalities' of human bodies, the merits of technological investigation, assessment treatment and interventions are given considerable emphasis. As a health (sickness) professional, the doctor is vested with great power to examine the body and tackle the 'mechanical' troubles of the human body caused by disease, and to further develop clinical knowledge within the hospital setting through the identification and localisation of pathology in passive bodies (Armstrong, 1987).

Reductionism Another important characteristic of clinical medicine or biomedicine is its reductionist account of disease in that explanations of disease focus mostly on biological pathology of human bodies to the relative neglect of socio-environmental factors (Atkinson, 1988). Disease is seen as an outcome of a biological or physiological abnormality, and the focus is on the immediately observable factors: malfunctioned organs, parasite, bacteria, virus, etc. Disease can ultimately be traced to the pathology of bodily structures or even specific aetiology which assumes that disease is caused by a specific, identifiable agent. The proposition of individual pathology and specific aetiology has placed sickness in the centre of the clinical or medical system in that sickness 'could be subjected to (a) operational verification by measurement, (b) clinical study and experiment, and (c) evaluation according to engineering norms' (Illich, 1975:112).

As a Scientific Approach to Medicine Viewed from the clinical perspective, disease and its manifestations in human bodies are recognisable by a natural science methodology (Boorse, 1977). Its conceptualisation of disease is in nature positivistic, which can be assessed by scientific methods and objective criteria, and which in turn involves empirical observation and induction. The development of medicine is presumed to be based on a scientific discipline that is considered to be a valid response to the understanding of disease (Rhodes, 1985; Gerhardt, 1989). The assumption of the objectivity of medical knowledge incorporates a view of medical practice performed by the medical profession as an applied science that is 'value free' (Mishler et al., 1981) and highly technological (Nettleton, 1995). This lends support to the claim that the clinical perspective of medicine provides a body of universally valid knowledge that can inform, assess, and evaluate the practice of medicine. This helps to justify the further expansion of scientised medical knowledge that can be translated into medical practice. Within the framework of the clinical perspective, medical practice is then defined primarily in terms of dealing with technical problems, and the direction of medical development is framed in terms of technical criteria, such as validity of diagnosis, scientific application of medical treatment and procedures, symptom relief, and removal of malfunctioned body parts that lead to disease. In this way, the medical-scientific assumptions of the clinical perspective serve to legitimate the doctors' control over medical diagnosis and treatment.

The clinical perspective of Western medicine is characterised by the medical profession investigating human bodies and diseases through a 'clinical gaze'. Under this perspective, doctors are regarded as trained and qualified professionals who can apply scientific biomedical principles in order to 'effectively' manage health problems, or more exactly, to tackle disease problems. This can explain why doctors sometimes show more interest in diseases themselves than in those persons or patients suffering from having diseases (Davies, 1989). Nevertheless, the clinical gaze is more flexible than static in viewing things and permitting new objects to be viewed (Nettleton, 1995). For example, within the professional circle, doctors nowadays are encouraged to be more sensitive to social, cultural and psychological factors behind seeking medical consultations and treatment, and the patients' interpretation and experience of their disease (Nettleton, 1992). In spite of the flexible application of the clinical gaze, Western medicine is still largely dominated by the medical-scientific assumptions of the clinical perspective which is used to legitimate the doctors' control over medical diagnosis and treatment on the one hand, and their shaping of health care policy in general and health care delivery approach in specific (Jones, 1994; Lupton, 1994).

Clinical Orientation to Health Care

Under the penetrative influence of the clinical perspective of medicine, the medical profession is oriented to applying and reinforcing curative and high-tech approaches to health care characterising the delivery of health care in developed capitalist societies.

Curative Approach to Health Care As Kennedy (1981:28), in *The Unmasking of Medicine*, puts it the medical profession 'tend[s] to just look for cures and the image created of medicine has increasingly been that of a curing science in which the model of the doctor is that of the engineer/mechanic curing a sick engine'. This suggests that the medical profession regards itself as a dispenser of cures even though many of the diseases that kill us nowadays are not curable. Within the framework of curative medicine, medical practice concretised into various sorts of surgery symbolises an advanced translation of biomedical science into clinical or highly technical services.

Backed by the 'ideology of cure' (Kennedy, 1981), a curative approach to the organisation of health care predominates in hospitals with its emphasis on the treatment of the acute conditions of diseases. The importance of the medical attention given to cure should not be denied. But the overemphasis on curative medicine will easily lead to the underestimation of the needs of the patients other than curing of the acute conditions of diseases, and in reinforcing the bias towards allocating resources to curative rather than preventive, rehabilitative or long-term health care.

The predominance of the clinical or curative approach lies in part in the overwhelming clinical emphasis of medical schools which play a significant role in professional socialisation (Joseph, 1994). Medical schools in Hong Kong, like elsewhere, are located in teaching hospitals that are acute and general hospitals. Although medical education nowadays pays more attention to behavioural sciences, such as psychology, sociology and other more socially and psychologically oriented specialities, such as psychiatry, community medicine, family medicine and geriatric medicine, social aspects of health, and preventive and rehabilitative medicine are still placed in a relatively marginal position compared to other clinical subjects. Medical education is controlled by the medical profession, from which the faculty is drawn, which designs the curriculum that places much greater emphasis on clinical subjects than in social and preventive medicine. Similar to the health workforce awarding the highest prestige to surgeons in hospitals, medical students tend to rank clinical subjects higher in prestige than social and preventive medicine (Open University, 1985b).

High-tech Orientation Hospitals provide an ideal setting for the application of high-tech medicine. The success of modern medicine in combating certain diseases has persuaded doctors that what is needed is further development of medical science, more advanced equipment, more improved technology, and more effective drugs (Roth and Ruzek, 1986). The high-tech orientation of medicine has speeded up the proliferation of medical technology, like CT scanners, magnetic resonance imaging, organ transplants and so on. New medical innovations and procedures open up new areas of medicine, say, cardiac cathetherisation units, coronary care units, bone marrow transplantation units and so on which are all very expensive.

In addition to the ideology of cure promoted by the medical profession, the media have, to some extent, contributed to the public interest in and appreciation of high-tech medicine (Ginzberg, 1990). The media's reporting of the 'wonders' of high-tech medicine is often incommensurate with its success in treating many incurable diseases. However, the public in general, and patients in particular are, to some extent, convinced by the medical profession as well as the mass media in viewing the high-tech orientation as a right one to make breakthroughs or miracles in medicine.

The medical profession's interest in clinical research and scientific medicine is entirely understandable from the clinical perspective. Nevertheless, this could mean that the clinicians or doctors tend to look more for exceptional clinical or pathological conditions to which sophisticated technology can be applied. After all, clinicians or doctors find the diagnosis and treatment of rare cases most fascinating since all this is closely connected with the further development of their medical knowledge and expertise.   The application of high-tech medicine to clinical cases or conditions also represents the specialised clinical peak in medical care, which is a key to greater prestige and income (Konner, 1993).

Moreover, the increasing concentration of high-tech medicine in hospitals cannot be separated from the capitalist expansion into the health sector that provides fuel for profit making (Caplan, 1989; Light, 1995). The quest for high-tech curative medicine is closely related to the medical-industrial complex, which involves research laboratories, and large corporations producing and marketing electronics, computers and expensive medical equipment and drugs. The fact is that advertising of sophisticated medical technology and drugs is usually targeted to doctors themselves (Open University, 1985b). Thus, the pressures originating in the supply industries further reinforce the development of high-tech medicine.

From a clinical perspective, quality health care is largely portrayed as being equivalent to the use of high-tech and sophisticated surgery and medicine. Consultants and surgeons have an embedded interest to adopt this definition since the mastery of high-tech medicine can further boost their image and status.   Thus, an increasing use of expensive and sophisticated medical technology can mutually benefit the medical profession and the health care industry. In some sense, these two parties are mutually interdependent. The quest for high technology in Western medicine is therefore closely connected with the quest for profit by the medical-industrial complex, and the quest for power and privilege by the medical profession. All this does not deny the effectiveness of certain medical technology in the diagnosis and treatment of certain diseases. However, such a trend of development in most developed societies has resulted in the concentration of attention on the medical problems of the few that simply cannot be equalled to meeting the health needs of the wider community.

Functions and Inherent Characteristics of Medicine: the Basis of Medical Power?

After reviewing the major characteristics of Western medicine and its clinical orientation to health care, this section discusses whether its functions and inherent characteristics are the basis of the dominant power enjoyed by the medical profession before making a critical examination of the various dimensions of medical power.

The Functionalist Approach

This approach attempts to account for the power of the medical profession in terms of the positive contributions of medicine. The functionalists are optimistic and confident about the intrinsic value of medicine in performing the vital health function for the society as a whole (Parsons, 1951; Barber, 1963). Viewed from the functionalist approach, good health is highly valued not only for its own sake, but also for its contribution to the maintenance of social order and development of a society. Western biomedicine is viewed as a response to the system's requirements for good health; to control the potentially disruptive nature of illness to the social order; and to hold the promise for eradicating and controlling existing and any new diseases in a scientific and rational way as well.

A Critique of the Functionalist Approach   Nevertheless, the value of medicine in promoting good health has been subject to much criticism. McKeown and Record (1963) convincingly argue that the major reasons for the decline of mortality in England and Wales during the 19th century are more to do with environmental health control of housing, nutrition and water supplies than with vaccinations, treatments or other modes of medical interventions. A similar study of European countries also shares the same conclusion that social and environmental changes form the predominant causes of the decline in mortality rates (McKeown, et al., 1972). These studies suggest that the positive health impact generated by medical intervention was relatively restricted.

Moreover, chronic illnesses that presently account for the major causes of mortality and morbidity in developed societies are most often alleviated rather than cured by high-cost medical intervention and technology (McKinlay et al., 1989). Some academics suggest that biomedicine is only capable of rendering successful treatment in only 10 per cent to 15 per cent of illness episodes (Wildavsky, 1977; Gill, 1980). Although the estimation may not be accurate enough, it at least shows that biomedicine is inherently fraught with limitations. The limited efficacy of Western biomedicine has been used as an argument against the functionalist point of view which regards the predominant power of the medical profession as being for promoting good health and thus consequently being functional for the maintenance of the social system as a whole.

The Trait Approach

The trait approach argues that the medical profession's command of medical science and knowledge acquired through academic training and clinical experience engenders a 'competence gap' between the medical profession and the public (Rayack, 1967). Accordingly, with the further development of medicine, the competence gap would be widened despite increasing health consciousness among the public. Given the lack of ability on the part of patients to adequately understand or evaluate medical knowledge and medical practice, they have to depend on doctors to give advice once they decide to consult them for treatment. Patients have to rely on the doctors as their agents to accumulate knowledge and information and prescribe treatment because of their competence in medicine and because of their supplying technical expertise in the best interests of the patient.

Underlying the formation and the further widening of the competence gap is the scientisation of medicine that serves to justify the dependence of the public on the medical profession in all questions having to do with health care. That is, the power enjoyed by doctors in health care is simply a result of their competence derived from their education and training, and the consequent asymmetrical power relationship between the medical profession and the public (Haug, 1981).

Rather than placing emphasis on the competence gap between the medical profession and the public in explaining the power assumed by the medical profession, Freidson (1970) focuses on the professionalisation of medicine which is characterised by state-backed monopoly. He argues that state support given to medicine would not be possible if it did not inherit and expand a body of scientific and esoteric knowledge. The conception of professionalisation as the unfolding of esoteric knowledge, and as the exercise of technical autonomy is used to characterise the essential character of professions. On the contrary, the essential explanation for the failure of occupations to develop into a profession is their inability to command an esoteric knowledge in a particular field, which in return could not back their demand for a state-supported license.

A Critique of the Trait Approach Nevertheless, the trait approach is criticised for being inattentive to the socio-historical context of the development of medical power (Alubo, 1986). The medical profession does not acquire traits naturally but in a given historical and socio-political circumstance. Nettleton (1995:7) argues that: 'what counts as legitimate medical knowledge and practice is decided through social process rather than being shaped by natural objects of which the profession has an accurate knowledge'.

Critics have further argued that the medical profession actually makes use of medical science to facilitate their strategies of occupational closure (Larson, 1978). The application of scientific principles has been so extensive and 'successful' in solving problems in recent centuries that science has emerged as an ideology (Sorell, 1991). The ideology of scientism has promoted the belief that science is valid and true and that the application of science will result in progress and development. Backed by such an ideology, the medical profession has been active in ascertaining its significant or paramount position in translating medical science and knowledge into medical practice, and also in monopolising medical practice (De Kadt, 1982). That is, medical power in health care is neither natural nor automatic but has to be attained, maintained, or even perpetuated through reducing or resisting challenges directed to the medical profession, and through political processes (Friedson, 1970; Coburn, Torrance and Kaufert, 1983).

Freidson is right to point out the significant role played by state-backed license in accounting for medical professional power. However, a major weakness of such an account is his contention that the medical profession has enormous power by virtue of the inherent characteristics of medicine itself but without emphasising the specific socio-political and historical context within which medicine developed itself into a profession. According to Abbott (1988), the medical profession has not achieved its dominant position because of its inherently superior expertise, but because it has managed to create and maintain the control over and the demarcation of medical tasks in relation to other health occupations. Far from avoiding politics by way of the establishment of technical autonomy of a neutral stance, the medical profession is continuously engaged in making claims and expertise for jurisdictions in health care, resulting in a competitive struggle and political conflicts with other health workers or health occupations.

Changing Boundaries of Health Care Politics   However, in Abbott's analysis, the state is largely conceived as a passive audience for competitive struggles between health occupations for jurisdictional claims, rather than as an active actor throughout the whole process.   In his analysis, the state does not take part in the jurisdictional claims until legislative measures are called into play. Although Abbott has recognised that the jurisdiction of professional expertise is an outcome of a political process rather than the product of a body of esoteric knowledge, he does not well appreciate the role played by the state. According to Starr and Immergut (1987), the sphere of health care politics is amenable to both contraction and expansion.   They emphasise not only the potential conflicts between various players or actors of different interests in health care politics, but also the changing boundaries of health care politics. In their own words, the boundaries are not fixed but are in reality 'ambiguous, multiple and overlapping' (Starr and Immergut, 1987:251) and are subject to manoeuvring or shaping in the sphere of politics. The state is vested with relative autonomy to define and redefine what is within its responsibility and competence and what is not, what kind of health care should be provided and what should not, and so on (Chapter 2). The power and autonomy enjoyed by the medical profession is but politically contingent, and may be constrained as a result of changing health care priorities, and in periods of health care reforms. The medical profession is however active rather than passive, and may seek to shape the uses of medical professional power in reproducing the predominant clinical approach to medicine and safeguarding their own interests. Terry Johnson (1995) suggests that the state, as an active actor, is usually engaged in conflicts and tensions with the medical profession, which results in the shaping and reshaping of the boundaries of health care politics.

Different Dimensions of Medical Power and their Implications

Medical professional power includes both professional autonomy and professional dominance. Professional autonomy and professional dominance are interrelated and mutually reinforce each other in the way of strengthening the power of the medical profession. Elston (1991) distinguishes between three types of professional autonomy: clinical autonomy, economic autonomy and political autonomy. Clinical autonomy refers to the autonomy of the medical profession in the organisation of clinical work, and the right to set standards and control clinical performance; economic autonomy to the right to determine the level of fees; and political autonomy to the right to make health policy decisions stemming from the position as professional monopoliser of scientific medical knowledge and experts on health matters. Friedson (1970), however, uses political power (which I prefer to use) rather than political autonomy to refer to the exercise of the medical profession's influence over health policy making and health care arrangements. Professional dominance primarily refers to the superior relation of the medical profession to other allied medical occupations in the division of labour (Friedson, 1970; 1985).

Clinical Autonomy

Clinical autonomy is closely related to the success of the medical profession in monopolising medical practice (Berlant, 1975). Doctors are not allowed to practise in health care unless they get a license from the state-recognised professional medical body on the grounds of 'life-and-death' issues and patients' limited knowledge about health care. So, a license system is supposed to safeguard the benefits of patients. According to Johnson (1972), doctors operate a collegiate type of occupational control. That is, the medical practitioners determine how much, how often and what kind of services will be rendered. In addition, it is also the doctors who make the referral to other medical specialists. Doctors can function as both providers and evaluators of medical care in which they are accorded a wide range of clinical or technical freedom and autonomy in determining medical treatment and procedures. But the clinical autonomy enjoyed by the medical profession also results in advancing its own interests, and in further enhancing the power of the medical practitioners in exercising control over recruitment, medical education, training and research activities, clinical performance and standards, and the regulation of members' conduct.

Economic Autonomy

In the health care market, the medical profession enjoys considerable economic autonomy in determining their remuneration. It is especially the case of those services provided on a fee-for-service mode. Friedson (1983) developed the idea of a 'market shelter', provided by legislative controls, which minimises internal competition between doctors themselves. Like many other societies in the world, doctors in Hong Kong have to refrain from advertising the fees for their services, and this has provided them an opportunity to maximise their income as a result. A representative of the Hong Kong Medical Association asserts that 'confidence [on the part of the patients] will make the operation more successful, less painful, explanations more communicable, side-effects more acceptable...' (Fung, 1991). The asymmetry of power as well as information permits doctors to exploit the advantage of practising price discrimination (Enthoven, 1988). The Health and Welfare Branch of the Hong Kong Government, in a consultation paper on health care, has reflected that:

> ...the lack of a fee schedule and the perceived excessive charging tend to be the focus of criticism by the public...While it may not be appropriate for Government to set fees for the private sector, there appears to be a case in the interests of consumer protection for the profession to publish a fee schedule. (Hong Kong Government, 1993a:para.2.16)

While it endorses the idea of doctors listing charges, the Health and Welfare Branch wants the initiative to come from the medical profession and does not wish to legislate for it. In other words, the state intends not to regulate the charges or put an upper limit on medical fees. In response to the overcharging issue of private medicine, the vice-president of the Hong Kong Medical Association has plainly expressed the 'market-shopping' idea that '[i]f doctors overprice, then people will not visit them. It just depends on what you care about - personal benefit or purse benefit' (Murphy, 1994). According to the market-shopping idea, it is the joint responsibility of the doctor and the patient to talk about charges before consultation and treatment. However, it is clear that patients are not in a bargaining position at the time they are ill or injured. They should not be viewed as free and rational buyers in the market, being able to choose intelligently among the providers of health care available to them. Regarding the patient as a free buyer is largely a fiction (Churchill, 1987). However, perpetuating such a myth is entirely favourable to maintaining the economic autonomy enjoyed by the medical profession in Hong Kong. Further, within the context of Hong Kong, the absence of a fee schedule has also made it very difficult for the medical insurance industry to 'monitor' the abuses of medical practitioners in overcharging patients who in turn can claim reimbursement from the insurer, and to devise a standard premium schedule (Hay, 1992) (See Chapter 8 for a detailed discussion of the conflicts between the medical profession and the medical insurance industry).

Compared to their counterparts in the private sector, public doctors (especially those who are salaried) are deprived of economic autonomy in determining their remuneration within the context of Hong Kong. For example, in the British NHS, doctors are salaried employees and do not enjoy the same economic autonomy as their counterparts in the US, where doctors play an important role in resisting the implementation of any national health scheme that may frustrate their professional and economic autonomy (Heung, 1990).

However, the socialisation of health care provision does not directly imply the corresponding reduction of medical power. Elston (1991) argues that the salaried status of doctors and the state intervention in the British NHS in the past forty years are found to be compatible with a high level of professional power in determining access to medical care and organising health care resources. Compared to their counterparts in the US, the salaried hospital consultants in the UK have been given more clinical autonomy pertaining to the diagnosis and treatment of disease, and to the allocation of resources within the health services (Schulz and

Harrison, 1986), despite the fact that the sum total of the financial resources available for public health care is determined by the state. For example, in the US, the implementation of a case-mix management based on diagnosis related groups (DRGs) integrates clinical data with financial data. A systematic peer review system, based on DRGs is organised for monitoring the appropriateness of admissions, surgical procedures, drug uses, and length of stay (Lichtig, 1986). Public hospital doctors both in Hong Kong and the UK do not face such a close monitoring of their clinical or medical activities even though more emphasis has now been placed on using more cost-effective means to treat patients (Abel-Smith, 1992; Hong Kong Hospital Authority, 1994).

Political Power

Politically speaking, doctors form powerful groups, notably national medical association and medical specialist associations, which act like trade unions to defend the self-interest of members. They make use of their position as professional experts in and monopolisers of scientific medical knowledge to justify their power and influence over health policy making. In the formulation of health care policies, the government of Hong Kong normally consults the two major medical professional associations: the Hong Kong Medical Association and the Hong Kong Branch of the British Medical Association. For example, in the preparation of the second or the most recent medical white paper which provided the plans for health care development between 1974 and 1984, the Governor of Hong Kong, in early 1973, appointed a Medical Development Advisory Committee to make recommendations. (This advisory body continued to function but was renamed as the Health and Medical Development Advisory Committee in 1992).

However, the state is often far from always happy with the medical profession. An event which took place in Hong Kong can help to illustrate how the medical profession may be in conflict with the state over the issue of medical personnel. In 1987 the government of Hong Kong was considering altering the Medical Registration Ordinance to admit a number of Belgian doctors not registrable with the Hong Kong Medical Council to practise in the Vietnamese refugees camps. The original idea was to make some medical care available to Vietnamese on site especially in view of the difficulties in recruiting Commonwealth or locally-trained doctors to provide health care services. However, the ex-President of the Hong Kong Medical Association made very strong remarks as follows:

> [t]he profession must forcefully object to this at all cost - for although waiving the registration required for a few Belgian doctors may appear a minor matter, this move may well open a floodgate for medical graduates from other parts of the world to seek similar favours, making thus a mockery out of our attempts to maintain a high standard of medical practice and service to our community. (Leong, 1987:12)

Confronting such a forceful objection from the medical profession, the idea raised by the state could not be realised until May 1992 (Hong Kong Medical Association, 1993:36). This case can show that the local medical profession was a barrier to the state's plan to satisfy the basic health care needs of the Vietnamese refugees as early as possible. The issue of medical manpower is not a new one. As will be discussed in Chapters 4 and 5, the relationship between the state and the medical profession was in much tension over the supply of 'qualified' doctors, and over the jurisdictions of expertise claimed by the medical profession. Matters which Freidson might identify as of purely technical concern erupted into political 'controversy' in the early decades of health policy formation in Hong Kong between late 1950s till mid-1970s.

Sophisticated Technology Partly because of its preoccupation with scientism and partly because of the political power of the medical profession, it has played an important role in shaping the development of high-tech orientation in health care. Unlike what is happening in other fields, the adoption of sophisticated technology in medical care appears to be both capital-intensive and labour-intensive. Capital equipment in medicine is not invariably labour-saving. Indeed, in most instances, it is not. The application of new technology and equipment often necessitates more personnel to install, maintain, operate and monitor the new technologies. Moreover, with the application of new sophisticated technologies - though they may be cheaper than those they replace - they will invite new demands for diagnosis and treatment that was not possible before. This will end up with requests for more well-trained or well-qualified staff to cope with the situation. As a result, unless there are sufficient economic resources together with active political support from the state, the high-tech orientation of scientific biomedicine is bound to be limited. The use of global budgets is a popular strategy adopted by the state to control the spread or development of sophisticated medical technology. In recent years, the role of the medical profession within the sphere of medical control and its high-tech approach to deal with diseases has been vigorously challenged (Gabe et al., 1994). It takes place within the context of rising expenditure on health.

Curative Approach to Health Care   As discussed earlier, with an ever increasing prevalence of chronic illness in developed societies, the curative approach seems to be only partly relevant to the many non-medical aspects of chronic illness. Unlike acute diseases, chronic illnesses usually last for life. The needs of patients and their families encompass far more than the treatment of acute conditions of chronic illness, and include ancillary services and various long-term care support.   A continuing emphasis placed on acute hospital care tends to neglect care when cure is impossible.

Under such circumstances, other non-acute-care approaches may be promoted instead especially in an era emphasising cost containment in health care (Chapter 2). It is generally believed that chronic patients and their family benefit most from long-term care rather than expensive hospital medicine (Wilkin and Hughes, 1986). Although the curative approach is only partly relevant to the many non-clinical aspects of chronic illness, its continual acceptance can however justify the predominant position and vested interest of the medical profession (Ham, 1985). How do recent health care reforms deal with chronic illness within the context of the constraints imposed by the acute care and high-tech approaches to medicine? How does the medical profession react to and involve itself in the transformation of health care delivery approach? How would all this redefine the role of the family in taking care of the sick, or redefine the boundaries between acute and non-acute care to the management of chronic illness? These important questions will be critically examined in Chapter 9.

Professional Dominance

Friedson (1970; 1985) considers the medical dominance enjoyed by the medical profession as a manifestation of its assuming a dominant position in the division of labour within the health care system. As a group, doctors rank higher than all other health workers, even though their numbers are relatively small. The dominance enjoyed by the medical profession over other health care profession highlights their differential access to powers, privileges, resources and other benefits within the formal health care system.

In assuming its dominance, the medical profession is eager to safeguard not only the autonomy to regulate itself and determine remuneration and its influence over health policy making, but also the authority to define the boundaries of and its leadership over other health care professions according to two types of medical dominance strategies: subordination and limitation (Turner, 1988). The subordination strategy characterises the efforts made in subordinating nurses and midwifes by the medical profession; whereas the limitation strategy is characterised by limiting the work of other health care professionals either to specific part of the body (e.g. dentistry) or to a specific therapy (e.g. occupational therapy, physiotherapy, pharmacy). For example, within the context of Hong Kong, the medical profession is allowed by legislative provisions to nominate its own representatives in the respect boards of the allied health professions, but not vice versa, however. In addition, a medical doctor does not permit any diagnosis and treatment of patients by these professions without his/her supervision or referral. In the eyes of the medical profession, such leadership can serve to defend the health of the public (Leong, 1987:13). However, such an assertion and exercise of leadership serves to justify the power of the medical profession in its control and authority over allied health professionals (Stacey, 1988).

According to Turner (1988), in addition to the subordination and limitation strategies in protecting its medical dominance, the medical profession also dominates health care work by means of marginalising rival health care occupations. Within the context of Hong Kong, this type of domination strategy is particularly relevant in explaining the medical dominance of the medical profession over traditional Chinese medicine practitioners who are excluded from the formal health care system. To better examine the political economy of medical power in Hong Kong, questions about the professional inequality between doctors and traditional Chinese medicine practitioners, and their relations to the state cannot be overlooked.

Marginalisation of Chinese Medicine and its Practitioners

As long as Chinese medicine practitioners pay a commercial registration fee, they are allowed to practise Chinese medicine. Nevertheless, the traditional Chinese medicine practitioners compete with the Western medical profession on a widely unequal basis (Lee, 1975; 1981). The Medical Council of Hong Kong, established by the government, is the only statutory body legitimating and supervising medical practice in Hong Kong. All the Council members are however qualified 'Western' doctors, and traditional Chinese medicine practitioners are excluded from the Council. The services of traditional Chinese medicine practitioners are not recognised by the legal authority as duly qualified.

Moreover, the state subsidises only the training of Western doctors, from a start of 1887 when the Hong Kong College of Medicine for Chinese was opened. This medical college later became the Faculty of Medicine, the University of Hong Kong in 1912 (Evans, 1987). Hong Kong has only two University medical schools that are heavily subsidised by the state. The graduates of these two medical schools are entitled to be registered with the Medical Council of Hong Kong. The two University medical schools play a role to legitimate the technical competence of the medical profession through its academic 'authority'. This further marginalises the position of traditional Chinese medicine and its practitioners. If state support in education and training, and in recognising the professional qualification of the traditional Chinese medicine practitioners were provided, there might be much more room for their development and the integration of traditional medicine and Western medicine. This is entirely possible as the People's Republic of China and Taiwan have witnessed such a scenario (Chi, 1994; Wong and Chiu, 1997).

Compared to the Western medical profession, the traditional Chinese medicine practitioners have a much lower degree of technical autonomy. If any practitioner of traditional Chinese medicine is found to possess any antibiotics, poisons or dangerous drugs, he or she will be charged for offence against the provisions of the Pharmacy and Poisons Ordinance or the Antibiotics Ordinance. Also, it is illegal for them to undertake surgery and the treatment of eye diseases for their patients, or use western methods for treatment, such as giving injection, using inoculation instruments, X-ray facilities, etc. Chinese medicine practitioners will be charged under the provision of the Medical Registration Amendment Ordinance if they are found to do so. Moreover, law also prohibits traditional Chinese medicine practitioners from using the English name of 'doctor', or any Chinese name or title which may induce the patients to believe that they are qualified to practise Western medicine. All these legal constraints serve to protect the economic interest and medical dominance of the medical profession both in the market and the public health care system.

Despite their very limited political power and constrained technical autonomy, the Chinese medicine practitioners can exercise their own economic autonomy in setting their level of fees. Also, unlike their counterparts practising Western medicine, they can freely advertise themselves and offer their services like any other goods provided in the market. Partly because of the exercise of medical professional power, and partially because of the legitimation and subsidisation of Western medicine by the state, the status of the traditional medicine system has been undermined. All this creates new forms of commodification and marginalisation of Chinese medicine within the context of Hong Kong (McDermott, 1986).

The state has legitimated Western medicine and regarded it as being relevant to health objectives, but refused to legitimate Chinese medicine in the same way. Because of the interplay of the politics of medical jurisdictional claims and government health care policy formation, the medical profession has heavily influenced the social organisation of health care, and commanded the trust of the public in relation to health matters. However, this does not lead to the elimination of traditional Chinese medicine in Hong Kong. The discussion of Chapters 4 and 5 will show how the government of Hong Kong gradually recognised and continued to maintain the role played by Chinese medicine in meeting part of the health care needs of the population.

Promotion of Traditional Chinese Medicine The above discussion has already pointed out that the marginalisation of traditional Chinese medicine has not led to the exclusion of its continuing practice in the health care market, even though it has not been incorporated into the official health care system. In short, state intervention in the field of health care has been biased against traditional Chinese medicine and biased in favour of scientific biomedicine. Compared to the medical profession, the practitioners of traditional Chinese medicine have obtained no control over health affairs, no economic subsidy from the state, but much greater restriction in respect of technical autonomy.

However, alongside the recognition of the limited efficacy and the cost implication of Western medicine, there has been an increasing interest in traditional medicine in many nation states (Hyma and Ramesh, 1994). Hong Kong is no exception to such a trend. In view of the need to contain the cost of health care, traditional medicine may be recognised by the state as a valuable resource to supplement scientific biomedicine. Certainly, in examining the promotion of traditional Chinese medicine in Hong Kong, the shaping and adoption of an 'appropriate' strategy must be examined in relation to the reality of medical professional power and the existing organisation of the formal health care system in the local context.

Conclusion

The clinical view of health has reinforced a health care system in which hospitals and clinics become the central workplace attracting most resources for dealing with health and diseases.   Above all, this clinical model has elevated the status of medical specialists and experts to a central position in the treatment of diseases despite their limited contribution to the achievement of health. The clinical approach to health care has important implications for the organisation of health care and the use of health care resources, which are all biased for interests of the medical profession.

However, the relationship between the medical profession and the state is a mixture of collaboration and tensions. According to changing health care objectives and socio-economic environment, the state may adopt a different mix of interventions to redefine the responsibility of the state and the public/private mix in health care.   It may also play a politically contentious role in reshaping the boundaries of health care politics and thus undermine the autonomy enjoyed by the medical profession. Precisely, the realities both of medical professional power and of the relations between the medical profession and the state have to be well appreciated in examining health care development and its reforms in the context of Hong Kong.

4　Health Care Development, 1945-1966

Introduction

The civil order, infrastructure and economy of Hong Kong were severely damaged during the Second World War and the concomitant Japanese army occupation of the territory for three years and eight months until August 1945. When the Communist Party took power in China in 1949, a huge wave of immigration took place in Hong Kong. The population of Hong Kong grew from 600,000 in 1945 to an estimate of 2,360,000 in 1950; that is, almost a four-fold increase within a short period of five years. This swollen population put a severe strain on the Colony's resources, of food, water supply, sanitation and medical services (Endacott, 1958:205).

In the immediate post-war years 1945-1949, Hong Kong society was still unstable, and its health care policy was also a reflection of such a situation. Since 1950, immigration from China was subjected to restriction and strict control by both China and Hong Kong, even though there were still three more surges in 1951-1952, 1957-58 and 1962 - all of them closely corresponding with the political ups and downs in China (Brown, 1971). Between 1950 and 1963, there was a more stable population and the take off of industrialisation took place. The year 1964 is an important milestone in the post-war health care history of Hong Kong, since the first Medical White Paper was released then. This White Paper covered ten years up to 1973 before the publication of the second Medical White Paper in 1974. However, since the 'rioting years' of 1966 and 1967 had significant implications for social service development in Hong Kong, the development between 1966-67 and 1973 will be discussed in Chapter 6. This chapter will particularly focus on how the government defined its role and boundary of intervention in health care and how it utilised the different major societal resources in response tothe changing political and socio-economic context of Hong Kong between 1945 and 1966.

Hong Kong's Political Context: an Alliance between Capitalists and Colonial Bureaucrats

During the seven years between 1945 to 1952, there were five different plans drawn for constitutional reform in Hong Kong (Miners, 1989). However, the only change which came out of the long-lasting and heated constitutional debates was just a modest increase in the number of elected seats on the Urban Council from 2 to 4 out of 15 (Endacott, 1964). Tsang (1988) argues that if any one of these plans had been successfully implemented, democracy would not have been shelved as a result, and the alliance formed between capitalists and colonial bureaucrats might then have been subjected to more challenge.

The debates over constitutional reform were overshadowed by the start of the Communist regime in China in 1949. The unofficial members of the Executive and Legislative Councils, who were mostly representatives of big businesses, requested that the constitutional reform be abandoned (Endacott, 1964). They were afraid that a more democratic government would lead to much public participation in the central decision-making body and much public discussion of various sorts of policies, and would give an opportunity to disruptive elements, in particular the Communists and the Nationalists in the Colony. Because of the political uncertainty of Hong Kong after 1949, what the capitalists wanted most was to exploit the cheap labour and the laissez-faire environment to accelerate the speed of capital accumulation. A more democratic government would mean a great obstacle to their exercise of influence over the economic and social policies implemented by the state.

Not only the capitalists but also the top-level colonial bureaucrats lacked enthusiasm for constitutional reform. The colonial bureaucrats were afraid that if a more democratic Legislative Council were set up instead, it would become a battlefield for fractional political interests which would then be too difficult for them to manage. The colonial bureaucrats were therefore unlikely to support reforms which would eliminate their political power and influence in the Colony. Although their arguments against the whole scheme of constitutional reform were different, colonial bureaucrats and capitalists formed themselves an alliance to safeguard their political status and interest in the post-war years.

Because of the setback in constitutional reform, Hong Kong's power structure was still characterised by the domination of a small group of elites comprised of high-level colonial bureaucrats and capitalists, both Chinese and European, as it was before the outbreak of the Second World War (Davies, 1977).   Such an alliance was by no means in perfect harmony, but it gave the very first priority to economic development, and strongly supported the principle and practice of laissez-faire policy characterised by a balanced-budget, a low-tax policy and incremental expansion of government expenditure in line with the overall rate of economic growth (Rabushka, 1976). Close working relationships and interdependence developed between colonial bureaucrats and capitalists in the Colony (Rear, 1971).

The capitalist class constituted itself as an important power group in Hong Kong with which the state had to reckon in formulating and implementing its policies (Leung, 1990).   The broad confluence of interests between the colonial bureaucrats and the capitalists contributed to an overall policy of supporting economic development, notably private enterpreneurship. However, to paraphrase Miliband (1977), the colonial state of Hong Kong was not acting at the behest of the capitalist class. Because of its exercise of relative autonomy, while the colonial state would provide a most favourable environment for the capitalists to make profits, including the provision of basic infrastructure and services, it would also consider the overall social and economic needs of the population in the Colony.

Health Care Development, 1945-1949

Control of Epidemics and Trade Restoration

Because of its endowment with few natural resources and mineral deposits and arable land, and because of its very embryonic stage of industrial development, the maintenance of port facilities and a general healthy environment were deemed essential by the government to the survival of the economy of Hong Kong in the immediate post-war years. During the immediate post-war period, 1945-1949, the health services development strategy was no different to that adopted prior to 1942: most of the state resources devoted to medical and health services were concentrated on the control of communicable diseases, particularly the formidable epidemics of small-pox, cholera and tuberculosis (Hong Kong Government, 1964). The underlying purpose of such a strategy remained the same: the maintenance of healthy conditions for the development of entrepot trade which remained active and well until 1949.

Overloaded Curative Care

On the curative side of health care, no new hospital was built during the period 1945-1950 (Hong Kong Government, 1964). Many patients were even refused admission on account of the overcrowding of wards (Tung Wah Group of Hospitals, 1961). The extent of overcrowding could well be illustrated as follows:

> [d]uring the period of 1945 to 1958, it was not uncommon to find two patients sharing a bed. A maximum record showed that even five patients shared a bed, which was of course not only against the principle of medical treatment but was also absolutely inhuman. (Tung Wah Group of Hospitals, 1971:48)

Both the accommodation and medical equipment of Tung Wah hospitals were inadequate to meet the sudden increased medical demand generated by the very large number of immigrants. In the words of the Board of Directors of Tung Wah, the number of patients they had to cope with had 'broke[n] the record in the Tung Wah history of the past 80 odd years' (Tung Wah Group of Hospitals, 1971:57).

Recruitment of Unregistrable Doctors

In addition, the government also experienced great difficulties in recruiting enough registered doctors to serve even the most basic medical needs within this period. Compared to private practitioners, who could make a good profit in the market, government employment proved unattractive to both overseas and local registered doctors. At the same time, the University of Hong Kong was experiencing considerable difficulties in getting into full swing after the end of the Second World War. In fact, the Medical Faculty of the University did not restart its training of post-war medical students until 1947. As it took five years until 1952 to have the first batch of post-war medical graduates serving as interns for a year in government hospitals before they could register with the Medical Council of Hong Kong, the severe shortage of registered doctors could not be immediately tackled. Confronting the strong opposition of the medical profession, the government decided to appoint doctors who had qualified in China and other non-Commonwealth countries but who were not eligible for registration in Hong Kong in order to maintain the most basic medical services.

These government-recruited doctors were exempted from registration and were legally entitled to call themselves 'Western doctor' (*sai-i*) along with the registered. They could work in the British Forces, in university teaching and government service (Topley, 1978). However, because of professional opposition, the appointment of unregistered doctors in government services could only be made on a temporary basis. The report of the Director of Medical and Health Services for the year 1948/49 states that 'The policy is to replace these [unregistered] doctors by those eligible for registration when the opportunity arises' (Medical and Health Department, 1949:28). The attractiveness of government employment could have been enhanced by means of significantly improving the salary and fringe benefits of government doctors. Certainly, such an exercise would be much more costly than the appointment of unregistered doctors who could not be promoted to the rank of Medical and Health Officer (the initial entry point of registered doctors) until after four years' satisfactory services (Working Party on Unregistrable Doctors, 1975). Even though the exercise of state power was against the wish of the medical profession, the state could make use of the available supply of unregistered doctors to serve its needs in medical care. Without the supply of unregistered doctors, the government could not maintain essential measures for the prevention and control of communicable diseases and to provide basic medical care for the poor. The medical profession was not passive at all; it continued to keep an eye on this issue which might threaten its interest. This will be further discussed in the chapter.

Measures Used to Discourage the Settlement of Refugees in the Colony

Overall, the government was reluctant to make any long-term social policy planning to cater for the new demands generated by the influx of immigrants. It was afraid that the better the facilities provided in the Colony, the more refugees would be attracted to Hong Kong (Hong Kong Government, 1949).

Even after 1949 when the Communist Party came into power in China, some government officials still believed that the immigrants would return home to China and the problems would be solved. The government just performed the role of trouble shooter. 'Whatever was most urgent was done in the easiest and quickest way...[N]o question of long-term policy was even considered unless an irrevocable decision could no longer be postponed' (Hong Kong Government, 1950:2).

Moreover, the government feared that any move to significant improvement of social services would result in attracting even larger number of immigrants from the Mainland (Hodge, 1976:6). Thus, during the period 1945-50, state intervention in social policy, including curative health services, was kept to a minimum so that both immigrants and potential immigrants might be discouraged from coming to or staying in Hong Kong.

Rather than expanding the provision of social services, the government used repatriation as a means to solve the problem of immigrants during the late 1940s just as it did prior to 1942 (Tung Wah Group of Hospitals, 1971:29). After the Second World War, the Board of Tung Wah was again entrusted by the government to form an association to persuade those unemployed and discharged patients to return to their places of origin. In 1947, more than eleven thousand people were repatriated either at the request of the government or at the discretion of Tung Wah (Tung Wah Group of Hospitals, 1961). However, the immigrant population was too large to be repatriated on any significant scale. Moreover, repatriation work could no longer be carried out ever after the start of the Communist regime in Mainland China about the end of 1949.

Health Care Development, 1950-1963

Changing Socio-economic Context in the Post-embargo Years

When the Communist Party came into power in Mainland China at the end of 1949, most of the immigrants in Hong Kong did not return to the Mainland as they had done prior to the outbreak of the Second World War. The United Nations' refugee report on Hong Kong published in 1955 estimated that about 99 per cent of refugees would not return to China (Hambro, 1955). In the past, repatriation was used as a means to reduce the number of immigrants. However, different political ideologies between Communist China and the Western World justified the immigrants' claim to stay in Hong Kong under the British colonial rule. In the words of the Hong Kong governor Sir Alexander Grantham (1965:112), the large influx of immigrants could no longer be viewed as a transient population but had to be integrated into the Colony as 'permanent citizens'.

In addition, the change of government in China in 1949 and the imposition of the United Nations embargo on trade with Communist China in 1950 brought fundamental changes to the economic policy of Hong Kong. These changes led to a drastic reduction in the volume of trade between China and the non-communist world, and in turn, the entrepot trade volume in Hong Kong (Cheng, 1986). As pointed out earlier, Hong Kong had always lived by entrepot trade. The stopping of the flow of goods through Hong Kong to China and the rest of the world was a tragedy to Hong Kong especially at a time when the Colony was burdened with a million refugees.

Nevertheless, the influx of refugees also brought to the Colony the necessary capital, knowledge, skill and technology which were essential for the development of manufacturing industry. In the years since 1950, the Colony successfully restructured its entrepot economy to a manufacturing economy which exported some 80 per cent of her industrial output mainly to the developed economies of the West (Hong Kong National Committee, 1966). Post-war immigration also brought a large volume of cheap labour to the Colony. These immigrants had little choice but to sell their labour for a low wage. Unlike the pre-war labour force that could return to Mainland China in order to escape poor living conditions, the post-war immigrants had no 'rural safety net' to catch the casualties of the industrial system (Owen, 1971:150). The political turmoil in the Mainland strengthened the discipline of the labour force and made it easier for them to accept low wages and very harsh working conditions. With the growth of manufacturing industry, a substantial proportion of the labour force could be absorbed into the manufacturing sector. Yet, the unemployment rate was still very high. It was estimated that in the financial year 1952-53, there were about 160,000 unemployed people (Hambro, 1955:47). Because of low wages, and because of the serious problem of unemployment, widespread poverty was evident. According to Hambro's estimation, the minimum income for a family with two children and two adults should be HK$120 to HK$150 per month. But he found that many families had incomes lower than HK$100 (Hambro, 1955:48).

Utilisation of Charity Efforts to Expand the Provision of Medical Care

Realising that a very large number of immigrants were going to settle in the Colony, the state was anxious to make use of charity efforts to meet the very basic social needs of the 'immigrant' society (Hodge, 1981).   In fact, in the immediate post-war period, Hong Kong was officially designated an area deserving of international aid.   Most of the work of these international aid organisations was concentrated on relief work and injection of funds into indigenous voluntary relief agencies.   In addition to relief work, some small-scale foreign missionary bodies were also involved in the provision of subsidised outpatient services to the general public.   But as will be shown later, these 'charity clinics' could only be run with a modest budget as a result of the availability of unregistered or unregistrable doctors in Hong Kong.

Some international missionary bodies, notably Caritas, were also involved in building private non-profit hospitals in the more deprived areas to provide hospital care (Chu, 1988).   However, in view of the rising demands for curative care, most of these hospitals had to apply for financial subvention from the government.   Prior to qualifying for state subvention and then turning into a subvented hospital, a hospital had to satisfy the government that it was capable of efficiently using financial resources.   Through giving annual subventions, the government could capitalise the infrastructure set up by these private non-profit hospitals and could therefore save expenses on building and other capital expenditure as well.   Besides, it was also a faster way to develop the basic health care facilities to meet the growing demand of the population for health care. Since these hospitals had to rely heavily on subvention, the role of the government was becoming increasingly important.

Within the local context, Tung Wah Hospitals became one of the focal points for the government's mobilisation of societal resources to cope with the rising medical demands of the population.   Moreover, the Tung Wah was an important mechanism in selecting Chinese elites for the top decision-making bodies of the Colony: the Executive and Legislative Councils. During the period 1946-60 five Chinese people were nominated into the Executive Council: 'all five are on the permanent board of directors of the most prominent charity organisation [i.e. the Tung Wah] in Hong Kong' (Topley, 1969:213).   In the same period, nine Chinese people held office in the Legislative Council and six of them were members of Tung Wah.   In addition, all members of the Tung Wah's Board of

Directors were non-official Justices of the Peace. The Tung Wah was thus an important mechanism for the Chinese elites to turn wealth and charity efforts into status and political power in Hong Kong. Being aware of the political ambitions of the leading Chinese elites, the government could make use of the appointment system to 'encourage' their contribution to meeting the needs of the community, including medical care.

The government's utilisation of charity efforts was also extended to the district level via its encouragement of the setting up of Kaifongs (or neighbourhood associations) which boomed especially after the imposition of United Nations embargo on trade with China (McDouall and Keen, 1955). Although Kaifongs had existed before the war, they all disappeared after the Japanese occupation of the Colony. It was not until 1949 that a first Kaifong was founded (Wong, 1972). Again, Kaifongs were conceived as a mechanism for the seeking of prestige and status among the Chinese. The main differences between Tung Wah and Kaifongs were that: first, the elites of Tung Wah were the most influential figures in the Colony, while the members of Kaifongs were prominent elements in a district; second, the work of Tung Wah was implemented on a community-wide basis, while the work of the Kaifongs were confined in a specific district. The Kaifongs were regarded as charities at neighbourhood or district level tapping and mobilising local resources and support for 'communal' welfare. As of 1966, among all the 29 Kaifongs established in Hong Kong, nearly all of them (96%) were engaged in the provision of medical services.

As a result of the booming of Kaifongs during the 1950s, the number of outpatient attendances provided at Kaifong-run 'charity' clinics as a proportion of those provided by outpatient clinics of ex-government and ex-subvented hospitals increased from 1 per cent in 1950 to its probable historical peak of 5.33 per cent in 1958 (calculation based on the data provided in Wong, 1972:264, and Census and Statistics Department, 1969). The contribution of Kaifongs could therefore help to supplement some of the work of the Medical and Health Department. Since the Kaifongs ran their services on a self-financing basis and on a smaller scale than the larger charitable organisations, it is not difficult to understand why they could not run hospitals to cater for the medical needs of a district. But because of their medium-size and their proximity to the local population, the Kaifongs could do something that Tung Wah might not be able to offer, for example, the provision of more accessible outpatient care, and the mobilisation of local finance and voluntary efforts for their work.

In addition to Kaifong associations, most of the district associations, clansmen associations, village associations and rural committees formed by Chinese people of different places of origin or different localities were also involved in the provision of low-cost outpatient care to their respective members (Hong Kong Government, 1967). As some of these were too small to finance their activities, the government also used other charity resources to finance their work. For example, 'Surplus moneys from the Chinese Temple Fund are paid into the general Chinese Charities Fund from which grants are made to various deserving Chinese charities and institutions' (Secretary for Chinese Affairs, 1952:3). In this way, community resources were further mobilised for the sake of strengthening a sense of charity among the Chinese population.

The Limitations of Charity Efforts   However, the fund raising capacity of Tung Wah was far from adequate to exempt the government from heavily subsidising its medical work. For example, Tung Wah Group of Hospitals received donations totalling HK$1,724,324 for the financial year 1958-59, which was 5.6 per cent of the subvention it received from the government (Tung Wah Group of Hospitals, 1971). Its financial dependence upon the government made it very difficult for Tung Wah to have a stronger bargaining power to make room for the practice of Chinese medicine within hospitals. Accompanied by the government's identification with Western medicine as a 'scientific' and 'modernised' way of healing was also an exercise of strong control of medical work by the medical profession. Within such a context, herbal medicine and acupuncture could not be used as an alternative or be integrated with Western medicine, which might help to limit the cost of inpatient treatment. Simply, in the case of acupuncture, the use of just a few needles was not an expensive medical procedure or treatment. In the post-embargo years when there was a severe lack of health care resources to deal with the very large population, the official decision to continue to marginalise the practice of traditional Chinese medicine outside the 'official' health care domain not only limited the health care resources available to hospital care, but also constrained the role of Tung Wah in developing traditional Chinese medicine.

Besides, the charity work of Kaifongs and other district or clansmen associations was largely confined to the provision of low-fee outpatient services augmented with assistance to immunisation campaigns and health education activities mainly targeted to women. However, because of their overall modest budgets, these associations were often under financial pressures, which ultimately led them to change their emphasis from welfare work, such as free education, medical services and relief work to community organisation and women's and youth work. Because of such a change of emphasis, and because of the lack of means of finance, the relative proportion of outpatient services provided by Kaifongs' clinics in relation to those subsidised by the government had dropped from the peak of 5.33 per cent in 1958 to 3.3 percent in 1963 and then to 3.2 per cent in 1966 (see Wong, 1972; Census and Statistics Department, 1969). But as will be further discussed later, because of the availability of unregistered doctors, the Kaifongs together with other missionary bodies, trade unions and employers (the latter two are non-charity-based) could still provide a considerable proportion of outpatient services to the working class or the poor.

Plans to Expand Subsidised Medical Care, 1957-1963

In 1957, an outline of a 15-year development plan for medical and health services was submitted to the government for consideration. From a historical point of view, this document had a special meaning because this was the first time the colonial government ever had a long-term outline plan for medical care. This plan outlined the desirable development of comprehensive medical services and the financial resources required. However this 15-year plan was not approved by the government for two reasons. First, it was prepared in the absence of factual census data upon which population projection could be based. Second, because of uncertain economic trends and changing patterns of demand for medical and health services, such a long term programme covering a period of 15 years was not regarded to be flexible enough (Hong Kong Government, 1964).

In 1959, a plan covering the years 1960-1965 was prepared by the planning unit of the then Medical and Health Department. This represented a more detailed plan for a segment of the 15-year outline proposal submitted earlier in 1957. Two points are worth highlighting. First, the plan accepted that the overall medical facilities provided by government, voluntary and private agencies existing at that time were insufficient to meet the medical needs of the community. Within this context, many poor patients who could not afford private medical care had to suffer as a result of the inadequacy of subsidised medical care. Second, it was recommended that the government should play a significant role in funding hospital and clinic services due to the fact that a very large proportion of the population could not afford to pay economic charges for the services provided in the private sector (Hong Kong Government, 1964:para.19).

The plan was approved in principle by the Executive Council in 1960, subject to provision of the necessary funds by the Finance Committee and further detailed consideration at all stages of development. It recommended a target of 5.75 hospital beds per 1,000 population. This plan also emphasised that greater effort should be concentrated on building new clinics because outpatient facilities could be provided more quickly than new hospitals and that they could play an important role in controlling and preventing communicable diseases. It was stated in the Annual Report of Hong Kong for the year of 1960 that:

> ...the policy of government is to provide, directly, indirectly, either free or low cost, medical and personal health services to that large section of the community which is unable to seek medical attention from other sources. (Hong Kong Government, 1961:213)

Such a policy statement was stated in subsequent annual yearbooks and further reaffirmed in the first Medical White Paper released in 1964. Moreover, the 1961 census in Hong Kong provided for the first time some basic data for planning purposes. This prompted the Hong Kong government to set up a Working Party to revise the 1960-65 plan in 1963. As a result of the government's decision to revise the medical plan endorsed in 1960, it had never been fully carried out. The Working Party produced a White Paper on the development of medical and health services in Hong Kong, which was accepted by the government in 1964. This first Medical White Paper considered the standards to be adopted in the planning of medical and health facilities, and set up the requirements of medical and health facilities for the 10-year period of 1963-1972. To facilitate the implementation of this 10-year medical development plan, the government also set up a Standing Committee in 1964.

The government, however, did not regard it desirable at all to plan to provide comprehensive medical services for the entire population. The reason stated by the government was lack of adequate resources (Hong Kong Government, 1964:para.18). As far as policy objectives were concerned, the government did not intend to provide medical care for those who could buy it in the private sector. In other words, the government's immediate role was defined as providing health care for the poor, not the whole community; and it had never entertained the idea of nationalising the health care system in Hong Kong. Private practitioners and hospitals were to continue to play a role in meeting the needs of those who could afford economic fees.

An Emphasis on Public Health Care, 1950-1963

During the period 1950-1963, major health services were developed along three lines. Firstly, similar to the medical strategy adopted between 1945-50, priority was given to the development of quarantine and epidemiological services dealing with epidemic diseases, particularly the formidable epidemic diseases of cholera which struck Hong Kong most severely in 1961 (Mackenzie, 1961). With regard to actual practice, the inoculation and immunisation schemes and the treatments of almost all communicable diseases were free of charge. The development of public health measures benefiting the whole community was also considered by the government as being important for providing a healthy environment for economic development (Hong Kong Government, 1964).

Secondly, compared with 1945-50, a new emphasis had been placed on maternal and child health services to combat the high maternal and infant mortality especially in view of the large natural increase of population. There was no charge for inpatient treatment or accommodation in the maternity wards of government hospitals although when food was provided there was a minimal maintenance charge (Hong Kong Government, 1960). The maternal and child health clinics were considered by the government to play a strategic role in supplying 'a healthy adult population of the future...[as a result of] the early diagnosis and treatment of those childhood illnesses which if allowed to progress can lead to permanent disabilities' (Hong Kong Government, 1964:para.62). Again, the priority given to the development of maternal and child health services was shaped by their contribution to economic development. The poor health and permanent disabilities of children as a result of poor access to health care was perceived to be an eventual burden on the health care resources of the Colony. A good healthy build-up of this segment of population was considered an important source of healthy adults in the future. As discussed earlier, no social assistance was given to the able-bodied adults because of unemployment.   Thus, within the context of Hong Kong, healthy adults were equivalent to healthy workers who had to work hard to make a living.   In Marxist terminology, the provision of maternal and child health services was aimed at the reproduction of future labour force (Chapter 1).   Pregnant women and mothers were targets for health education not only for their own health, but also for the health of their child(ren).   In feminist terminology, women's caring labour was exploited on the basis of their gender.   Indeed, child health services rely upon the basis of informal health care which is largely dependent on the unpaid labour of women (Stacey, 1988).

Thirdly, health services also included the institution of measures to control the major health menace of tuberculosis. The BCG immunisation scheme for preventing tuberculosis directly benefited those new-born babies in government hospitals and clinics. Besides, the BCG vaccine was also provided without charge to doctors and midwives working in the private and voluntary sectors throughout the whole Colony. During 1962, more than four fifths (82%) of new born babies were vaccinated with BCG within 48 hours of birth (Hong Kong Government, 1963). Free inpatient and outpatient treatment was free to tuberculosis patients. The outpatient clinics handled quite a number of tuberculosis patients who could continue to work without danger to others (Hong Kong Government, 1964). The provision of free or low-fee treatment contributed to the reproduction of the labour force for the expanding industrialising economy. As most of the light manufacturing industries established in Hong Kong were labour-intensive, the demand for healthy workers was great. In fact, by 1960, a shortage of young workers was reported by the Labour Department (1960).

Unregistrable Doctors and Charity Clinics: Conflicts between the State and the Medical Profession

Unregistrable Doctors Employed in the Public Sector

The two major professional associations, the local British Medical Association and the Hong Kong Chinese Medical Association (now known as the Hong Kong Medical Association) did not accept doctors trained in China for membership. The main criterion for recognition is that the relevant college or university should be open to inspection by the General

Medical Council in the UK. To achieve such a purpose, the Council should have right to access to the college or university, and that it should teach in a language the Council could understand (Topley, 1978). All this was very difficult to achieve especially when a closed-door policy was adopted by the Chinese government with the start of the Communist regime in Mainland China.

However, as discussed earlier, this did not prevent the government from employing these unregistrable doctors. Most of these doctors worked in ex-government hospitals, and if needed, some of them would be seconded to ex-subvented hospitals since the latter were not permitted to recruit unregistrable doctors by themselves. It was recorded that there had been a major intake of unregistrable doctors in 1963 following a large number of resignations from Tung Wah hospitals. Most of the recruited unregistrable doctors were immediately seconded to replace the many registered doctors who resigned from Tung Wah hospitals that year (Working Party on Unregistrable Doctors, 1975). During his governorship in Hong Kong between 1947 and 1957, Sir Alexander Grantham (1965:160) described the problem as follows:

[a]s we were very short of private practitioners, it seemed ridiculous to deny ourselves the services of these men [unregistered doctors]. To enable them to practise privately would have required an amendment to the law. The local medical profession was, however, strongly opposed. Throughout my service in Hong Kong and elsewhere, I have noticed that the medical fraternity is a past master at restrictive practices.

In the immediate post-embargo years, many local registered doctors left the Colony fearing that Hong Kong's socio-economic situation would get worse as a result of the drastic reduction of entrepot trade. Because of such a large-scale emigration of local registered doctors, the government found it very difficult to recruit enough registered doctors for its needs. Again, as it did in the immediate post-war years, the government continued to appoint unregistered doctors on a temporary basis, and had them accommodated within the 'exempted' category. The supply of unregistered doctors trained in Western medicine was further increased in 1949 with a large influx of these doctors. By 31st March 1950, when the total departmental staff was 127 doctors, 36 (28.3%) were unregistrable doctors (Medical and Health Department, 1951). A year after the imposition of the embargo in 1950, the proportion of unregistrable doctors within government service even increased to 49.6 per cent: of a total of 125 Medical Officers, Assistant Medical Officers and House Officers, 62 were unregistrable. The departmental report of the then Medical and Health Department (1951:32) for 1950/51 clearly states that without them 'it would have been impossible to maintain the medical services in the Colony at their present standards'.

The medical profession viewed this policy with dismay, but recognised that the government could not provide basic preventive and curative services without drawing on this 'reserve'. Yet the medical profession was very active to prevent the 'legal' practice of unregistrable doctors from becoming a permanent policy in Hong Kong. The Hong Kong Chinese Medical Association held an extraordinary general meeting on 14 July 1955 specifically discussing the question of licensing of unregistrable doctors. It came up with a resolution that 'All non-registrable doctors who wish to practice in Hong Kong must conform to the regulations of the General Medical Council of Great Britain' (Chow, 1956:1). In response to the practice of recruiting unregistrable doctors in government service, the local British Medical Association and the Hong Kong Chinese Medical Association jointly requested that they should be replaced by registered doctors as soon as possible (Working Party on Unregistrable Doctors, 1975).

Unlike their registered counterparts, the unregistrable doctors employed in government service could not practise privately. After several years of practice in government service, a registered doctor might resign and make more money by working as a private practitioner. As shown above, they might even emigrate to other countries in case of political and/or economic instability in the Colony. Compared with registered doctors, unregistrable doctors had much less choice and this is a significant reason to explain why they were a stable workforce in government service. Irrespective of the supply of local medical graduates by the University of Hong Kong since the early 1950s, the proportion of unregistrable doctors in the Medical and Health Service Department still formed about 18 per cent (18.12%) of the medical staff in 1963 compared to 49.6 per cent in 1951 (Advisory Committee on Reviewing the Doctor Problem in the Hong Kong Government Service, 1969).

Moreover, because of their limited bargaining power, they were often assigned to fill 'undesirable' posts: these include general outpatient clinics, family health service clinics, tuberculosis and chest clinics, the floating clinics, the Prisons medical service, and clinics in outlying islands of Hong Kong, like Lantau and Cheung Chau. The fact is that those doctors who were assigned to clinics of these sorts had no opportunity of specialist training that could lead to the development of expertise in certain areas (Advisory Committee on Reviewing the Doctor Problem in the Hong Kong Government Service, 1969). Through the utilisation of unregistrable doctors, the government could stabilise part of the medical workforce by placing them in unattractive posts which were deemed necessary for the prevention and control of diseases and for a more precise selection of patients admitted to hospital beds.

The 'problem' of unregistrable doctors, to a great extent, resulted from the shortage of registered doctors in Hong Kong, and their unwillingness to work in government service because of lower income compared to private practice. To increase the ready supply of registered doctors, the government took the initiative to invite the Society of Apothecaries of London to hold examinations in Hong Kong to allow the unregistrable doctors to sit for the qualifying examinations for the LMSSA (Licentiate in Medicine and Surgery of the Society of Apothecaries). It was finally resolved that the qualifying examinations would be held in Hong Kong on an once-for-all exercise for three consecutive years from 1958 to 1960. However, not all unregistrable doctor with Chinese medical qualifications were eligible to sit for the examinations: only graduates from 12 known Chinese medical schools, qualifying before 1953, were accepted. Finally, only 126 out of 177 sitting candidates could be admitted to the register (Advisory Committee on Clinics, 1966). As a consequence of the strict conditions required by the LMSSA, many unregistered doctors, including those employed in government service, were not qualified to sit for the examination. Because the General Medical Council of Britain would not welcome any further examinations for the unregistrable doctors, no further examinations were held after 1960. Such a decision had made it difficult for the government to significantly enlarge the pool of registered doctors for its recruitment exercises. But this did not result in the discontinuation of the employment of unregistered doctors in government service.

Unregistrable Doctors and 'Charity Clinics'

Since a large number of unregistrable doctors came from China after 1949, not all of them could obtain employment in government service. However, from the end of the Japanese occupation of the Colony, until it was amended in 1964, the Medical Registration Ordinance of Hong Kong provided that only a registered medical practitioner might practise medicine for gain. It could therefore be implied that any unregistered medical practitioner (or indeed anyone at all) could practise Western medicine if he or she did not do so for a profit. Many of the unregistrable doctors turned to the 'charity clinics' in an 'honorary' capacity. It was not said in the Ordinance, for example, that these doctors could not receive a 'donation' from the sponsoring bodies of the charity clinics. This class of unregistrable doctors was legally recognised but could not take the title 'Western doctors', practise privately, or join the major medical associations.

The charity clinics were set up with the objective of providing free or low-cost medical attention for the poor. The sponsoring bodies of the charity clinics were usually missionary societies, Kaifongs and other district associations, trade unions and even employers themselves. As discussed above, the first two types of sponsoring bodies were truly charitable. The third one was run on the basis of mutual help with financial contributions made by union members. The final one was in fact run by employers, and medical care was provided to employees as fringe benefits. To save expenses, and to run their clinics within their limited budget, almost all of these sponsoring bodies employed unregistrable doctors.

During the 1950s charity clinics rapidly increased in number. The Director of Medical and Health Services stated in the annual departmental report that 'hundreds of patients...[had]...literally to be turned away daily from Government outpatient clinics in the urban areas' (Medical and Health Department, 1957:7). The government was well aware that there was a need for the charity clinics to provide low-cost outpatient services to the sick poor. During the late 1950s and early 1960s, most of these charity clinics were staffed by unregistrable doctors (Advisory Committee on Clinics, 1966). Without the supply of unregistrable doctors, the sponsoring bodies could not run their own clinics within their limited budgets, nor could the government effectively utilise the charity or mutual-help efforts of the Colony in terms of providing low-cost medical attention for the poor.

In light of the interpretation of the Medical Registration Ordinance mentioned above, no effective control could be exercised over such clinics or the unregistrable doctors working in them. The numbers of charity clinics further increased and some of them were even found to be run by nurses, dressers or persons who had no qualifications whatsoever. In

1957, the government attempted to introduce a roll of licensed assistant medical practitioners to control unregistered doctors employed in charity clinics (Advisory Committee on Clinics, 1966). An appointed Board would hold examinations for admission to this roll on an once-and-for-all exercise. In response to this, it was stated in very strong wording in the annual report of the Honorary Secretary to the Hong Kong Chinese Medical Association that 'Both BMA and CMA are firmly convinced that while the registration of clinics is long overdue, the formation of a roll of licensed "Assistant Medical Practitioners" by a local examination board is *totally unacceptable*' (Kuan, 1958:para.Ic, my emphasis). The two major Associations objected to this scheme although it did not propose to allow the 'licensees' to have the right to private practice. Neither did the government give in to the Associations' wish to stop the unregistrable doctors from continuing their practice in charity clinics. For a short time the problem as well as the proposed solution were shelved.

Again in 1960, the Director of Medical and Health Services proposed the registration of clinics and the establishment of a list of assistant medical practitioners who might be permitted to practise medicine. An important reason underlying such an attempt made by the government was to turn unregistrable doctors into assistant medical practitioners, which would then expand the pool of medical workforce available for recruitment in government services or charity clinics. However, the two major medical Associations once again strongly opposed the proposed list of assistant medical practitioners. The Associations were of the view that 'those persons who failed the LMSSA examination or had not been eligible to sit for it should not be allowed to become assistant medical practitioners' (Working Party on Unregistrable Doctors, 1975:37). Their concern was not just on the continuing existence of charity clinics and their right to employ unregistrable doctors, but also on turning unregistrable doctors in government service into a permanent team of assistant medical practitioners. The underlying fear of the medical profession is that the setting up of a two-tier system of medical practitioners and assistant medical practitioners would be a threat to their own interests, both in terms of economic interest and their exclusive power to perform medical activities restricted to the medical profession only.

Because the government was unwilling to confront the strong opposition of the medical profession, neither proposal suggested above was pursued. Following further discussions and debate between the government and the medical profession, the Medical Clinics Ordinance was enacted on 5 September 1963. The Ordinance required that all registered clinics be supervised by a registered medical practitioner. Clinics already in existence might continue to employ unregistrable doctors if they passed an interview and could be classified as 'exempted clinics', but new ones had to employ registered doctors. Since the scheme was an once-and-for-all exercise, the legal 'loophole' would be closed but without losing charity clinics and their unregistrable doctors all of a sudden.

It was recognised that exemption - at least temporary - must be allowed in view of both political and practical difficulties. If all the unregistrable doctors were banned from practising medicine in charity clinics, not only would these doctors hardly make a living, but most of the charity clinics would also find it financially difficult to replace them with registrable doctors. Such an exercise would immediately pose political difficulties to the government itself. Practically speaking, a sudden discontinuation of employing unregistrable doctors in charity clinics would mean that lots of poor patients would be deprived of the provision of low-cost medical attention from these clinics, and their demands might be turned to government outpatient clinics as a consequence.

The Medical Clinics Ordinance which was enacted on 1st September 1963, finally came into force on 1 January 1964. Of the 801 who applied for exemption (disregarding those who did not apply), 482 unregistrable doctors were accepted as fit to practise Western medicine in 387 exempted clinics. So, the number of unregistrable doctors was drastically reduced after such an exemption exercise. To the medical profession itself, the Ordinance represented at least a significant measure to control the further expansion of charity clinics and unregistered doctors working in them. As the registration of charity clinics was an once-for-all exercise, there would not be any additional charity clinics or unregistrable doctors working in them after the enforcement of the Ordinance in 1964. In this way, the economic interest of private medical practitioners could be protected without facing increasing competition from the charity clinics that charged lower fees.

Report of the Advisory Committee on Clinics, 1966

An Advisory Committee was appointed by the government to review the operation of charity clinics in June 1965 to consider the future of unregistrable medical practitioners permitted to practise medicine at registered (supervised by registered doctors) and exempted clinics. As regards this matter, the two medical Associations considered that the number of exempted clinics was more than necessary to give low cost medical care to those in need, and that some of these clinics' standards were below what was acceptable (Advisory Committee on Clinics, 1966: para.111). The Associations recommended to the Advisory Committee that:

> ...after 31st December 1966, all clinics should be under the supervision of a registered medical practitioner, that unregistrable medical practitioners should be permitted to practise medicine at clinics only under the supervision of a registered medical practitioner, and that the geographical locations of clinics should be controlled. (Advisory Committee on Clinics, 1966:para.112)

Thus, the Associations did not object the continued medical practice of unregistrable medical practitioners already limited in numbers as long as they were bought under the immediate supervision of a registered medical practitioner. This recommendation could indeed reveal the interest of the medical profession in maintaining their own medical authority and their control over unregistrable medical practitioners. Besides, this also represented a very good economic opportunity for the medical profession to expand their market in medical care. However, such a recommendation was not feasible, since most of the sponsoring bodies would stop running their charity clinics if they had to recruit an extra registrable medical practitioner. This was in great contrast to the purpose of the government in keeping the charity clinics to serve its needs. The Advisory Committee (1966:para.158) clearly stated that:

> ...no sudden change should be made in present arrangements in regard to clinics at the end of 1966. If the Ordinance was allowed to stand as it is, most clinics employing unregistrable medical practitioners will have to close, and we do not agree that there should be any sudden closure of a large number of these clinics.

The Advisory Committee found that exempted clinics accounted for some 37 per cent of all clinic attendance in the Colony (para.93). The government well recognised the role played by charity clinics in terms of providing low-cost outpatient services especially at a time when it was estimated that about half of the total population could not afford to consume unsubsidised outpatient care. The medical facilities provided at government clinics and government-assisted clinics were still inadequate to cope with the rising medical needs in outpatient services. Further, queues were long and that it required even about half a day to obtain treatment at these outpatient clinics. Industrial workers could not afford the loss of earnings occasioned by the waiting time. The charity clinics were particularly useful to the working class for three reasons. First, the charges of these clinics were low. Second, there was little waiting time at them. Third, they were of considerable convenience as they were open at times at which government or government-assisted clinics were closed. In view of the advantages of the charity clinics which could not keep on running without the employment of unregistrable medical practitioners, and in view of the political difficulties brought about by the termination of the services of charity clinics, it was finally resolved that the exemption period of charity clinics be extended until 31 December, 1969 (para.201).

Proposal on Initiating a Roll of Assistant Medical Practitioners   The Advisory Committee still pursued the old idea of adding a roll of assistant medical practitioners as a long-term solution to the problems of unregistrable doctors and charity clinics. According to their recommendation, unregistrable doctors had to sit for a qualifying examination before the end of 1969. If they could pass the examination, they would be given a title of assistant medical practitioner, and would then be permitted to practise medicine at any medical clinics, registered or exempted. That is, if such an idea could be realised, after 31 December, 1969, the distinction between registered and exempted clinics could be abolished. Their recommendation went one step further that an assistant medical practitioner should be permitted to practise at any hospital approved by the Director of Medical and Health Services. Apart from engaging in private practice for gain, and from signing certificates as to the cause of death, an assistant medical practitioners was recommended to be granted all of the rights and privileges of a registered medical practitioner. In other words, this type of doctor could also work in ex-government or ex-subvented hospitals as well.

To the government itself, the roll could help to supply a more stable and yet cheaper source of medical personnel for its medical services on the one hand, and on the other, to effectively maintain the efforts contributed by charity clinics for the sick poor, and particularly for the industrial workers who supplied cheap labour for the expanding manufacturing economy. Indeed, there were shortages of registered medical practitioners in some particular fields which did not provide any specialist training. In 1966, most of the 116 medical practitioners without registrable medical qualification were assigned to fit in those less desirable posts in government service, some in government hospitals and clinics and others on secondment to subvented institutions. This represented almost one fifth (19.9%) of the total medical workforce employed in the service of the government (Advisory Committee on Reviewing Doctor Problem in the Hong Kong Government Service, 1969). The new roll was an attempt made by the government to meet the problems of doctor shortages in its own services and in private services aimed at the poor in poorer or deprived areas, by turning unregistrable doctors into assistant medical practitioners in the medical structure.

To the medical profession, such a new roll was a nightmare: it was contrary to their own interest in monopolising the right to practise medical care both in hospital and clinic settings. Unlike the temporary exemption given to charity clinics and unregistrable doctors, the implementation of the roll would permanently institutionalise a two-tier system of doctors and assistant doctors of which the latter could be given much power and autonomy in medical work. At this stage the strategy adopted by the medical profession was to tolerate the continuing but temporary existence of charity clinics, but to mobilise every effort to turn down the implementation of the roll. The medical profession was able to prevent the government from taking measures or attempts leading to the accommodation of unregistrable doctors in the medical structure until such an idea was again raised in 1969. However, it was not able to prevent the government from taking on some unregistrable doctors itself, or force them to be examined by the profession. The power to discipline these doctors was still vested on the government rather than the medical profession as in the case of unregistrable doctors in charity clinics.

Responses of Unregistrable Doctors

The sponsoring bodies of charity clinics and different associations formed by unregistrable doctors strongly opposed the Medical Clinics Ordinance 1964 by means of organising petitions and press conferences in which they tried to involve trade unions, clansmen associations, Kaifong Associations, and other community institutions. The legislation was not withdrawn. After the review on charity clinics was completed in 1966, the law was further tightened. Exempted clinics were required to register annually, and new clinics were required to be managed by registered doctors only. But their exemption was extended until the last day of 1969. After the clinic legislation, and after the review of charity clinics, a number of unregistrable doctors either engaged in black-market practice or called themselves 'herbalist' or 'Chinese practitioner'. They were mostly concentrated in poorer areas where the registered doctors did not like to go. For example, a survey of Kwun Tong, a new industrial town, revealed that in 1970 there were only 53 registered doctors working as private practitioners and 16 unregistrable recognised doctors working in charity clinics. However, there were some 230 unregistrable doctors, of which about 31 were believed to be illegal Western medicine practitioners, while the rest describing themselves as some sort of 'Chinese practitioner' (Sub-Committee of Task Force on Community Health, 1970).

As long as traditional Chinese medicine practitioners get a business license, they are legally allowed to practise traditional Chinese medicine. A number of unregistered doctors did it this way to avoid the pressure imposed by the medical profession against their practice of Western medicine. The government did take some measures in the post-war period against treatment of eye diseases and uses of some dangerous drugs by traditional Chinese medicine practitioners. In 1949, a committee set up to investigate infant mortality mentioned the 'belief in aged and harmful customs...and Chinese medicine' as contributory factors. But it did not think it 'advisable at this stage, to speak directly of the errors of...belief...[and]...we could achieve our aim by making known to the Chinese...the recent advances of Western medicine' (Medical and Health Department, 1949:76). Essentially the aim of the government was to entice people away from traditional Chinese medicine, and consequently traditional Chinese medicine practitioners by health education, and by subsidising Western medicine only.

In 1962 the Secretariat for Chinese Affairs, which was responsible for protecting Chinese customs, said that while there was still an *enormous* demand for herbal medicine, the herbalists were increasingly facing more and more difficulties from different sources (my emphasis).   First, increased costs of herbs and other Chinese medicine ingredients made the consumption of Chinese medicine increasingly expensive.   Second, competition was sharpened with more and more traditional Chinese practitioners engaging in private practice (including unregistrable doctors formerly practising Western medicine in charity clinics). Third, there was a growing belief in Western medicine, and more hard-selling marketing techniques of Western patent medicines (quoted in Topley, 1978:131). However, rather than diminishing, traditional Chinese medicine continued to prosper in spite of its marginalisation in the health care system and its total exclusion from the health care policy-making circle. The Western medical profession was concerned about the use of 'dangerous' herbs or medicinal ingredients by traditional Chinese medicine practitioners, but such a concern was much less in depth compared to that on unregistrable doctors, charity clinics and the proposed new roll of assistant medical practitioners. In short, the legal practice of traditional Chinese medicine was a shelter for those unregistered doctors who had formal training or some knowledge in Chinese medicine to practise privately.

Private Low-cost Clinics

The attractiveness of charity clinics to the working class was closely related to the relative unattractiveness of private clinics run by registered doctors. First, they charged much higher medical fee, ranging from HK$5 to even HK$50 for each consultation. Whereas, the charity clinics usually charged the patients HK$2 to HK$3 for each consultation. Second, the distribution of their clinics was uneven, and there were few clinics located around or at the resettlement estates or low-cost housing estates which were used to house the working class. All these housing estates were near to the factories which provided job opportunities for the nearby residents.

To attract registered practitioners to run clinics at low medical fee for patients, the Advisory Committee recommended the provision of clinic facilities charged at reasonable rent for registered practitioners to run their private clinics in public housing estates. The Committee even proposed the medical profession charging a fee of HK$3 per consultation, including medicine and treatment. The bargaining power of the Committee was enhanced by emphasising the needs of the majority of the sick poor. This is indeed the first time for a government-appointed committee to advise the medical profession over the practice of fee charging. In the eyes of the medical profession, this could represent a threat to their economic autonomy. However, the response of the medical profession to this idea was quite positive. As early as 1967, some such clinics were established in the housing estates with each housing-estate clinic serving 6,000 residents nearby. This move could be seen as a concession on the side of the medical profession to the proposal of establishing a new roll of assistant medical practitioners on the one hand, and an action to engage in direct competition with charity clinics and unregistrable medical practitioners by means of providing 'qualified' professional services on the other.

The highly interrelated issues of unregistrable doctors and charity clinics presented an opportunity for the state to tackle the problems of doctors' shortage in its service and in charity services as well as low-cost medical attention aimed at the poor. They presented as potential threats to the interest of the medical profession, however. So rivalry between the state and the medical profession still continued. This will be discussed in further detail in next chapter.

First Medical White Paper 1964

This White Paper described the minimum ratios of provision necessary for hospital and clinic services to meet the most urgent medical and health needs for the ten years from 1963 to 1972. It stated that by 1972 there should be provided in Hong Kong 4.25 hospital beds per 1,000 population; one standard urban clinic to 100,000 urban population; one standard rural clinic to 50,000 rural population; and one polyclinic constituted of a variety of specialities for every 500,000 population (Hong Kong Government, 1964). Whereas in the 1960-65 medical plan, the 'predecessor' of the Medical White Paper 1964, the ratio of hospital beds proposed was 5.75 per 1,000 population. Thus the target to be achieved had been significantly reduced by 1.5 beds per 1,000 population. From the viewpoint of the government, such a reduction could however help to make it easier to achieve the planned ratio ten years later on the one hand, and to reduce the expectation of the public upon itself in the provision of hospital care on the other. Yet, if the target ratio of 4.25 could be achieved in 1972, it would still stand for an increase of 1.12 as compared to 3.13 as at December 31, 1963.

Moreover, in view of the high fees charged by private hospitals and clinics and of the prevailing wage levels in Hong Kong, it was conservatively estimated in the White Paper that:

> ...unsubsidised general outpatient medical care is not economically feasible for 50 per cent of the population, and that for inpatient treatment this figure rises to a minimum of 80 per cent. (Hong Kong Government, 1964:para.26)

The White Paper not only reaffirmed the state policy of continually providing highly subsidised or even free medical care to the section of the population who were unable to seek medical attention with their own means, but also specified how large such a section was.   This also indicated the estimated extent of state intervention in formal health care in the Colony.   In a reversed sense, 50 per cent of the population were supposed to consume outpatient care with their own means; while 20 per cent of the population were expected to go private with respect to the consumption of hospital care. Thus, the provision of highly subsidised medical care was not developed on the basis of providing health care to the whole community, but with respect to the practical constraints of the majority of the population in having their medical need satisfied on their own means. When the practical constraints were reduced, the state might then ask the patients to pay more, or limit its scope of intervention in health care.

Alongside the expanded provision of health care facilities, there were also two other   factors which could help to enhance patients' access to subsidised public medical services. First, patients were only required to pay a nominal fee for using public medical services. The fees were not charged on a cost-recovery basis, nor regarded as a means to raise revenue to cover the cost of production. Some health and epidemiological services for the prevention of diseases were even provided free.   In case of economic hardship, patients could have their fees partially or completely waived although they had to go through means-testing procedures often associated with stigma (see Chapter 2).   Second, the community could have access to virtually free medical care without any testing of means as far as they did not have any difficulties in paying the hospitals or clinics the nominal fees. Since a very great majority of the patients could afford the nominal fees, a relatively small proportion of them had to be means-tested as a result.   This could serve to encourage people to have early consultation with doctors.

The government could in theory means test the patients so as to reduce the chances of public medicine being 'abused' by those 50 per cent and 20 per cent of the population who were supposed to consume private outpatient service and hospital care respectively. According to this policy ruling, the principle of selectivity, instead of universality, should serve as the guiding principle underlying the provision of medical care. However, in reality, such a practice was not very feasible since it would be a very expensive exercise to means test all patients of which a majority could not afford to consume private medicine. Doing away with the means-testing procedures could then encourage the patients to consume medical care in case of need, and save administrative expenses in identifying the most needy. In theory, public medicine was not delivered to the whole community, but to those who had no choice but to depend on subsidised medical care. But in actual practice, every patient including those who could afford to go private could go public if they wish.

Expansion of Health Care and Economic Productivity

The Medical White Paper 1964 was aimed at adequately providing comprehensive services to those who could not afford private medicine. The scope of state intervention in formal health care was very significant as the provision of services was planned to meet the medical needs of a very large proportion of the population in the Colony. However, from the following paragraph quoted from the Medical White Paper 1964, it can be seen that the government was well aware of the economic cost incurred for both individuals and the community at large if urgent medical necessity was not met in a rapidly expanding economy.

> In Hong Kong, where admissions to hospital are for the most part governed by urgent medical necessity and where the bonds of family and of local community...are being subjected to increasing strains by a rapidly-expanding and highly-industrialised society, the economic loss due to sickness or disability, both to the individual and to the community, should not be underestimated. (Hong Kong Government, 1964:para.107)

The government was aware that the economic loss due to sickness was not only incurred to individuals, but also to the whole community as well. As shown from the following quote, the rationale underlying the provision of low-cost or even free medical care was clearly spelled out in a very economically utilitarian manner.

> A good general standard of health throughout a community is an economic asset to it and helps to condition the levels of energy and initiative which determine productivity, particularly in a free enterprise economy such as Hong Kong. (Hong Kong Government, 1964:para.89)

Put in other words, the guarantee of public health and the restoration of the sick to health were believed to be important in contributing to the increasing level of economic productivity in terms of healthy environmental conditions and healthy labour. Probably there were three more reasons accounting for highlighting the relationship between the provision of public medical services and economic productivity. First, Ng (1994) pointed out that tightened immigration controls erected at the border with China had literally halted the main exogenous source of inflow into the domestic labour supply pool by the end of the 1960s. The supply of local healthy labour was thus important for the expanding labour-intensive manufacturing industries. Secondly, since China did not open its door for trade and economic development until 1978, this had ruled out the possibility of importing cheap labour from China or making use of cheap labour in China by moving some of the manufacturing line or procedures from Hong Kong to the Mainland. Thirdly, 'non-restricted' immigration of Chinese people from the Mainland might have provided more cheap and healthy labour to the expanding manufacturing economy. However, a loose control over the border might give a wrong message that illegal immigrants were most welcome to settle in the Colony. A large influx of immigrants from the Mainland would have posed a serious problem to the political stability and residual welfare system of the Colony.

The idea of supplying sufficient amount of healthy labour was close to the concept of manpower investment adopted in an official education document released in 1966. It stated that '...bearing in mind the inherent limitations, the manpower assessment is the first step in formulating a strategy for a national programme of developing human resources...' (Rodrigues et al., 1966:2). An Education Department's paper published in 1971 also stated that education in Hong Kong should fulfil the function of skill-training to ensure economic viability (Education Department, 1971:1218). Such a social investment objective was also echoed in the White Paper on Social Welfare released a year later in 1965.

> [The] explanation of the need for social welfare services may appear to place rather more stress on the economic returns to the individual and the community of effective services than on the humane and charitable considerations that should motivate a community in providing for its less fortunate citizens,...this emphasis is unavoidably necessary in the special conditions of Hong Kong...and in this context Government's first emphasis must be placed on encouraging and developing those social welfare services that most directly contribute to the *economic well-being* of the community. (Hong Kong Government, 1965:para.6; my emphasis)

Within the context of Hong Kong, economic returns versus humane considerations were not given equal weight by the government. Instead, the major emphasis was placed on developing those social services that were most contributory to the economic well-being of the Colony. Viewed in this light, it is no wonder the Social Welfare White Paper 1965 claimed that the aims of provision should be to 'help individuals to become independent and productive citizens and to progress rapidly from independence to self-sufficiency', and 'to those temporarily incapable of maintaining themselves as a result of illness, misfortune, etc.' (Hong Kong Government, 1965:9-10). Productive citizens were considered being equivalent to the healthy labour force whom they could make a living through their labour wage earned. To concentrate state resources on those individuals who can benefit the most from social services, 'the most receptive, adaptable and responsive, e.g. children, young people, those of the handicapped who can be readily rehabilitated and the temporarily dependent' were given priority (Hong Kong Government, 1965:10). An expanded provision of personal medical care and maternity and child health services could be understood in relation to the role of health services in economic development. In Marxist terminology, the provision of such health services was mainly for the purpose of reproducing healthy labour for capitalist exploitation both at present and in the future. In other words, those services that could not contribute to the economic well-being of the Colony would be given a lower priority. As will be discussed later, most older people or geriatric patients were deprived of domiciliary medical and nursing services, and the task of meeting their long-term health care needs was expected to be the responsibility of the family.

Moreover, the government suspected that a good standard of health care provision might threaten the work ethics of inpatients whom they might prefer to stay in convalescent beds than return to work. The following quote from the 1964 White Paper could well illustrate this point.

In convalescent and long stay wards, floor areas may be reduced...[and] the whole atmosphere should be...designed to encourage activity and self help towards early restoration to daily life and the family environment. Otherwise, the incentive to return to work is diminished or lost, the accommodation tends to be used as hostel rather than a hospital and, inevitably, turnover dwindles. (Hong Kong Government, 1964:para.95)

In the 1960s, overcrowded housing conditions were the norm of the society. Within such a context, reducing the floor space of convalescent and long stay wards were conceived by the government as desirable so as to encourage patients to return to work as soon as possible. However, such a worry was used more as an excuse to keep the standard of provision low. Moreover, most of the workforce was unskilled or semi-skilled and was on hourly and daily rates of pay. Hence, it is very unlikely for them to stay in hospital beds to 'maximise' their benefits without having their private wage reduced as a result. After all, the emphasis laid on work incentives could well reflect the government's anxiety to minimise the undesirable effects of subsidised health care in affecting the economy. Such an emphasis is consistent with the purpose of social welfare in 'helping to alleviate or prevent the causes of dependency...[and doing] everything possible...to enable [the destitute] to fit themselves for, and to find and to retain, suitable employment' (Hong Kong Government, 1965:para.10).

Promotion of Family Responsibility in Informal Health Care

According to the 1961 Census, 61 per cent of the population was aged 29 or below, while less than 5 per cent (4.8%) aged 60 or above. It was projected that by the year of 1971, the respective percentage for these two age groups would reach to 61.7 per cent and 6.6 per cent (Census and Statistics Department, 1961). Thus, there would be envisaged an ageing of a relatively young population in Hong Kong. The Medical White Paper 1964 (para.41) pointed out that the majority of deaths for the age group aged 60 and over resulted from 'chronic or protracted diseases'. The White Paper further stated that there were two cases where the taking care of geriatric patients would be unsuitably placed within home circumstances:

> [O]ne consists of those requiring some continuous but basic form of nursing care during the terminal stages of a chronic fatal disease such as cancer; the other category comprises persons suffering from severe disabilities resulting from disease or accident whose return to a comparatively normal life is impossible due either to the degree of incapacity or to completely unsuitable domestic conditions or to a combination of both these factors. (Hong Kong Government, 1965:para.15)

Because of the gradual ageing of the society, there was a growing need for geriatric beds and especially long-term care for older people. Long-term care was mainly provided to deal with the chronic conditions of geriatric patients, while geriatric beds for acute conditions or inpatient medical rehabilitation. However, the government just aimed at providing long-term care for only two types of geriatric patients: those who were at the terminal stage of disease and those with severe disabilities. Certainly, beyond these two groups of geriatric patients, there were still many of them requiring long-term care. However, the Medical White Paper 1964 (para.40) emphasised that it was impracticable to provide 'any government domiciliary medical or nursing services' at the present stage. Then, within the home context, the burden of taking care of geriatric patients would solely be placed on the family without getting any state assistance in the form of domiciliary nursing care. It is but a utilisation of unpaid labour of the family in the provision of informal health care for its elderly member(s).

Family Responsibility in Tending Care While recognising the disruptive social influences which tend to accompany urbanisation and industrialisation in Hong Kong, the 1965 Social Welfare White Paper argued that family responsibility should be encouraged and enforced.

> In Chinese tradition, social welfare measures which individuals may need on account of poverty, delinquency, infirmity, natural disaster and so on are regarded as personal matters which at least in theory ought to be dealt with by the family...It is clearly desirable, on social as well as economic grounds, to do everything possible in Hong Kong to support and strengthen this sense of *'family' responsibility*...The constant endeavour should be to rely to the maximum extent on the natural family unit, to strengthen the help the family to cope with its members rather than removing them to institutional care. (Hong Kong Government, 1965:paras.7&10)

However, the Director of Social Welfare had observed that '...the traditional family obligation to care for the weaker members, whether handicapped children or the aged and infirm, is perhaps somewhat less binding, though still remarkably strong' (Social Welfare Department, 1960). The government was aware that there was still widespread poverty in Hong Kong society on the one hand; however, it still strongly urged the family to shoulder the responsibility to take care of its members on the other. The government's determination to refrain from giving domiciliary medical or nursing services to geriatric patients can thus be seen as its desire to maximise the unpaid resources contributed by the family in the area of informal health care. Such a practice made it very difficult for the family to have access to state subsidised domiciliary health care for its infirmed members. In short, the provision of domiciliary care was largely considered as the responsibility of the family rather than the state.

In the words of the government, the strengthening of the sense of family responsibility was incompatible with measures taken to remove the 'needy' family members to institutional care. So, within the ambit of state policy, geriatric patients could only be provided with institutional care in terminal or severe cases. Realising that it may be necessary to increase 'provision of long-stay infirmary patients', the government still emphasised that 'care will need to be taken, in making such facilities available, that family ties are not disrupted as has occurred in other social systems. In providing such geriatric services...elaborate standards of accommodation and nursing care will not be required...' (Hong Kong Government, 1965:para.103). Thus, every effort or measure was made to ensure that subsidised institutionalisation was used as the very last resort and that the standard of long-term geriatric care should be kept at a modest level.

As stated in the Social Welfare White Paper 1965, 'social welfare services should not be organised...to accelerate the breakdown of the natural or traditional sense of responsibility - for example by encouraging the natural family unit to shed on to social welfare agencies, public or private, its moral responsibility to care for the aged or infirm' (Hong Kong Government, 1965:para.7). All this implied that the family was seen as the 'natural' unit to shoulder informal health care work necessitated to take care of its sick and infirm members. Thus, despite an expanded provision of formal health care, the ideology of family responsibility was strengthened and reinforced. To the government, the emphasis placed on family responsibility was but to reduce its efforts made in delivering long-term health care support to the sick and the infirmed, notably geriatric patients.

Women's Responsibility in Health In Hong Kong society, concern for the health of the family is seen as a prime duty of women. As discussed in Chapter 1, prevention of symptoms or disease is brought about by taking regular herbal teas or soups. Further, it is usually the mother's responsibility to know about the body constitution of her family member(s), and to prepare regular brews appropriate to one's constitution. For example, 'purifying-cool' herbal teas (*leung-chai*) for 'hot' constitutions and herbal tonics to build the blood (*po-huet*), or strengthen the ether (*po-hei*) (Topley, 1976; 1978).   In case of illness, it was believed by the respondents of a research project in 1965-66 (living in two Chinese communities in Castle Peak Bay, the rural New Territories of Hong Kong) that 'Western medicine is best...at fighting the invaders of the human body, the bacteria, parasites and so on....[But]...Chinese medicine seeks to strengthen the patient (so he can fight off disease or whatever insult he has sustained), while Western medicine seeks to deal with the insult' (Anderson and Anderson, 1975:163).   These cultural beliefs on the usefulness of traditional Chinese medicine both in prevention and treatment of disease prevailed among Chinese irrespective of their background (Topley, 1978).   Again, it is most often the responsibility of a woman to take care of her ill family member(s), and spend lots of time in preparing herbal medicine after consulting a traditional Chinese medicine practitioner.   Indeed, the above research further commented that:

> [i]t must be remembered that the traditional system had accumulated a lot of chaff - Lu Hsun's classic story 'Grandma Takes Charge' is all too accurate a picture of family medical practice. (We have seen women very much like the Grandma of the story, doing things not significantly different from what Grandma did). (Anderson and Anderson, 1975:161-2)

'Grandma Takes Charge' is a vivid description of the heavy and yet taken-for-granted burden of women's responsibilities in taking care of their members' needs.   The above research project reaffirmed such a description of the place and role of women in family health care.   The prevalence of Chinese cultural beliefs not only generates a heavy demand for traditional Chinese medicine, but also adds further burden on women themselves to take care of their family health.   Through emphasising family responsibility in taking care of its aged, sick or infirm members, women's unpaid caring labour continues to be taken for granted.   In a way, the government would like to protect, though not promote, traditional Chinese medicine, because it was recognised that traditional physicians took some of the strain off Western doctors, (including state-subsidised service of course) in dealing with diseases (Advisory Committee on Reviewing the Doctor Problem in the Hong Kong Government Service,

1969). Such a protection served to make use of women's caring labour in the area of informal health care.

Constraints on Fee Charging Practices and Expansion of Health Care Facilities

As regards the provision of highly subsidised health care for the next ten years until 1972, priority was given to those services which could contribute to the economic well-being of the Colony, and which would not disrupt the 'moral' responsibility of the family in taking care of its chronically sick and infirm members. Nevertheless, the practice of nominal fee policy had placed medical consumption outside of the commodity form and outside the sphere of market exchange through an indirect, administrative means (Offe, 1984). State intervention effected a process of decommodification of medical care where patients could have access to virtually free medical services provided by the government. When projecting into the next ten years, the Medical White Paper was of the idea that 'it is unlikely that living standards will improve so materially as to make full economic charges for health services realistic within the period under review (until 1972)' (Hong Kong Government, 1964:para.89).

The practice of nominal fee charging policy was partly based on the criteria of the affordability of the public and its implication or contribution to economic productivity. The following quote is a clear illustration of these underlying considerations.

> Some increases in fees may be possible but the resultant revenue is unlikely to be significant in relation to the total cost of the services. If the prevention and control of disease and the restoration of the sick to health and productivity are to be continued at present levels of efficiency, increasing subsidy from public funds will therefore be required unless the standards of the services are reduced. (Hong Kong Government, 1964:para.89)

That is, the practice of nominal fee policy was conditioned by economic considerations. It does not mean that the political factor was not given consideration at all. A Working Party appointed by the Hong Kong government stated in its 1967 report that 'it is only because injured workmen are treated at a nominal charge (or free in cases of need) at government hospitals and clinics that hardship has not resulted and strong protest has been avoided' (Hong Kong Government, 1967:para.31). Thus, the Working Party was also well aware of the stabilising effects brought about by the provision of low-fee public medical services. Moreover, an over-exploitation of the working class and the 'natural' units of the Chinese family but without giving them some state support may result in political and social unrest, especially in a society like Hong Kong where the majority of the population could not afford going private in case of medical need. As far as hospital care is concerned, the role played by voluntary agencies, though significant, was still heavily dependent on financial subvention from the state. As stated in the Medical White Paper 1964 (para.108): 'Although the extent to which voluntary agencies will be willing or able to participate in providing both capital and recurrent expenditure is uncertain, it is clear that the burden will fall mainly on public funds'.

Even though the increased contribution of the public in the form of fees was predicted to be insignificant, the Medical White Paper 1964 reminded the public that:

> [i]t will be necessary, therefore, to keep under constant review the charges levied on patients for such services to ensure that, subject to economic conditions, the cost is borne as equitably as possible by all sections of the community. (Hong Kong Government, 1965:para.108)

One of the premises for forward planning of public medicine was based on the estimation of the proportion of the population who could not afford unsubsidised outpatient and inpatient care respectively. The provision of public health care facilities does not directly imply that the government would not charge the patients a fee for the consumption of public medicine. Theoretically, those who could not afford full economic charges might be able to pay some fees for consuming public medicine. As can be shown from the above quote, the extent of medical subsidy was no minor concern of the government: it can be ranged from full subsidy to no subsidy at all. The government did not regard it desirable to abandon the use of fees and charges in reflecting individual responsibility in sharing some of the cost of health care provision. Access to almost free public medicine was therefore conditional and subject to the evaluation of the economic situation of the average service recipients.

Throughout the whole Medical White Paper 1964, access to highly subsidised public medicine was not mentioned as a social right enjoyed by the citizens of Hong Kong. This could explain why the Working Party mentioned above suggested that arrangements should be made to collect realistic charges, more closely related to the economic cost of treatment, from those persons who could afford to pay, and in respect of cases where there was a clear obligation on another party to pay for the treatment (Hong Kong Government, 1967).

Conclusion

From the mid-1950s, the state was active in initiating long-term health care which finally led to the release of the first Medical White Paper in 1964. However, the seemingly universalist practice of providing low-cost medical care was conditional and was constrained by the priority given to economic development. This was entirely understandable since the period was characterised by the alliance formed between capitalists and colonial bureaucrats which supported the principle and practices of laissez-faire policy. Whenever conditions allowed, cost recovery of public medical services was deemed important by the state to prevent abuse of services. Further, the state did not hesitate to utilise charity efforts of organisations or bodies, like international aid, Tung Wah Hospitals and Kaifong Associations. Nevertheless, as seen above, international charities and Tung Wah hospitals had to depend heavily on state subsidy or subvention; while the Kaifong Associations were constrained by their limited budget in the provision of health care. Thus, in spite of the state's utilisation of charity efforts, its role in health care was becoming increasingly important.

In addition, the government also made use of the available supply of unregistrable doctors to supplement its medical work force, and to staff the charity clinics in the provision of low-cost outpatient services. However, because of the strong opposition of the profession, the state's attempts to properly accommodate unregistrable doctors within the medical structure with the establishment of a new roll of assistant medical practitioners were futile. If professional opposition had not been that great, the state's utilisation of unregistrable doctors would have become even more important.

To reduce its financial commitment, the government much emphasised the promotion of family responsibility in health care. The promotion of family reliance or family responsibility by the government was a great strain on women themselves since the health of the family was regarded as their primary responsibility. The government's protection of traditional Chinese medicine was not only amenable to reducing a significant demand for public medical care, but also to strengthening the concept of regarding women's caring labour as something taken-for-granted. One of the major tasks of the next chapter will discuss whether these major features would be changed or maintained in the period between 1966 and the mid-1980s.

5 Health Care Development: from 1966 to the Mid-1980s

This chapter is devoted to examining health care development between the years 1966-67 when the riots took place and the mid-1980s in Hong Kong. It provides a critical review of the context and practices of public medical services prior to analysing the health care reforms started with the publication of the Scott Report in 1985.

The Riots of 1996 and 1967: Implications for Social Service Development

The mid-1960s was characterised by the publication of various White Papers on health care, social welfare and housing. All this had significant implications for improving the low living standards of the majority of the population despite the further economic development of the Colony. As discussed in Chapter 4, the major emphasis was still placed on developing those social services that had the biggest impact on the economic well being of the Colony. The Chinese family was still considered by the government as an ideal unit to provide caring and welfare functions. Although the government was becoming more directly involved in the provision of social services, its commitment remained uneasy and hesitant. Nevertheless, as will be discussed below, the riots of 1966 and 1967 forced the alliance of colonial bureaucrats and capitalists to realise the significant inequilibrium between economic development and social order, and the importance of internal security to the further development of the economy (Chow, 1986b; Scott, 1986).

In April 1966 a protest against fare increases on public transport led to the outbreak of riots. After the suppression of the riots, a commission was appointed to look into the causes of the rioting. It was officially acknowledged that the poor social and working conditions of the Colony were contributory factors in these public disturbances. In spite of this acknowledgement, the Report of Commission of Inquiry into the 1966 Kowloon Disturbances stated that:

> [b]ut legislation alone is unlikely to provide a solution to this problem since the major contribution to the improvement in conditions must come from a continuing growth of our economy and the capital necessary for growth will not be retained in or attracted to Hong Kong unless the rewards for investment are better here than in other places....(Commission of Inquiry, 1966:124)

So, capital accumulation was still considered as an important factor for generating the necessary resources for improving the social conditions of the population. Accordingly, social services could only be improved as long as the economy of Hong Kong continued to grow. Viewed from the perspective of the ruling class, those favourable conditions for attracting capital investment to Hong Kong would be threatened if such a rule was not well observed or practised.

The suppression of the 1966 riots by the Hong Kong police could neither address the underlying social causes, nor lead to a period of stability in the Colony. Inspired by the 'revolutionary spirit' of the Cultural Revolution which took place in Mainland China, Hong Kong was rocked by territory-wide rioting as evidenced by anti-colonial demonstrations, widespread strikes, a bombing campaign and serious social unrest for nine months between March and December 1967 (Waldron, 1980). The Colonial government used force to try to restore public and social order: mass arrests, detentions and deportations were resulted. The riots of 1967 finally ended with suppression by the government.

The 1967 riots focussed the attention of the international community and the world's media on the poor working and social conditions in Hong Kong. Within the local context, the government realised that Hong Kong was no longer a simple society but was full of all sorts of conflicts, contradictions and instabilities, like the disparity between the rich and the poor (Hong Kong Government, 1967). The 'gap' between the ruling elite and the ruled was more than a political issue, but was also concerned with the social dimension of meeting the needs of the people of Hong Kong. While there could not be an easy solution to all the social problems of the Colony, the government realised that better social and working conditions among the working class could serve to lessen underlying contradictions, and therefore be contributory to maintaining stability and government legitimacy in Hong Kong.

Because of the low unionisation rate of the workforce, and because the labour legislation was biased towards protecting the benefits of employers, the vast majority of the working class had no access to the welfare provided by trade unions or employers. In the aftermath of the riots, the need for changes was recognised within the administration. Immediately following the 1967 riots, an Employment Ordinance was introduced to improve basic employee rights. For example, this Ordinance reduced the legally permitted working hours for women and juveniles from 60 to 48 a week, though this reform was only to take effect four years after. Over the lengthy process lasting for next eight years after the end of 1967, the Ordinance was followed with subsequent amendments to those aspects related to sickness allowances, severance pay and compensation for industrial accidents (Miners, 1991:217-8).

The 1966 and 1967 riots enabled the government to understand the danger of remoteness with the general public. Instead of accelerating the democratic processes, the riots were followed by a series of reforms of the consultation system and communication channels with the public. During the MacLehose years of governorship from 1971 to 1982, rapid economic growth and attendant social changes helped to stimulate aspiration for wider and more public involvement in the policy process (Tang and Ching, 1994). Irrespective of more public participation in the political process, the Hong Kong polity throughout the late 60s and early 80s was identified as an 'administrative state' as all important decision-making processes were much dominated by government officials (Harris, 1978; Mushkat, 1982). The political interest of the alliance of capitalists and colonial bureaucrats could still be well protected as public participation in the central government, i.e. the Executive and Legislative Councils, was not enhanced to any significant extent. In addition to this, the government still exercised much political control and surveillance in various areas, like public order and activities of pressure groups and trade unions (Lo, 1988; Leung, 1994).

Despite the awareness of the underlying social causes of the 1966 and 1967 riots, and despite the increasing attention drawn to the significance of improved social conditions in enhancing the political stability of the Colony, the state did not hesitate to cut the budget for social services when the economic future of Hong Kong was not so certain. For example, the government still made cuts in social services in 1966 and 1967 (Sung,

1986) when Hong Kong was in an unstable situation, socially and politically.   About a year after the 1967 rioting, Sir David Trench, Governor of Hong Kong 1964-1971, emphasised that:

> Hong Kong's generally laissez-faire economic policies have always been based on considered decisions, not mere paralysis of mind and will...But this does not mean that measures of direction and control would not be restored if circumstances changed and the need arose.   Hong Kong thinking in the management of its affairs is always pragmatic and intensely realistic. (Economist, 2 November, 1968:4)

This does not imply that the provision of social service was not deemed important by the government in strengthening its political legitimacy and enhancing social stability, but that the improvement of social conditions was still constrained by the 'necessity' of complying to the laissez-faire economic policies and creating a favourable environment for the purpose of capital accumulation.   An important major implication of the 1966 and 1967 riots was that social services could be used as a pragmatic tool to 'close the gap' whenever the economic situation of the Colony allowed rather than viewed as a manifestation of the pursuit of equity.   As will be discussed later, the further development of social services in the 1970s was still underpinned by this pragmatic or utilitarian concern.

Review on the 'Doctor Problem', 1969-1975

Review on the 'Doctor Problem' in Government Service, 1969

An old issue of the shortage of registered doctors working in government service was getting more serious with the outbreak of riots in 1966 and 1967. The doctors were politically sensitive to these riots as much as they were pessimistic towards the circumstances of Hong Kong after the imposition of the United Nations embargo upon trade with China in 1950. This time, history repeated itself: many doctors left government service for fear of the unstable political and economic conditions of the Colony. Most of the doctors in the Colony either made as much money as they could by practising as private medical practitioners while preparing for emigration should the political situation of Hong Kong get worse, or even immediately emigrate to other countries for settlement (Advisory Committee on Reviewing the Doctor Problem in the Hong Kong Government Service, 1969). During the years 1966, 1967 and 1968, 160 government doctors left Hong Kong. Following the riots in 1967 the government made a major intake of unregistered doctors in 1968 to replace the many registered doctors who resigned (Working Party on Unregistrable Doctors, 1975). As a result, there was a corresponding increase in the proportion of unregistered doctors in government service, and they formed more than 25 per cent of the medical staff (Advisory Committee on Reviewing the Doctor Problem in the Hong Kong Government Service, 1969).

In view of the 'already serious and getting worse' situation of the shortage of doctors in government service, a Committee was appointed by the government (Advisory Committee on Reviewing the Doctor Problem in the Hong Kong Government Service, 1969: para.1). The Committee was assigned the tasks of recommending measures to recruit and retain doctors in government service, and to examine whether para-medical persons can be trained and/or utilised for duties which do not require registered doctors. Indeed, the shortage of doctors in government service had made it difficult to develop the basic medical and health services according to the plans laid down in the first Medical White Paper released in 1964.

The Committee finally recommended comprehensive measures to enhance the attractiveness of working in government institutions, including increases in salary and allowances, and an increase in senior posts and training opportunities. If fully implemented, the immediate and additional annual financial commitment would total HK$16.5 million which represented 8.6 per cent of medical expenditure spent in the year 1968/69 (Advisory Committee on Reviewing the Doctor Problem in the Hong Kong Government Service, 1969; Census and Statistics Department, 1972). Most of these recommended measures were accepted and implemented almost immediately with the wish that registered doctors could be better recruited to and retained in government service.

Nevertheless, the Committee suggested that the possibility of creating and training a new grade of medical assistant (equivalent to the list of assistant medical practitioner discussed in Chapter 4) deserved further study and that a team should be sent to Fiji and East Africa to study the function and training of the grade. The treatment which such an idea received remained the same during the last 12 since years since 1957:

deserving further study and met with strong opposition from the medical profession. For example, the Dean of the Medical Faculty of the University of Hong Kong, a member of the Committee, disassociated himself from the recommendation because he was fully convinced that there was no place for such a grade in Hong Kong and that its establishment would be a retrograde step (para.111). However, the Medical and Health Department did not further pursue the issue of medical assistants, and no team was sent to Fiji and East Africa for investigation or study (Working Party on Unregistrable Doctors, 1975). In fact, no further study on the issue of medical assistants was made until a Working Party was appointed by the government to review the issue of unregistrable doctors in September 1974. There are probably two major reasons for the 'non-action' of the Medical and Health Department. First, the Department, headed and administered .by doctors themselves, identified itself with the interests of the medical profession. Second, after 1969 the political and economic situation of the Colony became more stable, and the rate of losses of doctors was reduced.

Upon the recommendation of the Committee, temporary exemption for charity clinics employing unregistered doctors was further extended. However, the number of charity clinics was reduced from the original 482 to 347 in 1969. In spite of this, the charity clinics and unregistered doctors working there still played an important role in the provision of low-cost medical care to the working class and in deprived areas. For example, as in 1969, some 3,750,000 patients were claimed to be seen in charity clinics, while the number of attendance at government outpatient clinics was about 7,000,000. In other words, charity clinics provided more than half (53.6%) of the total volume of outpatient medical care provided by government clinics (Advisory Committee on Reviewing the Doctor Problem in the Hong Kong Government Service, 1969). If temporary exemption for charity clinics was not further extended, and government clinics were to replace, the government had to open more clinics and employ more doctors, registered or unregistered, to cope with the unmet demands of the working class. Such a sudden change would have imposed a significant financial cost to the government and made the shortage of doctors a much more serious problem. Nonetheless, the once-for-all exercise also paved the way for the gradual diminishing role of charity clinics in providing low-cost medical attention to the working class living in more deprived areas of the Colony. Such a scenario might not have happened if the proposal for a list of assistant medical practitioners could be realised, which would then enable the sponsors of charity clinics to recruit low-pay doctors but without being required to apply for temporary exemption from the government.

Review on the Issue of Unregistrable Doctors, 1975

A Working Party on Unregistrable Doctors was appointed in September 1974 after the second Medical White Paper was tabled in the Legislative Council in July 1974. The government recognised an urgent need to tackle the problem of the shortage of doctors in government service especially in view of the further development of public health care outlined in the White Paper. It was stated in the second Medical White Paper that:

> ...in the case, for example, of non-Commonwealth graduates, it is understood that there is no possibility of any examining body coming to Hong Kong from the United Kingdom to conduct qualifying examinations which would lead to registration with the General medical Council of the United Kingdom...However, the Director of Medical and Health Services can offer employment to non-Commonwealth graduates whose training and experience is acceptable to him. (Hong Kong Government, 1974:para.9.7)

In fact, the Medical and Health Department undertook a major but what proved to be the last intake of unregistered doctors to staff the department's expanding service before the appointed Working Party coming to any recommendations. In October 1974, 132 or 17 per cent of government doctors were unregistered doctors (Working Party on Unregistrable Doctors, 1975:22). In addition to reviewing the issue of unregistrable doctors, the Working Party was also asked to look into the possibility of initiating 'a new list of unregistrable doctors licensed to practise in Hong Kong' (Working Party on Unregistrable Doctors, 1975:iii). Again, the issue of assistant medical practitioners or medical assistants was put on the agenda.

The Working Party recommended that 'those [non-Commonwealth] doctors whose qualifications are not recognised by the General Medical Council of the United Kingdom should be given an opportunity to achieve registration in Hong Kong'. The Working Party further recommended that those doctors who wanted to gain full registration in Hong Kong were required to sit for an examination and complete a clinical attachment, to be known as 'externship', which would not be less than 18 months. The government finally endorsed the recommendation of the Working Party, and the mechanism is still working today. However, the Working Party did not recommend a new roll of assistant medical practitioners nor any further study on this matter.

Although the 1974 Medical White Paper endorsed the establishment of a new medical school to train up more local doctors, the supply could not be suddenly increased. Thus, the establishment of the recommended mechanism not only enabled non-Commonwealth Doctors to gain full registration in Hong Kong, but also expanded the potential pool from which the Medical and Health Department could seek appropriate medical personnel to staff its expanding health services. Secondly, such an expansion of the potential pool for recruiting public doctors does not incur any extra government expenditure since it is not involved in the subsidisation of the training of non-Commonwealth doctors. Thirdly, the period of 'externship' is half a year longer than the 'internship' that local graduates have to fulfil in public hospitals before they could gain full registration. This could increase the number of provisionally registered doctors available for work in public hospitals.

The reaction of the Hong Kong Medical Association towards the recommended mechanism was not so positive. It strongly stated that 'it is the firm belief of the Hong Kong Medical Association that even if a shortage of doctors does exist in Hong Kong, such shortage is only in the public sector but not in the private sector' (Working Party on Unregistrable Doctors, 1975:47). It can be seen that the Hong Kong Medical Association wanted to play down the problem of the shortage of doctors in Hong Kong. The underlying reason for this reaction might be due to the medical profession's eagerness to protect their economic interest in the health care market since competition between doctors would become greater following an expanded supply of doctors in Hong Kong. Although the Hong Kong Medical Association still agreed with the setting up of the recommended mechanism, it emphasised that 'those who pass the examination must serve a certain mandatory period of years in public service in order that the community will be benefited' (Working Party on Unregistrable Doctors, 1975:47). Although the number of years was not specified, it appeared that the Hong Kong Medical Association wanted to confine the non-Commonwealth doctors within public institutions longer before they could gain full registration and be allowed to practise privately in Hong Kong.

The Hong Kong Branch of the British Medical Association was also eager to play down the problem of the shortage of doctors in Hong Kong by pointing out that 'in Hong Kong many patients consult one doctor after another for the same illness (thus creating a false impression of shortage), and moreover that there are still very many people who make no calls at all upon Western-trained doctors since they prefer practitioners in traditional Chinese medicine' (Working Party on Unregistrable Doctors, 1975:50). The Association was even more negative towards the recommended mechanism. In its submission to the Working Party, it recommended instead the extension of the period of internship to two years so as to double the number of provisionally registered doctors available at any one time (1975:50). To the medical profession itself, it might be seen as a much better way to do away with the recommended mechanism and to protect its existing economic interest in the health care market.

As regards the issue of initiating a list of assistant medical practitioners, the opposition of the medical profession was much more evident. The Hong Kong Medical Association felt 'very strongly that there should not be two standards of medical practice' (1975:47). But on the other hand, it also recognised the role played by unregistered doctors in Hong Kong by pointing out that:

[t]here are some avenues whereby unregistered doctors can already practise, namely either to be employed by the Hong Kong Government or by the University of Hong Kong (in which cases, they are deemed to be registered) [but are not allowed to practise as private medical practitioners], or to practise in exempted clinics under the Medical Clinics Ordinance, Chapter 343. (1975:47)

So, the Association was much more committed to opposing the formalisation of a list of assistant medical practitioners whom they would be allowed to practise in the health care market than to realising their claim to maintain their expected standard of medical practice in Hong Kong. In fact, those unregistered doctors working in government services or in the University of Hong Kong would continue to be confined to public institutions unless they gain full registration in Hong Kong. Besides, the once-for-all exercise had already limited the further growth of unregistered doctors working in charity clinics, and thus effectively constrained their base to compete with private medical practitioners. In 1975 the number of clinics registered with exemption was 337 as compared to the original 387, and the number of unregistered persons authorised to practise in these clinics was 304 as compared to the original 482 (1975:39). Charity clinics were given further extension of exemption until the end of 1977. As at 1 June 1995, 'temporary exemption' for 124 charity clinics is still given (Hong Kong Government, 1995a). The number of these charity clinics will gradually reduce, as the unregistered practitioners authorised to work in these clinics will retire one day.

With the publication of the Report on Unregistrable Doctors in 1975, the dual issues of unregistered doctors and a list of assistant medical practitioners came to a final 'resolution'. The state gained from the review by increasing the supply of doctors within a short period of time but without incurring itself extra expenditure. Viewed from this point, such an outcome could be considered as a cost-effective solution to tackle the shortage of doctors in the public sector. However, the publication of the report in 1975 also represented an end to the state's recruitment of unregistered doctors into its health services who were more willing than their counterparts to fill those posts with no or less training opportunities. In other words, the state's exploitation of unregistered doctors to maintain or further develop its health services could not be expanded since the mid-1970s. Because no more unregistered doctors would be recruited since then; their role in government services would be gradually reduced as time went by. Such a scenario was similar to what had happened to the charity clinics and the unregistrable doctors working there since the end of 1963. The state might continue to recruit unregistered doctors alongside the operation of the mechanism to facilitate the registration of non-Commonwealth doctors in Hong Kong. Nevertheless, such an option would most probably invite severe criticism from the medical profession to whom the state had, to a great extent, to rely on to deliver public health services. Moreover, the state incurred a potentially significant financial loss over the final dropping of the idea of a new roll of assistant medical practitioners who were deemed capable of replacing some of the less sophisticated work done by fully trained higher salaried doctors.

On the other hand, the gains and losses of the medical profession appeared to be exactly the opposite to those of the state. Firstly, the exclusion of the idea of preparing a list of assistant medical practitioners beyond the official health care agenda represented a final victory for the medical profession in a battle that had been fought for more than twenty years. If such a list were realised, assistant medical practitioners would have replaced some of the medical work of government health services, and in the long run, this might have reduced the government's demand on fully trained doctors. In addition, the realisation of such a list might immediately impose a threat to the economic interest of private practitioners. The Hong Kong Branch of the British Medical Association also implicitly sounded out such a worry.

> If some relatively simple avenue is provided for unregistrable doctors to gain registration, it is pointed out that there will be an inducement for more such persons to make their way to Hong Kong...into private practice where there is no real shortage. (Working Party on Unregistrable Doctors, 1975:50)

It seems that the idea of initiating a new roll of assistant medical practitioners was considered by the Association as a relatively simple means to legitimately absorb the unregistered doctors into the medical workforce and induce more such persons to compete with them in the health care market. These might be the major reasons underlying the medical profession's opposition to such a 'retrograde' idea.

Secondly, the approval of the idea of allowing non-Commonwealth doctors to fully register in Hong Kong (on the condition that they pass required examinations and externship) also expanded the pool of fully registered doctors, which would then in the long run increase mutual competition within the medical profession. However, confronting the need for further development in government health services in the mid-1970s which was outlined in the 1974 Medical White Paper, the medical profession's opposition to such an idea would make the proposed list of assistant medical practitioners a much more attractive solution to the shortage of doctors. Therefore, it is not difficult to explain why the medical profession could come to accept the reality of establishing a mechanism for registering non-Commonwealth doctors even though they did not initially or wholeheartedly buy the idea.

Second Medical White Paper, 1974

In view of the continuing growth and internal movement of the population, the rapid pace of industrialisation and urbanisation, and the period covered by the 1964 Medical White Paper coming to an end, the government appointed the Medical Development Advisory Committee (MDAC) in March 1973 to advise the government on the further development of medical and health services in Hong Kong for the next ten years (Hong Kong Government, 1974:v&para.2.8). The publication of the second Medical White Paper in 1974 had started another phase of the development of public medical services in Hong Kong.

Open Access to Public Medical Services Charged at Nominal Fees

The 1974 Medical White Paper started off by stating the two main principles of government policy in public health services are:

> to safeguard and promote the general public health of the community as a whole and the need to ensure the provision of medical and personal health facilities for the people of Hong Kong, including particularly that large section of the community which relies on subsidised medical attention. (Hong Kong Government, 1974:para.1.1)

In addition to the provision of general public health services in terms of public goods, the policy ruling governing the provision of heavily subsidised medical care for the great majority of the population of Hong Kong was once again reaffirmed. Besides, the definition of the persons eligible for heavily subsidised public medicine was so vague that it did not preclude those who could afford private medicine from using public medical services. The public health care system was in actual practice open to all, and was not restricted to those who had to rely on subsidised medical attention. However, unlike the first Medical White Paper, the second one did not make an estimate of the proportion of the population which had to depend on subsidised medical care nor of the proportion which could afford private medicine.

Further, the charging practices of public medical care remained unchanged. It was symbolic or nominal in nature, and the patients would not be means-tested unless they could not afford the nominal fees. The full cost of a hospital bed in a public ward was about HK$100 a day in

1973. The patient just paid a daily maintenance charge of HK$2 a day, which was first instituted in 1961. The MDAC recommended that the charges should initially be increased from HK$2 to HK$3 a day and then to HK$5 a day at a later stage. Finally, the daily maintenance charge for using a public-ward bed was set at HK$5 per day with effect from April 1, 1977 (Medical Development Advisory Committee, 1979:para.2.5). This showed that public medical services remained heavily subsidised, and not charged on the basis of cost recovery. Further, user fees were not used as a tool to ration public demand, or as a form of intervention aimed at redirecting users' demand from the public to the private sector. Judge and Methews (1980) argue that the financial exchange between the provider and the user could help establish a satisfactory relationship between them. In this sense charging the service users a nominal charge can be positive and healthy in promoting access to public medical care.

Measures to Improve and Expand Health Services

Moreover, the White Paper recommended the establishment of a second medical school at the Chinese University of Hong Kong, a third nurses training school, family planning clinics, drug addiction treatment centres, specialist treatment facilities for psychiatric cases, expansion of geriatric services, and other facilities to improve and expand health services. Most important of all, priority was to be afforded to medical facilities of the new towns, including hospitals and clinics, and through them to the remainder of the New Territories so as to reflect the distribution of the Hong Kong population (paras.7.9&7.10). In addition, it also established a goal of 5.5 hospital beds per 1,000 population as a long-term goal (this has not yet been realised).

However, the further development of health care in the public sector as outlined in the White Paper still had to confront many constraints, conceptual and practical, and had many loopholes. For example, economic development still subordinated social services development; much less emphasis was placed on developing rehabilitation and long-term care measures to meet the growing needs of patients in these areas. All of these will be discussed in detail in other sections of the Chapter.

Regional Approach to Public Health Care

Another significant feature of the White Paper was the introduction of a regional approach to medical and health services. Each region would be served by (a) a regional hospital equipped to treat patients requiring the highest level of specialist care; (b) one or more district hospitals playing the dual roles of referring patients to the regional hospital for more specialised treatment on the one hand, and receiving patients from the regional hospital for rehabilitation or convalescence purposes on the other hand; (c) one or more specialist clinics or polyclinics providing outpatient specialist services, including those for patients before and after any hospital treatment; and (d) a number of general clinics providing both outpatient and general public health services. The application of the regional approach to public medicine was considered necessary to meet the medical or health needs of the population living in the new towns or in the New Territories since most of the health care infrastructures or facilities were concentrated in the urban areas (Hong Kong Government, 1974:para.2.6). If the approach is well supported with government resources, the regionalisation of health care facilities could, in particular, help to enhance patients' access to comprehensive health care in a geographical sense.

The application of the regional approach to public health care started on April 1, 1977 (Tang, 1978). Initially, Hong Kong as a whole was divided into four regions. With the anticipated growth of population in the New Territories, a fifth region would be established. It was expected that the regional approach to public health care could ensure that 'patients are treated with facilities more appropriate to their ailments' (Hong Kong Government, 1974:para.6.7) and secure 'a more even use of the general beds available in government and government-assisted hospitals' (ibid:para.6.1). The problem is that while there was overcrowding in government hospitals, the occupancy rates in the majority of ex-subvented hospitals were much lower, and most of the latter type of hospitals was not equipped to provide highly specialised acute hospital care. There was little transfer of patients between ex-government/ex-subvented hospitals. As a result, many rehabilitating patients would still stay in very high-cost acute beds instead of being transferred to hospital beds with appropriate but simpler services. Such a practice was certainly wasteful of valuable health care resources.

Later development of public medical services showed that although the regional approach could serve as a good basis for health care planning for each region, the approach still failed to achieve the two desirable goals listed above. There were two important reasons for this. Firstly, there was a lack of rehabilitation beds within each regional hospital, and patients could not be readily transferred to low-cost beds after the acute phase of illness. Secondly, doctors working in regional hospitals did not want to shoulder the responsibility for any accidents that might take place during the transferral process or the worsening of patients' conditions after the transferral (Government Secretariat, 1987).

The Context of Health Care Development from the Mid-1970s to the Mid-1980s

Social Service Expansion in the 1970s

The planned expansion and improvement of public health care for the next years since 1974 and the continued practice of maintaining an open access to public medicine charged at nominal costs were consistent with social service expansion in the 1970s. The growing emphasis on social services in the 1970s was partly an antidote to the social grievances expressed in the 1966 and 1967 riots (Chow, 1986b; Scott, 1986). The Green Paper on Social Security published in 1977 was the first to employ the concept of social wage (see Chapter 1) to appreciate the positive function of social services in redistributing public resources to the lower income groups as follows:

> [a] social security system, and any proposals for its development, must be related to all social services available in the community...(known as the 'social wage'). The social wage provided through the social services is particularly important in those countries, like Hong Kong, where it is a major factor in income redistribution, since it benefits mainly the non tax paying lower income groups. (Hong Kong Government, 1977a:para.3.1)

The state obviously realised that in a capitalist society like Hong Kong, social services, including health, education, employment, housing and social welfare services, whether understood as the social wage or social welfare in general sense, had a positive function in income redistribution and meant a great deal to the beneficiaries, in particular the lower income groups who might have faced insurmountable difficulties if certain social rights were not guaranteed by the government.

Moreover, social goals seemed to have a place in the policy thinking when Sir Murray MacLehose (1971-1982) was Governor of Hong Kong (Hodge, 1981). Chow (1982) argued that the 1970s could be considered the golden age for social services development in Hong Kong, which was related to the governorship of Sir Murray MacLehose. In his first address to the opening session for the Legislative Council, Sir Murray (1973) appeared to give a green light for various social development plans and emphasised that social progress should go along with prosperity. Moreover, in his annual speech to the Legislative Council in 1973, housing, social welfare, education and medical service were regarded as the four pillars of the society, and as important measures to enhance community building.

> We thus now have four pillars on which the future well being of our community can be built. The concern of Government must now be to ensure that the plans do not slip and that they are carried out with the vigour that the community demands. (MacLehose, 1973:8)

The four pillars of the Hong Kong society were all largely supported by means of government revenue, and were thought of having the effect of cementing the bonding of the citizens within the society. This showed that the government was willing to provide social services and facilities to make Hong Kong a better place to live. But as will be shown below, state provision of social services was not unconditional, and the governorship of Sir Murray MacLehose still emphasised the importance of maintaining a low-tax environment for economic growth and paid great attention to the constraints of open economy and revenue in financing social services.

Conceptual and Practical Constraints Placed on Social Services Development

MacLehose's Governorship: Giving a Green Light to Social Services Development? Although the four pillars of the society were given emphasis in government's agenda, the philosophy underlying the provision of social services, in the words of Sir Murray (1973:16), was that 'social progress can only be based on prosperity'. That is, there was no unqualified right to welfare provision in Hong Kong, which had to be earned by means of further economic growth instead. The predominant concern of the state was not to pre-empt resources that otherwise could be used more efficiently by the private sector. Sir Phillip coined the phase 'positive non-intervention' during his office and stated that:

> [t]he plain fact is that a fiscal system which is pitched as low as possible as to minimise its impact on the supply of human effort and investment decisions cannot afford to finance costly overheads. For this reason, in a low tax environment, not only in the pursuit of equity...for its own sake unnecessary, it is also not possible. (Hong Kong Government, 1977b:19)

> Given the extent to which the Hong Kong economy is externally-oriented and subject, therefore, to turbulent market conditions, we take the view that there is a compelling need to keep the relative size of the public sector as small as possible so as to leave the private sector as much room as possible to react to changing trading conditions. (Hadden-Cave, 1980:vx)

While the Labour Government of 1974-1979 was in power, Sir Murray was pressed by the Foreign and Commonwealth Office (which was responsible for all matters relating to Hong Kong) to introduce a more progressive system of taxation. However, there was no change with the low-tax policy long practised in the Colony. The Governor and the Financial Secretary believed that maintaining a low-tax environment was in the best interests of the Hong Kong economy (Miners, 1991:142). Indeed, the dominance of business interests and the almost complete absence of representatives with a working class background in both the Executive and Legislative Councils tended to suggest that business interests had a powerful influence on government's policy making.

Moreover, Scott and Cheek-Milby (1986) argued that the government of MacLehose was more concerned about fiscal growth constrained by an open economy and a low-tax environment rather than accomplishment of programme goals. For example, although the economic recession in 1975 and 1976 did not lead to a serious reduction of public expenditure on social services, the expansion plans for social services were delayed or even indefinitely extended (Chow, 1982). During the last year of his governorship in 1981/82, Sir Murray MacLehose reiterated that '...it is still important that government expenditure should not fall far out of step with the growth of the economy'. All this indicated MacLehose's preference for a pragmatic decision making approach to planning for social services development, which paid great attention to the constraint of government revenue. Where long term plans did exist for medical care, social welfare, housing and education in the 1970s, there seemed to be an inclination to mistrust these plans and to favour ad hoc and incremental solutions (Lo-Cheng, 1990). Such a view reinforced the 'bureau-incremental' nature of planning (Walker, 1984b:71) biased towards the development of economy because the commitment of resources to social services depended on economic growth and any long-term planning would be constrained to reflect the financial constraints.   Walker (1988:10) further argued that such a pragmatic approach towards social services development in Hong Kong tended to be 'cost-oriented rather than needs-oriented'. It appears that MacLehose's government continued the welfare philosophy of its predecessors, though with a more human tone.

Subordination of Social Services Development to Economic Development
Under the policy of positive non-intervention, an increase in general revenue is dependent on further economic growth. This means that public spending in general, and social services spending in particular, would depend on increasing economic prosperity in Hong Kong.   However, giving the private sector more freedom means putting more constraints on government taxation and public spending.   In terms of public spending, the government consciously based its total spending in approximate proportion to the GDP.   In his first Budget Speech delivered in 1982, Mr. John Bremridge, the successor of Sir Philip Haddon-Cave, reiterated consistent government policy that Hong Kong should try to keep the growth rate of the public sector down to the growth rate of the GDP (Hong Kong Government, 1982:429). Table 1 shows that for the period 1974/75-1985/86, total public expenditure remained under 20 per cent of the GDP. As in the mid-1970s, the government also made cuts in 1983 because of economic recession (Sung, 1986).

The pattern of public expenditure in relation to the GDP is the result of the state policy of keeping public spending under control and to leave more resources to the market.   In the case of public health care, the 1974 Medical White Paper (para.13.2) clearly stated that 'any capital works programme of the magnitude suggested must take into account the economic circumstances of Hong Kong from year to year'.   This showed that expanded health care development must be constrained when the economic future was not so certain. The MDAC also foresaw that the full achievement of the White Paper for the next ten years since 1974 'would be likely to exceed the ability of the Government to build finance or staff the institutions that would be necessary' (para.7.8). This could explain why the bed to population ratio increased only slightly from 4.25 in 1973 to 4.5 in 1985, which was still far from the goal of 5.5 set in the White Paper.

Table 1   Total Public Expenditure and Public Spending on Social Services in Hong Kong between the Mid-1970s and Mid-1980s

Financial Year	Total Public Expenditure as a % of the GDP	Public Spending on Social Services as a % of Total Public Expenditure
1974/75	15.0	39.8
1975/76	14.2	43.7
1976/77	12.4	41.6
1977/78	13.3	41.8
1978/79	14.9	42.8
1979/80	14.6	43.6
1980/81	16.1	44.1
1981/82	17.8	39.3
1982/83	19.1	40.6
1983/84	18.6	42.4
1984/85	16.4	45.0
1985/86	16.0	45.3

Source: Chow, 1986b:143.

The government spent 8.8 per cent of total public expenditure on health care in 1972, and it amounted to 1.5 per cent of the GDP. But during the period 1980-1984, the government spent only about 7.2 per cent of total public expenditure or 1.3 per cent of the GDP on it (Wong, 1992). Nevertheless, because of the rapid growth of the economy, public health care still saw a real increase in actual spending during the period 1980-1984 (see Table 2 under the section of *Financing*). Such a growth pattern, which was directly linked to the state of Hong Kong economy and not paid for by increased taxation, was likely to be a painless process for the alliance of capitalists and colonial bureaucrats. The adoption of the positive non-intervention principle, though flexibly applied to the area of social services, still maintained the subordination of social services development to economic development. Such a neo-liberal policy stance places considerable conceptual and practical constraints on the financing or provision of social services in Hong Kong.

Utilitarian Purposes Underlying the Provision of Public Medical Services

Unlike the first Medical White Paper, the second one did not explicitly mention about the potential economic contribution of medical care. However, enhancing people's access to public medical services was still closely related to the notions of legitimation and accumulation. The four pillars of the society of Hong Kong identified by Sir Murray MacLehose represented an urgent need to address the underlying social grievances which might be brought into open conflict and social unrest if not handled properly. The continued economic growth of Hong Kong might further widen the gap between the rich and the poor if the state did not play a certain role in income redistribution.

Rather than developing the political system into a more democratic one the government sought its legitimacy via the development of social services. The fact is that until September 1985, all members, official and unofficial, of the Executive and Legislative Councils were appointed by the Governor of Hong Kong, and most of the unofficial members came from big business firms of the Colony (Leung, 1990). Table 1 shows that during the period 1974/75-1985/86, the government usually spent more than 40 per cent of its expenditure on social services. Such a figure was comparable to that of other Western developed economies although they have to spend considerably more on military and defence spending than required of Hong Kong. However, Scott and Milby (1986:172) argued that government's involvement in social policy was much more to do with maintaining 'economic prosperity and political stability' than with moves towards greater responsiveness and accountability. Promoting economic growth and ensuring stability were regarded as more important than 'social' objectives narrowly conceived by the state as solving social problems or soothing social grievances rather than further advancing the social rights of the citizens of Hong Kong.

In addition, the government also realised that '...occupational benefits have tended to be a bonus enjoyed by a minority of employees, often white collar workers or those employed by the Government or by quasi Governmental bodies' (Hong Kong Government, 1977a:para.7.2). For example, in 1984, the number of people working in the manufacturing sector was 955,746, more than one third of the total working population in Hong Kong. Most of the workers of this sector were mostly of lower income groups. The government might enhance the role of occupational benefits by legislatively requiring the employers to contribute more in this area. However, it was clearly that '...the Government does not expect occupational benefits to play an enlarged role in the formal structure of social security nor that employers will be required, by law, to provide any further type benefit' (Hong Kong Government, 1977a:para.7.5). The provision of the social wage, including health care, could therefore supplement the low private wage earned by these income groups in view of the less significant role played by occupational benefits as one of the components of the private wage (Chapter 1).

Some authors suggest that the state's minimum intervention in labour and industry have to some extent permitted capitalists or entrepreneurs to save on health and safety expenditures and occupational benefits and thus enabled them to extract large profits from the labour force (England and Rear, 1981; Woronoff, 1980; Youngson, 1982; Schiffer, 1991). For example, a government-appointed working party stated in its 1967 report that 'cases of employment injury are treated in government hospitals and clinics without any charge being made to the employer' (Hong Kong Government, 1967:144). The Working Party considered this practice as a misallocation of subsidy and recommended that 'the employer should be made liable for the actual cost of treatment - including hospital maintenance - in all cases of employment injury' (Hong Kong Government, 1967:145). Nevertheless, to the benefit of employers and capitalists, this proposal was not put into practice. Schiffer (1991) argues that insofar as non-market forces permit a smaller percentage of expenditure for basic social services, they provide the possibility for employers to lower the labour wage accordingly. Thus the reproduction of labour through social or collective consumption could play a role to facilitate capitalists' exploitation of cheap labour (Chapter 1).

Practices of Public Medicine before the Era of Health Care Reforms

After critically examining the broader context of health care development between the mid-1979s and mid-1980s, this section turns to discuss the specific practices of public medical care before the era of health care reforms (the discussion will, however, include some unchanged practices extended up to nowadays). The discussion will provide background to understand the changing practices of public medicine in the on-going health care reforms since the mid-1980s. This section is divided into three parts and discusses the three constituent elements of the public health care system, namely, access, financing and delivery respectively. Throughout the discussion, the public demand for private medicine and the relationship between public and private health care will be highlighted whenever necessary or relevant.

Access

In addition to the factors of doctors' assessment and the availability of services, patients' access to public medicine may be rationed by prices (fees or charges), queues or waiting time, means testing and any other forms of inconvenience (Chapter 2). It is evident that public medical services provided in Hong Kong is not 'free' but paid for either by general revenue or fees and charges. However, patients can have access to public medical care free at the point of consumption. Most of the preventive health care services could stand the challenge of health care reforms and remain free or nearly free at the point of consumption; they include health education and promotion, maternal and child care, immunisation, student health, and to treatment provided to patients suffering from certain communicable diseases at specialised clinics on tuberculosis and chest, leprosy, dermatology and verneral diseases. Even neo-liberals would not have objections to the free consumption of most of these public health services.

Fees and Charges On the other hand, curative services did charge a certain level of fees to public patients. There were three basic characteristics of the fee charging practices of public medicine before the health care reforms started. First, fees were set at a flat rate without regard to the service users' economic standing or purchasing power. Thus charges were not set on a sliding scale in relation to users' ability to pay. Second, fee income in most cases constituted a very small percentage of the cost of the services provided. In fact, hospital fees were charged on the basis of food expenses only. So, the deterring effect of fees and charges to universal use of hospital care could be largely reduced. Third, minor fee adjustments were mainly made to catch up the general inflation rate. Since the baseline of fees and charges was low, the increase of fees did not change the nature of nominal fee charging practices. Therefore, it is fair to say that fees and charges were not used to ration patients' access to public medicine.

Opportunity Costs   For public patients themselves, even though out-of-pocket costs may be nominal, inadequate health care facilities serving growing numbers of patients means incurring many non-monetary costs especially in view of the government emphasis placed on the control of public spending. (However, since the mid-1980s, some chronic patients have to pay expensive itemised charges for surgeries or medical equipment. This point will be discussed in Chapter 6).   Such costs manifest in the forms of waiting lists and short clinical consultation time. Once hospitalisation has been approved, except in the case of emergency situations, patients with relatively less urgent problems are put on waiting lists which may last for several months or even years (Hay, 1992). This problem is not just common among surgeries, but also other specialities and some diagnostic tests. A patient needing a special kind of X-ray may have to wait for months before receiving it.

Moreover, patients with chronic illness needing cold surgery may not receive an operation even if it is a simple one to perform. A relevant example is elderly male patients suffering from prostatic hypertrophy. Even though a simple operation would have much improved the situation, the patients are usually prescribed drugs which only relieve the symptoms. In general, patients with relatively less acute or urgent diseases, who should be hospitalised under ideal treatment conditions, are delegated instead to specialist clinics for outpatient treatment. As a result, those patients who should receive hospital care may suffer more inconvenience and pain because of inadequate facilities and medical personnel to perform surgery.

Again, as regards outpatient services, although the money prices are nominal, the time prices remain substantial. General and specialist clinics are open at 9 a.m. at which time a limited number of consultation permits for that day are handed out to patients. It is not unusual for patients to line up three hours earlier to make sure that they are sufficiently advanced in the queue to obtain a consultation permit. However, the average time per physician consultation is very short. According to the estimation of Chu (1992), in 1987 the average time per physician consultation in general and specialist outpatient clinic was just 3.8 and 1.8 minutes respectively. Because of the limited consultation time, only patients with obviously serious external symptoms would get the physician's attention. Others who have less obvious or internal and yet equally or even more serious symptoms may have easily been overlooked.

Size of Public Hospital Care and Outpatient Services In the late 1980s, public institutions were responsible for about 82 per cent of hospital admissions (Hay, 1992) and another 23 per cent of outpatient services (Census and Statistics Department, 1990; Working Party on Primary Health Care, 1990). While the private sector was responsible for the majority of outpatient services, and some 18 per cent of hospital care. The figure for public hospital admissions was very close to the 80 per cent estimated by the 1964 Medical White Paper. However, the figure for public outpatient services was far away from the estimated 50 per cent made in the same White Paper. It can be seen that up till late 1980s, health care consumption in outpatient services was predominantly private, and that in hospital care was predominantly public.

Such an uneven distribution of hospital admissions and outpatient services between the public and private sectors cannot be fully addressed without taking opportunity costs and monetary costs into consideration. By paying a monetary but an affordable cost, patients could jump off the public queue by visiting a private practitioner at clinic. Time costs can then be significantly reduced, and they usually get longer clinical consultation time than they do from public clinics. However, since private hospital care is very expensive, it is well beyond the ability of the general public to go private. So this could explain why most patients still have to use the public sector in the case of hospitalisation in spite of the significant time costs and inconveniences associated with public hospital care.

Unavailability of Health Services Chinese medicine was still excluded from the official health care domain, and the state was not responsible for subsidising any consumption of Chinese medicine (Chapter 4). Unless there was a demand in the community, practitioners of Chinese medicine could hardly survive. In September 1966, Choa (1967), who later became the Director of the then Medical and Health Department, asked his public-ward patients in a government hospital (Queen Mary on Hong Kong Island) if they had consulted a traditional practitioner in connection with their current illness. He found that 41 per cent of the patients (150) interviewed had attended practitioners of Chinese medicine either at the outset of illness (19%) or after they had taken Western medicine without improvement (22%). In the early 1970s, Lee's survey on Kwun Tong, a new town in the east of Kowloon, found that 36.2 per cent of his respondents had consulted a general practitioner of Chinese medicine in the past three years (Lee, 1981). Another survey done by Lee (1981) in the mid-1970s on a Hong Kong-wide scale also found that in the past three years, 2.4 per cent consulted Chinese medicine practitioners only, 52.8 per cent consulted both, and 44.9 per cent consulted Western-style doctors only. Thus, in spite of the dominance of Western medicine, more than half of the population of Hong Kong consulted both Western and Chinese medicine practitioners in the past three years. All the above statistics could show that despite the dominance of Western medicine, there was still a significant demand for Chinese medicine which was not supported and legitimated by the state as a formal medicine. (In Chapter 9, the change of the attitude of the state towards Chinese medicine and the implications of the recognition of the status of Chinese medicine practitioners and the further promotion of Chinese medicine will be examined in much detail).

In addition to the exclusion of Chinese medicine from the official health care domain, certain health services are simply unavailable in public institutions, and patients have to seek treatment or services from the market. For example, the government does not provide universal dental care for the population. Simple emergency treatment is available for the public at some district dental clinics. The so-called 'public' dental health service is only responsible for caring for civil servants and Hospital Authority employees, and their dependants (Huang, 1991). The case of optical services is similar, which have mostly been provided as a commodity in the market: the public has to pay for the check-up service for eyes and eyesight, and buy their own glasses entirely by their own means.

In the late 1980s, most patients had to wait for more than three months for an initial consultation at a public specialist clinic. Even now, the average waiting time for first-time consultation at specialist clinics is still approximately two months (Hospital Authority, 1995a). Moreover, day hospitals which could play an important role in supplementing the in-patient treatment by continuing to provide curative and rehabilitative services on a non-residential basis did not develop until the late 1970s (Hong Kong Government, 1979:para.4.8).

Access to Community Support Service In the Medical White Paper 1974, there was only very little emphasis placed on the development of long-term care, and nothing about the strategy adopted to improve this area in the long run. There was nothing wrong with the further development and expansion of acute care facilities especially in view of the growth and movement of population in Hong Kong. However, the bias towards acute hospital care would overlook the needs of the population in the fields of rehabilitation and long-term care.

The Hong Kong Methodist Medical Committee made a critical observation that the whole burden of sickness in the home rested almost entirely on family members with no formal support (Committee on Community Nursing Service, 1973:19). For example, the White Paper was still hesitant about developing community nursing service which was instituted on a very small scale by voluntary agencies in 1967. By 1973, services were provided by voluntary organisations to a limited number of patients through a total of 11 community nurses. The government did not subsidise the service until 1979 (Little, 1979:3). Because of the lack of formal support and domiciliary services, the vast majority of those discharged patients in need must remain in a community setting under informal care, in particular family care, or under private care.

A Working Party was appointed by the government in view of the growing elderly population in 1972 to study the issue of care for this group. The Working Party concluded that 'the right approach   is to concentrate on "care in the community" as the guiding principle for the provision of services' (Working Party on the Future Needs of the Elderly, 1973:4). The term 'care in the community' was officially used for the first time in Hong Kong. The main theme of this policy approach implemented in Hong Kong is to enable old people to live in the community for as long as possible, and to provide residential care when necessary. The 1973 report further emphasised that the approach '...make the least demand on community resources of finance, skilled manpower and accommodation...[and was] value for money' (ibid:4). The government in the Social Welfare White Paper released in 1979 formally adopted such policy approach. However, it must be emphasised that the approach is heavily dependent on the informal care provided by the family. The Green Paper on Services for the Elderly published in 1977 already clearly stated that:

> ...a caring Government on its own cannot be expected to provide an entirely satisfactory solution to the problems of old age...The community as a whole must be willing and able to preserve and foster the caring role of the family...[T]he provision of services...act[s] as support or reinforcement to the family when it is faced with the strain of looking after an elderly member. (Hong Kong Government, 1977c:3)

Community support services for old people and other vulnerable groups have slowly developed since the late 1970s. Indeed, the relationship between long-term care and health care did not attract the attention of the policy makers until the 1990s. This area will be examined in much more detail in Chapter 9, and I will discuss how the strategies implemented have further expanded informal health care, in particular family care.

Delivery Mechanism and Service Provision

Government's Taking Advantage of Ex-subvented Hospitals Before 1991, Hong Kong had three types of hospitals: government hospitals; subvented hospitals (or government-assisted hospitals) and private hospitals. Since the formal take over of public hospitals by the Hospital Authority in 1991, ex-government and ex-subvented hospitals are all regarded as public hospitals. But to the general public, these two types of hospitals had long been viewed as public hospitals as they could have access to highly-subsidised medicine there. It is important to highlight the similarities and differences between ex-government and ex-subvented hospitals since the latter constituted almost 50 per cent of public hospital beds in Hong Kong in the late 1980s, and to see in what ways the government could take advantage of ex-subvented hospitals.

Once a hospital was classified as a subvented hospital, it was subjected to a tremendous amount of direct and indirect control from the government even though it remained privately-owned. First, subvented hospitals had to abide by government rules regarding financial reimbursement. The then Medical and Health Department had the power to monitor the financial conditions of ex-subvented hospitals and make potential changes to the monthly or quarterly cash advances. Second, with respect to personnel policies, although the staff employed in ex-subvented hospitals were not civil servants themselves, the ex-subvented hospitals had to follow the same pay scales of the civil service, and were not allowed to exceed the quotas for new personnel approved. Third, the then Medical and Health Department also achieved *de facto* control over all capital acquisitions. The government might deny a capital acquisition even if it was funded from a private source on the basis of its concomitant annual operating expenses subsidised by the government.

Therefore, although ex-subvented hospitals were technically non-government hospitals and owned by the voluntary organisations concerned, they were under quite strict control, especially in financial terms, from the government. The financial relationship between the government and ex-subvented hospitals made the latter subversive to the control of the former. Because of their strong financial reliance upon the government, ex-subvented hospitals had been institutionalised as an arm of the government, acting its agents in providing health care in Hong Kong.

However, ex-subvented hospitals could exercise certain, though very limited, autonomy that their counterparts wholly owned by the government could not enjoy. Firstly, they could play the role of innovator since they were free to experiment new programmes and new projects without being restricted by the incumbencies of government bureaucracy (Hong Kong Government, 1973:para.2.7). Since any self-initiated innovations were not subsidised by the government, it could reap the benefit without incurring any financial implications and could wait and see before it found that an innovation was 'value for money' or worthwhile for government subvention. The community nursing service mentioned above was a good example.

Secondly, ex-subvented hospitals were also free to increase or reduce the level of fees and charges. In the case of increasing service fees, the extra fees collected were regarded as the hospital's income and would be deducted from the following year's budget allocation. So, although ex-subvented hospitals could enjoy certain autonomy in this area, there was no incentive for these hospitals to increase their incomes by raising fees. Fees were also kept low in ex-government hospitals as all revenue received from fees and other sources went directly to the Government Treasury. While in the case of reducing service fees, ex-subvented hospitals had to fund the extra subsidy by themselves. For example, the Tung Wah Group of Hospitals, which provided almost 50 per cent of all ex-subvented hospital beds (Census and Statistics Department, 1990; Tung Wah Group of Hospitals, 1990), had the tradition of providing a certain number of free 'charity beds' without requiring patients to go through any means-testing procedures. The government could again enjoy the benefit without paying the extra subsidy.

Finally, the staff of ex-subvented hospitals had enjoyed inferior fringe benefits compared to their ex-government hospital counterparts. Promotion opportunities were limited in ex-subvented hospitals since there were fewer senior posts in these hospitals (Cheung, 1994). All this could reduce the financial input of the government into the ex-subvented hospitals. In short, the incorporation of the voluntary organisations into the public health care system could enable the government to exercise strong control on ex-subvented hospitals on the one hand, and exploit the differences of fringe benefits between those working in ex-government and ex-subvented hospitals and the extra resources funded or mobilised by these hospitals on the other hand.

Tight Financial Control of Ex-government and Ex-subvented Hospitals
The Finance Branch is vested with the power to control resource allocation over all government departments; its primary responsibility is to fulfil government priorities and stay within the budget (Miners, 1994). The then Medical and Health Department, being a government department, had to negotiate with the Finance Branch with respect to the departmental budget. In turn, each ex-government hospital had to negotiate with the then Medical and Health Department for resource allocation. Within each hospital, there were a number of budget-holders who were heads of various administrative and clinical departments. Each budget-holder had to submit two budgets each year: a five-year forecast and an annual estimate. Should overspending occur after prior budget approval, the responsible budget-holder had to assume personal liability until subsequent approval was granted (Chu, 1992). In this environment,

ex-government hospitals were very unlikely to spend more than the budget limit.

As mentioned above, even though ex-subvented hospitals were privately owned, they could only enjoy very minimal financial autonomy. If a surplus existed at the end of a fiscal year, an identical amount would be deducted from the next year's recurrent subvention. But deficits were not automatically subsidised. Ex-subvented hospitals with deficits were required either to make cuts in existing expenditures or to request for extra government funding. According to the study of Chu (1988), it was rare to have the then Medical and Health Department approved extra government funding request from ex-subvented hospitals. The option left behind was to cut expenditures in other planned areas. Thus, there was no incentive for the ex-subvented hospitals to overspend or underspend.

The tight financial control exercised by the Finance Branch and the then Medical and Health Department could be better understood with respect to the government's consciousness to keep total public spending under its strict control. This is probably an important reason to explain why the idea of replacing government-financed services by individual cash subsidies was not welcomed by colonial bureaucrats. The 1977 Green Paper on Social Security stated that:

> ...it is difficult to be confident that services provided privately, without any overall planning, would provide as adequately for those in vulnerable groups, as services financed by the Government and provided either by Government directly or by voluntary agencies. Services provided by market forces will respond to demand and profitability, but would not necessarily be spread evenly throughout Hong Kong; nor is it likely that a full range of services would be provided, or that the charges made would be below those made for Government financed services...Altogether, a large private social welfare sector would make it significantly more difficult to secure the most effective use of available resources. (Hong Kong Government, 1977a: paras.11.12&11.15)

On the one hand, the government was not confident that the scarce public resources available could be effectively used by means of subsidising individuals to purchase services from the market. On the other hand, under the circumstances of seeking political legitimacy and social stability via the provision of social services, the government did not want to take the political risk of enhancing the market mechanism to play a significant role in providing basic services to the vulnerable groups. Put it the other way, the government was afraid that its tight or almost centralised control over social services spending would have been severely undermined if the combined system of direct provision and subvention were to collapse.

Lack of Interface between Public and Private Hospitals Private hospitals operate independently of public hospitals in every aspect insofar as they pay a small annual license fee. They can almost charge whatever fees they like as long as private patients are willing to pay. The two Medical White Papers made no mention about private sector activities. In 1979 the Medical Development Advisory Committee (1979:12) recommended that 'encouragement should be given to the development of more private non-profit making hospitals'. The government does give incentives for the development of private hospitals since it has provided land at designated sites at nil or nominal premium (Hong Kong Government, 1993a:10). Because of the very high prices of land in Hong Kong, such an encouragement is not insignificant. Nonetheless, there were only 11 private hospitals in 1993, and the number had not increased since 1971 (Hong Kong Government, 1993). Before the 1990s, public and private hospitals existed almost independently as different entities with little co-operation or competition. An important factor for this is that the price gap of the services provided between these two types of hospitals is very large. Those public patients who can afford to pay more may not be able to consume private medicine confronting such a price gap.

The lack of interface between public and private hospitals is also accounted by the fact that subsidised medicine has been provided in kind rather than cash or voucher. Public patients have to consume subsidised medicine in public hospitals since no subsidy would be given to them if they consume private medicine or purchase medical insurance in the market. If the manner of delivery were to be replaced by individual cash subsidies or voucher, and patients were allowed to purchase their health care or health insurance from the market, competition between public and private hospitals would have been facilitated, and the health insurance market would have further developed. But as discussed above, the government in the 'golden' age of social services expansion ruled out such an option.

Moreover, doctors in public hospitals are all salaried employees, and doctors or consultants are not allowed to have private practice either in public or private hospitals. If they were allowed to do so, they might have played a role either to develop a greater demand for private beds in public hospitals, or encourage their patients to opt for treatment in the private sector.   In both cases, private hospitals would have engaged in competition, or a closer interface with public hospitals for private patients.

Service Provision There are two dimensions of service provision: service quality and differentiation of products (Chapter 2). In addition to the significant time cost, there are also a few problems with the service quality of public medicine, which often create inconveniences to public patients.   As regards public hospital care, overcrowding in regional hospitals has long been regarded as a serious problem in Hong Kong (Hong Kong Government, 1964; 1974; 1993a; Lee, 1975; Scott, 1985; Hay, 1992).   Although the situation has been improved in the 1990s, occasional usage of camp beds is still common (Hong Kong Government, 1993a).   Moreover, public hospital patients do not have much privacy since no partitioning is installed between hospital beds located in public wards.   Some of the hospitals do not even have any air conditioning in public wards. Patients have to suffer much from the very high humidity and temperature in Hong Kong summer. In spite of all this, the majority of patients could not afford to go private because of the very high monetary cost.

As regards the quality of public outpatient service, the Working Party on Primary health Care (1990:para.8.19) commented that:

> [i]n most cases, little attention has been given to the development of doctor-patient relationship, continuity of care and education and counselling to help patients to manage their health problems.   The outcome of a medical consultation is usually characterised by a low level of investigation, a high level of medication and little acquisition of medical knowledge by the patients.

It was also observed in a survey that many general outpatient clinics processed the clinical consultations well ahead of closing time; in some cases doctors working in these clinics could even save one and a half hours before the end of the session (Hedley, et al., 1990). All this encourages patients to consume outpatient services in the private sector.

With regard to the differentiation of service products in public hospitals, there were three types of beds in public hospitals: first-class and second-class beds, and public ward beds before B-class beds (semi-private beds) are experimented in the 1990s. The first two types of bed are used predominantly by upper level government officials and private-pay patients referred for hospitalisation by their private physicians. After the establishment of the Hospital Authority, its top level employees are also entitled to use these private beds. Only a small number of such beds (about 2% of all beds in public hospitals) are available in Hong Kong (a total of 300 and 453 beds as of 31 December 1987 and 31 March 1993 respectively). The majority of hospital beds are found in third-class or public wards. Since first- and second-class beds are private beds, the patients are charged a per diem room and board fee plus fees for any ancillary services. Patients in second-class beds are charged the average daily cost of maintaining a hospital bed in all public hospitals. Patients in first-class beds are charged 1.5 times the average daily cost (Provisional Hospital Authority, 1989).

Even for those who can afford the dear price of first- or second-class beds, they may not have an easy access to such facilities. The main reason is that upper level government officials and Hospital Authority employees are given first priority. They like to choose to use these private beds in case of hospital treatment since they are entitled to enjoy this kind of fringe benefit provided by their employers at a highly-subsidised rate. Besides, they can jump off the waiting lists as they are given priority in hospital admissions (Chu, 1992). As private beds were few in number and mainly provided as fringe benefits for upper level civil servants and Hospital Authority employees, public hospitals were not intended to compete with the private sector for private patients.

Financing

Government Financing of Public Health Care Data in Table 2 show continuous real growth in government expenditure on hospital and health services. Despite this continuous growth in the actual amounts spent on public health care, the amounts as a percentage of total government expenditure were kept roughly between 6 per cent and 9 per cent throughout the 1980s. Moreover, within the same period, government expenditure on health care as a portion of the GDP was kept between 1.2 per cent and 1.5 per cent. These two statistics could indirectly indicate the effectiveness of the Hong Kong government's system of control over its spending on public health care in this period.

Table 2 Government Expenditures on Public Health Care, 1980-1989

Year	Real growth (%)	% of total government expenditure	% of GDP
1980	22.8	6.9	1.4
1981	13.5	7.4	1.2
1982	1.3	6.3	1.2
1983	3.6	6.4	1.2
1984	9.4	7.4	1.2
1985	17.1	8.4	1.4
1986	15.4	9.0	1.4
1987	4.4	9.0	1.3
1988	7.2	8.7	1.3
1989	17.0	8.9	1.5

Sources: Hong Kong Yearbooks, 1981-1990.

Another way to finance health care is social insurance. This is also one of the hot issues in the health care reforms. But colonial bureaucrats in the Hong Kong context did not regard social insurance as a feasible means to finance public services or social security. The 1973 Social Welfare White Paper explained that:

> ...social insurance should not be considered as suitable for Hong Kong, there are a number of practical objections...Foremost amongst these is the fact that a social insurance system is usually built round the payment of compulsory contributions by employees and employers. The Government does not believe that such a system would be generally acceptable to the people of Hong Kong. On the other hand, the alternative of making employers alone responsible for funding the scheme is not regarded as the right way...because it would concentrate the burden on only one section of the community. (Hong Kong Government, 1973:para.6.8)

If the social insurance approach were adopted, it might have increased the public's ability to express a clear preference with regard to public health care spending. As mentioned above in the Chapter, the polity of Hong Kong was still in nature an 'administrative state' before the mid-1980s. Colonial bureaucrats might not want to see a greater say of the public in the distribution and allocation of government funding in public programmes in general, and public health care in specific.

Because of the practice of charging public patients only a nominal fee in the use of hospital care and other health services, the overall role of out-of-pocket payment in financing public health care was small in the 1980s. For example, in the late 1980s, the income collected from fees and charges represented only about 4 per cent of the recurrent expenditure on public health care (Yuen, 1992). Since the fees and charges of public medicine were easily affordable, there was no incentive for the majority of the population to purchase health insurance for insuring themselves against the cost of going public.

The Role Played by Private Health Insurance and Employers' Fringe Benefits As private hospital care is so expensive, one might expect that a very large proportion of hospital patients going private in Hong Kong would carry with themselves private health insurance. However, such a scenario did not fit into the 1980s. A study in 1987 indicated that only 21 per cent of those who went to private hospitals carried private health insurance (Yuen, 1988a). This could explain why health insurance agencies only funded 12 per cent of private hospital care in 1984 (Scott, 1985). Because of an annual growth rate of about 40 per cent in the private health insurance market since the late 1980s, the per cent of the population covered by private health insurance was increased from less than 5 percent in 1987 to some 12 per cent in 1990 (either purchased on an individual basis or by the employer as a fringe benefit) (Yuen, 1988b; Hay, 1992). In short, it is fair to say that the role of private health insurance was not so significant in the financing of private hospital care in the 1980s, although its significance has been increasing since the late 1980s.

How significant is the role of employers' fringe benefits in financing health care? A recent government survey shows that 28.5 per cent of the population were either entitled to medical benefits from employers or covered by private health insurance in 1991. One point to be emphasised is that 30 per cent of this relatively privileged population were civil servants and their dependants. A great majority of this population could either receive subsidised or free outpatient service in kind provided by employers or have their expenses on clinical consultation reimbursed by employers or health insurers. In other words, more than 70 per cent of the total population of Hong Kong had to pay out-of-pocket for using outpatient service, both public and private, in 1991. However, within this relatively privileged population, about one third of them (32.5%) could not enjoy the coverage of hospitalisation as part of their fringe benefits provided by their employers (Hong Kong Government, 1993a). All these statistics show that the role played by health insurers and private employers in financing health care was not as significant as that played by general government revenue and individuals' out-of-pocket payment.

Within the context of the 1980s, general government revenue was a major means to finance public health care, especially expensive hospital care; while direct payment from households and individuals was a dominant one to finance both private hospital care and outpatient services. Probably because of the heavy involvement of the government in the provision of hospital care, the average household spent only about 2.44 per cent and 2.97 per cent of its bi-weekly expenditure in health care in 1984/85 and 1989/90 respectively (Census and Statistics Department, 1986; 1991). In addition, all different income groups spent more or less the same proportion on health care. Nevertheless, the escalation of health care costs and the increase in demand for public health care led to the call for the expansion of the private sector for the provision of inpatient services made by some appointed Legislative Council members in 1985 (Yuen, 1992). Later, the call also included the promotion of private health insurance and an increase of fees and charges in consuming public medicine. As will be discussed in Chapters 6 to 8, the trend towards further expanding the role of private spending in health care has become more evident as the momentum of health care reform starts.

Conclusion

This chapter has examined the development of public medical services in Hong Kong between the rioting years 1966-67 and the mid-1980s. The final settlement of the interrelated issues of the problem of unregistered doctors and the initiation of a new list of assistant medical practitioners represented an end to the state's further utilisation of these doctors or medical assistants as an 'alternative' medical work force to staff its expanding health services since the mid-1970s. In spite of the gradually diminishing role of unregistered doctors, the state could continue to take financial advantage of the differences between ex-government and ex-subvented hospitals before the establishment of the Hospital Authority in the early 1990s.

The expansion and improvement of public medicine in the period was still constrained by the priority given to economic development and the maintenance of a low-tax policy in Hong Kong. Moreover, the family was still expected to play an important role in providing care to its sick and infirm members, and there was a lack of emphasis placed on the development of long-term care in Hong Kong.

Partly because of strict control exercised over public spending on health care, and partly because of increasing public demand for health care, patients' access to public medicine was rationed by significant time cost and other forms of inconveniences. As regards health care consumption, the use of outpatient services is predominantly private; while hospital care is predominantly public. Out-of-pocket payment was the dominant means to finance outpatient services, and government general revenue was a major way to finance hospital care. The role played by private health insurance and employers' fringe benefits in financing or providing health care was less significant than that played by public spending and out-of-pocket payments. However, the expansion of the private health insurance market has become evident since the late 1980s. In short, the chapter provides the background for examining health care reforms started in the mid-1980s, which will be the focus of discussion in the following chapters.

6 Reducing Patients' Access to Public Medical Care

Introduction

After the publication of the Scott Report in 1985, a number of official documents appear to suggest that the financing and delivery of health care have become acute political and economic problems that need to be thoroughly addressed. Underlying such a concern has been the government's realisation of growing community aspirations to enhanced access to quality health care with its cost of provision rising faster than that of inflation and of most other public services (Scott, 1985; Provisional Hospital Authority, 1989; Working Party on Primary Health Care, 1990; Hong Kong Government, 1993a). Economically, the government was heavily involved in the financing of expensive hospital care. Politically, with the further development of representative government since the mid-1980s, the government had to face much more political pressure in relation to various social policies and social issues. It is within such a context that the objective of cost containment in public health care was given paramount importance.

Hong Kong developed over the past few decades a virtually free and practically universal service for all (Chapters 5 and 6). Even though such a seemingly universalist practice could serve different political and economic purposes for the state, it was also of 'undesirable' ideological significance in shaping the public health care system as a social welfare institution, in the conventional sense of the legal responsibility of the state to provide or finance universally free health care to the citizens. It is within such a context that the citizens' universal access to public medical services was perceived to be a political problem that would overload the health care system, and would finally defeat the objectives of health care policy if health care reforms are not persistently undertaken (Working Party on Primary Health Care, 1990). Such a worry is indeed consistent with the state's eagerness to place various political and economic constraints upon the development of public sector health system before the health care reform started in the mid-1980s (Chapters 5 and 6).

The political problem of reducing or redirecting demand for public medicine, I shall argue, cannot be separated from the ideological issue of coping with the growing expectation of social rights to public medicine. In what ways could the state seek to control or redirect the demand for publicly funded health care? In what ways should the competence and responsibility of the state be redefined? In what ways can new or extra non-public funding be tapped to finance expensive health care? Irrespective of which choice, or combination of choices the state makes, it has to deal with the political problems of how to manage the relationship between on the one hand the demands placed on it and the available resources defined by it; and on the other hand the relationship between the public health care system and the non-public sector of private finance and private provision.

This chapter is focused on critically examining two approaches adopted by the state in reducing and redirecting demand for public medicine: the safety-net approach and the shared care approach. The coming discussion will show how the former approach is used by the government to reduce the demands placed on it by redefining the scope of social rights to public medicine. Justifications made by the state to target heavy subsidy to the needy and to impose user fees to those who have the ability to pay will be discussed. However, I shall argue, the existing political pressures also make it difficult for the state to completely reform the pricing structure of public medicine in the short run, though the safety-net approach can form part of a long-term strategy of ideological and practice changes. Then the chapter will examine why and how the government shift or redirect public demand to the private sector by applying the shared care approach in the management of chronic illness.

Fewer Social Rights to Health Care

A 'Public Assistance' Approach to Public Medicine?

At the opening of the 1990/91 session of the Legislative Council, the ex-Governor Sir David Wilson (1990:para.45-46) made a very interesting statement about the approach underlying the provision of public medical services.

[W]e cannot continue to provide more and more sophisticated treatment or the choice of service that people increasingly want, unless we begin to move away from our traditional 'public assistance' approach to hospital care. This has tended to assume that the average in-patient is impoverished. In the Hong Kong of the 1990s, such an approach will be out of date.

The description of the 'public assistance' approach to public medical services did not appear before in any official documents. This may explain why the term 'public assistance' was bracketed with inverted commas, which was used to reflect the underlying assumption of policy makers on the impoverishment of the average in-patient in the past. Such a belief is similar to the principle of poverty discussed in Chapter 2 on which the state provides health care as a form of public assistance to those who are least able to help themselves. Although the actual contents of reform cannot be made clear out of these few lines, the government's discontent with the so-called 'traditional' approach and the 'misconception' of the socio-economic conditions of the average patients, and its desire to adopt an up-date approach to health care is unambiguous.

The Report of the Working Party on Primary Health Care (1990:para.4.4-4.5), which was released two months after the ex-Governor's address helped to clarify the actual discontents with the 'traditional' approach to public medicine.

[The objectives of health care have] been framed in terms so general and with the target population so vaguely defined that as a result, the public sector...is now providing a highly-subsidised service for all...While the provision of a heavily subsidised medical service for those who cannot afford to pay full fees is undoubtedly a suitable policy objective in the absence of some form of national health scheme, the lack of clearly defined target groups and objectives has turned the public sector health care system into one which is passive, reactive, overloaded and isolated from service providers in the non-public sector...With rising public expectations for better service, a 'public assistance' approach for all in the delivery of personal medical care services seems no longer appropriate.

This means that the continuing provision of heavily subsidised medicine has to be restricted to clearly defined target groups lest the public health care system should be overloaded. The 'public assistance' approach is deemed inappropriate in the sense that highly subsidised service is in actual practice provided for all as long as the patients are

willing to consume public medicine. The admission of the ex-Governor
and the elaboration made by the Working Party on Primary Health Care
made it clear to the community that the existing practices of providing
heavily subsidised medicine were not based on the ideal of social
citizenship, but on the assumption that the average patient was
impoverished. This means that such an assumption is in the eyes of the
policy-makers a necessary condition for the practice of universal
(virtually) free use of public medicine. Regarding this assumption no
longer appropriate does imply that the continuing practice of (instead of
belief about) universal free consumption is something 'historical' or
'traditional' and is not suitable any more in the 1990s. Put it in another
way, when the government's fear is translated into criticisms on the
underlying assumption, explicit policy objectives and inappropriate
practice of health care, one can see that the government is prepared to
persuade the citizens that they should not have additional social rights to
health care - contrary to the 'original' intention of the past several decades
in targeting heavy subsidy to the poor.

A Safety-net Approach to Public Medicine

It is stated in the 1990 Hospital Authority Ordinance that no one should be
prevented through lack of means from obtaining adequate medical
treatment. Such a policy enshrined in law is consistent with the 'original'
purpose of providing highly subsidised medicine to the needy. However,
the statement is somewhat put in a negative tone, and the positive meaning
of universal entitlement to free medicine is not promised or implied. Such
a point can be further substantiated by the following quote from the
consultation document *Towards Better Health*:

> [a]ll public health services [inpatient, outpatient and public health] are heavily
> subsidised by Government...The rationale is that the public sector acts as a
> safety net for those who are less fortunate [or less affluent, para. 2.1] and that
> no one would be denied adequate treatment through lack of means. In
> practice, even those who can afford to pay more than the token fee use the
> highly subsidised services, particularly hospital services. (Hong Kong
> Government, 1993a:para.2.13)

This statement can be considered as a redefinition of the rationale
underlying the provision of public medical services since the public

institution of health care was not mentioned as a safety net for the less fortunate until the release of this consultation document. This seems to be a determined move on the part of the government to prevent highly subsidised public medicine from becoming part of a citizen's rights or legal entitlement. The ex-Secretary for Health and Welfare stated that:

[i]t's our responsibility to provide a safety-net for our less fortunate citizens...The fact remains that a complete free-for-all service of this nature will send a wrong message to the public that we are running a 'socialised' medical system...We must determine who should be entitled to 'welfare', and who should pay more for using public services. (Interview)

Mrs. Katherine Fok Lo Shiu-ching, the current Secretary for Health and Welfare, also stated that:

[g]overnment has a responsibility to ensure access to adequate health care. It does not mean that everyone should be provided with everything for free. This means helping the financial needy to obtain treatment in the public sector. It does not mean that everyone should be provided with everything for free. (Hong Kong Standard, 1 June 1995)

The criticisms made on the current practice of public medicine represent the government's desire to reclarify its role in health care or the level of social rights to health care that the citizens of Hong Kong should enjoy. Providing highly subsidised medicine to practically everyone who likes to use public service, and keeping the rationale 'unambiguous' or 'unclear' would carry the message that the citizens of Hong Kong have a particular social right to it. In other words, the current practice of public medicine has to a certain extent acted as the material context which relates abstract values, like universalist principle and social right, with concrete experiences of medical treatment in the public health care system. The fear is that by extending the safety net beyond the financial needy would further reinforce community expectations for more social rights to health care. Such an 'unchallenged' growing array of social rights may then help to legitimate the political demands on the state in the provision or financing of health care. It represents the state's conscious attempt to place a limit on the 'undesirable' extension of social rights to health care.

The safety-net approach appears to be similar to that adopted in the provision of public assistance (now renamed as comprehensive social security assistance) in Hong Kong: needy families or persons have access to public assistance only if their family or personal income is found to be below a certain level. In short, public assistance is provided as the last resort, and to help those who are least able to help themselves (Chiu and Wong, 1998). In this sense, we can make no difference between the safety-net approach and the public assistance approach. That is, virtually free medicine or public assistance should only be restricted to the financial needy except that the former is provided in kind and the latter is provided in cash. However, the above quotes show no indication that the public sector will only be responsible for providing health care to the financial needy and that those who are not should use private health care. The key message of the safety-net approach is that every public-sector patient should not be provided with health care for free for fear that a wrong ideological message would be sent out and that political demands upon the state to fulfil the legitimate expectations of the citizenry would increase as a result. The state's proclamation of the safety-net approach to public medicine could, in ideological terms, serve to persuade all citizens that they should have fewer social rights to publicly funded health care as they may perceive or believe. This has formed part of the state's strategy to reform the pricing structure of public medicine and to reduce the increasing citizens' demands for virtually free medicine.

Justifications for Reforming the Pricing Structure of Public Medical Services: An Examination

Users versus Tax-payers

The Scott Report suggests that even if no improvements are made to existing services, the proportion of the total government budget devoted to public medicine will increase steadily, unless the resources deployed are utilised more efficiently and additional revenue is raised by the introduction of higher charges.

> [The] cost of providing medical services in hospitals is likely to continue to rise more rapidly than most other public services. Yet there is little evidence that the government will move to radically change its overall tax policy nor that the proportion of total public expenditure on medical and health services will be increased significantly. (Scott, 1985:para.3.6.2)

Based on such an understanding, the Scott Report recommends that the fees charged be linked up to a certain percentage of the cost of provision of hospital care rather than charging the users the catering cost as practised nowadays. To the government, the prospect of additional taxes would reduce the attractiveness of Hong Kong as an investment centre, and is inconsistent with its policies of encouraging the growth of Hong Kong as a low-tax trading centre favourable for maintaining its economic performance especially against the fierce competition from industrialising territories in the same region (Macleod, 1994). This means that the maintenance of the low-tax policy is viewed as a strong justification for the seeking of other measures to finance cost-escalating health care. The Provisional Hospital Authority (1990:para.12.4.2) puts this in the following manner.

> There appears to be a case therefore for a shift in the proportions of the cost of hospital services which are borne by patients and tax-payers respectively, provided that there is no abandonment of the basic Government policy of providing heavily subsidised public hospital services to the community and that no one would be deprived of hospital services purely because of a lack of financial means.

Thus, if the users of public medical services are not asked to pay more, the taxpayers would be the ones to suffer; and it is fair to increase the fees as long as the government does not abandon its safety-net approach in targeting heavy subsidy to the needy. However, it may be argued that taxpayers have already paid their due and it is unfair to charge them a higher fee if they choose to use public medical services. They may indeed query the rationale behind being charged twice for health care. However, a Legislator elected from the Medical and Health Care Functional Constituency is not optimistic about the prospect of a tax increase to finance social service in Hong Kong.

> Unless and until we change to a high tax structure; unless and until there are taxes designated for specific purposes, then tax revenue generated will definitely not be able to tackle the unsatiable appetite of next to nothing health care, free education, free transports, and so on and so forth. In the foreseeable future, you know, the government shows no intention at all to pay for health care cost via an increase of taxes. (Interview)

Another Legislative Councillor who is the spokesperson of the Liberal Party on health policy clearly expressed his objection to the idea of raising additional resources for health care from increasing taxes as follows:

> [w]e should provide high quality health care and we need additional resources. The additional resources should not come from higher tax. Patients who can afford to pay should pay for part, if not all, of the cost instead of just paying a nominal cost. If we treat medical care solely as welfare and take into no account of the patients' ability to pay, medical cost would have to be borne by taxpayers alone. Since we have to maintain a low-tax policy, it is neither fair nor prudent to accept this philosophy and maintain the current system. I must admit that those users who can afford must share the responsibility of paying for at least part of the medical cost. If not, the end result is an infinite increase in the burden on the public health budget to the extent that tax increases may become inevitable. (Interview)

The maintenance of the low fees policy not only signifies itself as a deviation from the 'original' objectives of public medicine, but also a 'potential' threat to the low-tax policy. As the low-tax environment is considered as the cornerstone of the success of Hong Kong's economy, increasing the tax rate to finance public medicine is not feasible, or not yet put on the political agenda. So, the low-tax policy has provided a 'solid' ground for justifying the partial shifting of the financing cost of public medicine from taxpayers to patients. It looks apparent that the state would continue to allow the universal use of public medicine rather than its universally free use: highly subsidised medicine should only be available to a targeted community rather than to the whole community. That is, the targeted community should continue to benefit from taxpayers' money, and the rest of the community who opt to use public medicine should share some of the cost by paying a user fee.

'Users Can Afford to Pay More'

The 1993 Medical Green Paper points out that there has been significant real increase in the incomes of the families in Hong Kong, while there has been no real increase in health care charges for many years. The Provisional Hospital Authority (1989:para.12.4.2) argues that 'the majority of Hong Kong people can afford to pay a significantly higher proportion of the total cost of hospital services than is now the case'. The 1991 Social Welfare White Paper also states that 'in an increasingly affluent society, the principle of asking those who can afford to pay for the service provided is not unreasonable' (Hong Kong Government, 1991:42). As discussed in Chapter 4, the 1964 White Paper also regarded it appropriate to increase fees and charges if the circumstances allow.

During the period 1981-89, the median household income of a four-member family has increased in real terms by about 37 per cent (Hong Kong Government, 1991:para.17). Median household income also grows in real terms by 3.8 per cent between 1993 and 1994 (Macleod, 1994:para.10). Moreover, about half (52.6%) of the inpatients in public hospitals are having a monthly household income higher than the median one (Census and Statistics Department, 1993). So, a real increase in household income has been used by the state as a strong justification to nullify the assumption of the impoverishment of the average patient and to increase health care charges accordingly.

As far as public hospital care is concerned, excluding those who are of low income, nearly 70 per cent (68.3%) of inpatients are economically inactive (Census and Statistics Department, 1993). Therefore, if only personal income is taken into consideration, it may not sound justifiable to increase health care fees and charges. However, in the local context, in addition to the emphasis placed on laissez-faire values, the government has long stressed the reliance on family in minimising its provision of welfare (Hong Kong Government, 1991). Taking into account household income could therefore re-emphasise the importance of the family in taking care of the health needs of its family members, whether they are infirm, children, old people or other economically inactive members. In this connection, to propose the shifting of the cost from taxpayers to users would imply the greater responsibility of the family in financing public hospital care. In other words, 'users can afford to pay more' should be read as 'family can afford to pay more'. The family has therefore become the basic unit of accounting in health care and public hospital care in particular.

By emphasising the family's ability to pay, the government can serve two purposes accordingly. First, it can legitimate a partial shifting of the cost of hospital care to the users or their family. Second, throughout the process of forcing the family to bear the family welfare responsibility, the government can seek to construct the family as a self-help or self-reliant unit on which individual welfare can and should count on. This can provide an ideological buffer for the state to reshift part of its responsibility in financing health care. As a result, the family is central to the state's efforts made in reforming the pricing structure of public hospital care both in practical and ideological terms.

Preventing Abuse by Users of Private Medicine?

The consultation document *Towards Better Health* has identified the large price gap between public and private hospital care as an important factor encouraging users of private medicine to go public. These patients are regarded as abusers of publicly-funded health care since they can afford but are unwilling to consume private medicine because of its much higher price. The ex-Secretary for Health and Welfare reflected her worry as follows:

> [t]he low price policy will lead to a never-ending absorption of patients who can afford and are willing to patronise private hospitals to take refuge in public hospitals. Public money may thus well be used to heavily subsidise many who can and should pay for their health care cost in the health care market. (Interview)

Without reforming the pricing structure or narrowing the price gap between public and private medicine, any improvements made in the public sector in terms of reducing barriers to health care, e.g. shortening the waiting queue, minimising inconveniences, etc. are believed to be susceptible to further aggravating the problem. *Towards Better Health* points out that 'paradoxically, these improvements may exacerbate old problems by causing a new influx of patients from the private sector' (Hong Kong Government, 1993a:para.2.10). The fear of the government is that the more improved the services, the more serious will be the problem. This implies that the private sector could be placed in a better position to meet the health care needs of the community if the public sector does not compete with it by charging patients a lower price. In other words, such a competition for patients is deemed undesirable in terms of encouraging the 'abusers' to use low-price public medicine. In its annual plan for 1995-1996, the Hospital Authority (1995a:21) also highlights the problem by stating that:

> [o]n the issue of waiting lists, the Hospital Authority is constrained by the current pricing structure. Our pledges and commitment to quality have attracted more patients to our service, as evidenced by a 10% increase in the

number of patients attending our specialist outpatient clinics and a 7% increase in admission of hospitals in 1993.

This points in the direction that the current pricing structure should be reformed lest more and more private patients should be attracted. In addition to charging higher user fees, there are indeed some other available options for the government to redirect patients' demand to private medicine. Firstly, patients with individual or family income above a certain limit may be totally excluded from using public services. But the government which is not unaware of the associated political cost has never raised such an option. Secondly, the public health care providers may continue to rely on using various non-price barriers, like waiting list, poorer non-clinical service quality and other inconveniences, to discourage private patients from using the service. However, stating the reality of the existence of all these non-price barriers is one thing, while explicitly using them as a policy tool to suppress public demand is another thing. Again, political pressure cannot be underestimated if the quality of services is drastically reduced. Indeed, *Towards Better Health* also emphasises that 'long queue...is a constant source of dissatisfaction to, and a point of complaint from, the public' (Hong Kong Government, 1993a:para.2.10). Thirdly, the public sector may redirect the demands to the private sector by means of transferring part of the responsibility of following up the discharged patients by involving private practitioners. This point will be discussed in more detail later.

If the government decided to make virtually free public medical services available to the whole community, the influx of private patients to the public sector would not have been considered as an abuse case. That is, it is up to the patients to opt for private health care if they are not satisfied with the minimum provided by the state. However, judged by the safety-net approach promoted by the government, the influx of private patients to the public sector is but an abuse of public subsidy.

Making the Pricing Structure More Equitable?

From the government's point of view, the existing fee charging structure of public medicine is basically a non-discriminatory system that cannot differentiate those who can afford to pay from those who cannot (Hong Kong Government, 1993a). This system is taken by the government as constituting a threat to the aim of equity. The current Secretary for Health and Welfare argued that an unreformed pricing structure 'would unfairly enable people who could afford to pay extra for medical facilities and treatment to enjoy a free service, while pushing up the total cost of medical care' (Eastern Express, June 1, 1995). In short, the government seeks to set up a discriminatory system to make the fee charging structure more fair and equitable so as to reflect patients' ability to pay a higher fee and to save resources for meeting the needs of the genuine needy.

To argue that differential fees should be used to protect the needy sounds vertically equitable in the sense that persons of unequal ability to pay make dissimilar payments for the same level of services (Wagstaff and Doorslaer, 1993). The 1985 Scott Report emphasises that by holding the principle of patients' ability to pay, a better redistribution of wealth or cost responsibility in the community can be achieved. However, equity in Hong Kong is narrowly defined by the safety-net approach. If the universalist approach was adopted instead, we can see a different picture of equity. Recent international research on the equity in the finance and delivery of health care of European countries has shown that tax-financed health care systems tend to be more equitable; while the predominantly private systems, like the US system, are particularly inequitable (Doorslaer et al., 1993). Unlike some of the European nation-states, the taxation system of Hong Kong is regressive, and the financing of public medicine is not, therefore, progressively linked up with the taxpayers' ability to pay. If the goal of user fees is income generation for health care, it is fairer to adopt a taxation system which is progressive. Hence, the official argument of equity fits in the safety-net approach rather than the universalist approach.

Promoting Health Consciousness?

The government identified low fees as an important factor not only in overloading the public sector, but also in reducing health consciousness in the community which in turn will reinforce the over-utilisation of hospital care. The Working Party on Primary Health Care (1990:para.1.31) expressed that:

> [w]ith public hospital care being available at highly subsidised charges, people in Hong Kong tend to pay less attention to preventive care and do not take adequate steps to maintain good health. This has resulted in a heavier demand for hospital services.

The discourse of health-consciousness places emphasis on the relationship between user fees and encouragement of a proper lifestyle: the lower the money cost, the lower the health consciousness; the higher the money cost, the higher the health consciousness. According to this logic, if individuals find it cheap to be ill, they tend to ignore health-induced behaviour and as a consequence place themselves in danger of illness, which incurs costs upon the public purse. Higher user fees would therefore help to promote healthy ways of life and reduce the chances of getting ill or using health services.

Although medical fees and charges are low, it is not 'cheap' to be ill at all. Because of the lack of a good package of fringe benefits provided by their employers, the working class usually have their earnings reduced when seeing a doctor or being confined to a hospital bed. Unlike their well-off counterparts, the lower income groups have to pay a higher opportunity cost for being ill (see Chapter 2). As a matter of fact, almost nobody would like to be ill simply because of the availability of free or virtually free services, although free services can help minimise the economic consequence of illness. Health is usually understood as a resource which is functional to serve one's general welfare. The absence of illness may not be a sufficient condition for health and welfare, but is surely a necessary condition. Being ill can thus be regarded as a welfare deficit. The use of hospital services is driven by many factors, the least of which may be patients' wishes.

Adopting a fee-charging approach on promoting improvements in lifestyle and health-induced behaviour thus places the emphasis upon self-control. Individuals in lower socio-economic circumstances generally have the lowest standards of health and a consequently greater need to use health services (Townsend and Davidson, 1982; Black, 1993). In addition, they usually have fewer resources to adopt a 'proper' and healthy lifestyle to prevent themselves from falling ill. Using price to 'ration' access to public medicine may achieve contradictory purpose of deterring their legitimate demand or postponing early treatment of diseases until it has become too expensive to deal with them.

Promoting Cost Awareness

Towards Better Health (para.2.13) criticises the existing fee structure as one that is 'not conducive to public awareness of the high cost of maintaining community health'. That is, the public is not cost-aware enough in the use of highly subsidised health services. In addition, the government also regards such an approach as having the advantage of making 'healthcare professionals more conscious of costs, which is conducive to overall cost containment' (Hong Kong Government, 1993a:para.4.7). The ex-Secretary for Health and Welfare elaborated that:

> [i]ncreasing the fees will make the users more cost conscious. When the fees increase, people will ask why the operating cost increase? In this way, consumers can participate then. The Hospital Authority and the health care professionals have to give the public a satisfactory answer on this...This will enhance the health care professionals' awareness of exercising a tight control over the cost of health care. (Interview)

So, as far as the issue of cost containment is concerned, the government is eager to place considerable political pressure upon public hospital doctors to avoid performing unnecessary expensive procedures or treatments. Such intent is not difficult to understand since the medical profession enjoys much clinical autonomy in the use of health care resources in spite of their status as salaried employees. It is however an indirect approach to modify the behaviour of public doctors to comply with the objective of cost containment since public pressure rather than direct state regulation is used. This also means that the government wants to involve the public in its attempt to shape the attitude and behaviour of doctors much oriented to the acute care or clinical perspective (see Chapter 3). In the eyes of the officials, charging the patients higher fees can serve to make the cost of provision more transparent, and heighten their awareness of the importance of placing increasing political pressure upon the health care professionals to provide health care in an efficient way. On the one hand, such a strategy can help to shift part of the responsibility from the government to the health care providers. On the other hand, this can justify the implementation of the demand-side strategy (i.e. on the side of the users) to contain health care cost by making use of the contentious relationship between the health care providers and the public.

Fee Charging Measures and Targeting of Subsidy

Towards Better Health recommends the use of higher user fees, itemised charges and fee-waiving measures to reflect patients' ability to pay and target virtually free medicine to the needy. All these are not new recommendations even though their proposed arrangements or formats have been modified from time to time.

Higher User Fees

Hospital Services The 1985 Scott Report proposed higher user fees based on the idea of cost recovery. Cost recovery in the public health care sector is generally understood as the pricing of health care services provided in public hospitals and clinics (Griffin, 1992) that can be either partial or full - patients pay a certain proportion or the full cost of service at the point of consumption. The Scott Report proposed to tie the basic charge for public-ward or third class beds to a certain percentage (proposed to be set at 3%) of the total running cost per hospital bed rather than to the cost of food as practised nowadays. The Provisional Hospital Authority Report 1989 even recommended tying the user fees of hospital care to 15 per cent to 20 per cent of the running cost per bed of the acute and convalescent beds. *Towards Better Health* released in 1993 also favoured the recommendation made by the Provisional Hospital Authority.

This recommended fee policy aims to fix a higher per diem rate for hospital care and outpatient service. Therefore, this policy does not directly link fees to household income in the sense that a progressive rate be based on income level. While this fee charging practice might appear to be 'equitable' judged by the safety-net approach, the administrative problems and costs associated with the implementation of such an arrangement would be considerable. This is probably an important reason for the government's preference of a simpler system of targeting subsidy.

Rather than employing the term cost recovery approach, *Towards Better Health* uses the percentage subsidy approach instead to set higher fees that the users have to contribute to a certain percentage of the cost of treatment. Moreover, a differentiation would be made between the different running cost per bed of the acute, convalescent and psychiatric beds. In 1992/93 figures, the operating cost for an acute bed is HK$2,150, convalescent bed HK$910, and psychiatric bed HK$429 (Hong Kong Government, 1993a:para.4.6). During the interview, the ex-Secretary for

Health and Welfare explained to me that such a differentiation would make sure that the high operating cost of acute beds would not pass on to psychiatric beds.   This supplements the point made in *Towards Better Health* that 'long-stay patients in psychiatric and convalescent/infirmary hospitals would be paying less than short-stay patients in acute general hospitals' (Hong Kong Government, 1993a:para. 4.7).

When explaining to the Health Panel of the Legislative Council, the ex-Secretary for Health and Welfare claimed that the concept of cost recovery approach was different from that of percentage subsidy approach. The former approach would require users to pay a share of their own expenses on a case-by-case basis, which could be high in the case of, say, an organ transplant.   While the latter approach would set the fee at a certain percentage of the hospital's average operating costs (Hong Kong Legislative Council, 1993).   However, such a definition is no different from that made in the 1985 Scott Report, the 1989 Provisional Hospital Authority Report and the 1990 Primary Health Care Report.   A significant difference between these two terms is just on the tone itself.   The cost recovery approach sounds quite negative: taking back some benefit the citizens presently enjoy; while the percentage subsidy approach is seemingly 'positive': ensuring a more equitable fee structure and giving the genuinely needy more protection.

In spite of the employment of a more positive tone, the ex-Secretary for Health and Welfare was still much aware of strong public's opposition to increase the public patients' burden by setting higher user fees. In a press release, she clearly pointed out that:

> [the Health and Welfare Branch] will also study the fee structure for general wards in public hospitals, having regard to public misunderstanding of the percentage subsidy approach, and having regard to the importance of maintaining the principle of cost awareness and the concept of price mechanism in the allocation of resources...At the same time, we should also be reviewing again the appropriate extent of subsidy and how best to target those most in need. (Wong, 1994)

General and Specialist Outpatient Services   As regards the per diem rate for outpatient service, it was proposed in the Primary Health Care Report 1990 that user fees should be eventually charged at cost.   But *Towards Better Health* eventually proposed to maintain the status quo by stating two points. First, some 55 per cent of general outpatients are old people or from the lower-income group with personal monthly income less than $3,000 at 1989 Hong Kong price. Second, the public sector attracts about 15 per cent of those in need of primary medical care while the bulk of services is provided in the market (Hong Kong Government, 1993a:para.4).

However, the government has not given up the attempt to persuade the public to accept a more drastic increase in hospital fees. Indeed, unlike outpatient care, hospital care is far more expensive, and nearly 90 per cent of hospital services are provided in the public sector. *Towards Better Health* emphasises that 'the public sector remains the major provider of hospital services. The ensuing [overloading and overutilisation] problems have made it necessary to concentrate reform in this area' (para.5.2). Compared to the cost of hospital care and its current predominantly public provision, the government's decision to abandon the use of higher user fees to ration patients' demand for general or specialist outpatient services appears to be a more economically and politically feasible option. Confronting strong political pressure, such a decision may also be regarded as a concession on the part of the government in view of the priority to reform the pricing structure of hospital care.

The maintenance of the low-fees policy applied to primary medical care is seemingly not consistent with the government's desire to reduce patients' demand for heavily subsidised health care. Nevertheless, as discussed in Chapter 2, pricing is only one of the barriers to access to health care. As regards the case of outpatient care, there is no sign of the government changing its long-practised policy of controlling the volume of services by means of prospectively setting a limit (see Chapters 4 & 5).

Itemised Charges

The practice of itemised charging means the imposition of a fee on certain procedures, facilities or services. Such a practice is in nature a fee-for-service system which requires patients to pay extra charges in addition to a fixed per diem fee for hospital care or outpatient services. *Towards Better Health* recommended several itemised charges: (a) admission charge in hospitals; (b) first referral to specialist clinic; (c) charges for drugs at specialist clinics and (d) use of accident and emergency service.

Hospital Admission Fees and First Referral Charges The 1985 Scott Report (para.11.3.7c) stated that charging a fixed admission charge to cover extra administrative and diagnostic procedures associated with formal entry to hospital can discourage patients from seeking hospital admission for a very short time when attendance at a clinic would be adequate. Instead of highlighting this point, *Towards Better Health* argues that hospital admission fee and first referral charges can help to reflect the additional cost incurred.   This argument is consistent with the government's objective, already discussed in the chapter, of instilling greater cost-awareness among patients.   In addition, the government may indeed want to use such charges to remind service providers to be aware of the financial implication of admitting patients to hospital especially in the case of 'foreseeable' short stay.

A Legislator elected from the Medical and Health Care Functional Constituency stated that:

> [r]equiring patients to pay an additional charge for hospital admission and first referral to specialist clinic would deter certain individual patients from access to health services, and force them and their family to carry an extra financial burden. It is not fair. (Interview)

The point is that these types of user fees may deter the sick and the poor from seeking warranted or legitimate demand for health care services. Further it is unjust that patients be asked to pay a hospital admission fee or first referral charge when service providers primarily make the decisions about admission or referral. Even though the hospital admission charge is unrelated to the length of hospital stay, and the first referral charge to specialist clinic is unrelated to the frequency of follow-up visits, public opposition is still strong.

Drug Charges Again, *Towards Better Health* admitted that one reason for charging for drugs prescribed by specialist clinics is to instil greater cost-consciousness among patients (para.4.14c).   However, the Health and Medical Development Advisory Committee did not endorse this recommendation. Without the support of the Committee, it is even harder for this option to survive public opposition. A member of the Committee explained to me that:

> [l]ots of specialist clinic patients are the chronically ill or the elderly. Besides, drug therapy is commonly used to monitor the conditions of these patients for a long time. Most of them could not afford the levy on drugs. So,

lots of them would require fee exemptions. It is not a sound idea to means-test the patients from a economic point of view since the administration cost will be very high. (Interview)

A User Fee for Using Accident and Emergency Service The 1985 Scott Report emphasised that charging a fee for attending a hospital accident and emergency service can deter people from abusing service. Thus, the Report recommended charging users a fee equivalent to that of specialist outpatient service. *Towards Better Health* also favoured such a recommendation.

However, as well as avoiding payment for treatment, there are a lot of other explanations for the use of the accident and emergency service. First, the supply of outpatient clinic service at the public hospitals cannot meet the demand, and it may indirectly encourage someone to use the emergency service for treatment. Second, there is no night clinic services and holiday clinic service in many districts. When someone is sick at night or in holidays, he or she cannot get service from a private practitioner or from public institutions in most occasions, and under such circumstances, the patient would probably seek help from accident and emergency service available in public hospitals. Third, many patients do not possess the medical knowledge and information to make a differentiation between emergency and non-emergency cases. When facing an 'emergency' - at least felt by the patients and/or their families, a secure course of action is to go the Accident and Emergency Department for medical treatment. Fourth, it was observed that many people went to an Accident and Emergency Department between 8 p.m. to 9 p.m. in the evening because they could not leave their work to attend clinics during the day (Government Secretariat, 1987:para.4.24). In this connection, there is a need to call for improved night clinic services or 24-hour clinic service in the regional hospitals and to promote the usage of night clinic services at the same time. Finally, if a fee deters the poor from demanding emergency service, their medical need would be overlooked. The promise made by the government that nobody would be denied health care because of the lack of means would be thrown in doubt. Probably because of strong public opposition to this user fee, accident and emergency services are still provided free of charge in public hospitals.

Charges for Specific Items In addition to the above recommendations made by *Towards Better Health*, the government has recently pursued standardised charges for specific items used in the treatment of patients. Charges for specific items, materials or accessories have been levied widely in ex-subvented hospitals since the mid-1980s. These items include joint replacements, orthopaedic implants, artificial limbs, artificial heart valves and so on. While the patients in the general wards are entitled to free surgery, they may come to realise, only too late, that in addition to paying a maintenance charge for hospital service, they are charged for specific items at the hospital's discretion from a hospital charging list.   In the words of the Hospital Authority, specific items have to be 'self purchased' (Hospital Authority, 1995b:2). Worse still, these charges are neither standardised nor uniformly applied, and different hospitals charge different rates for the same item. The ex-Secretary for Health and Welfare argued that the standardisation of itemised charges could reduce the patients' uncertainty and anxiety about them (Hong Kong Government, 1993b:110). A possible option for the government to achieve such a purpose is to eliminate all itemised charges if social rights to health care are to be further developed.   However, viewed from the safety-net approach, such an option is not deemed to be viable.

In light of the likely trend of 'formalising' and 'standardising' itemised charges for specific items, a Legislator elected from the Medical and Health Care Functional Constituency, Mr. Michael Ho Mun-ka, proposed to scrap all itemised medical fees and that 'patients and families should not have to pay more on top of taxes, [private] health insurance and hospital maintenance fees' (Eastern Express, 1 June 1995). His motion met with stiff resistance from the current Secretary for Health and Welfare who stressed that 'abolishing itemised charges would be to cast the safety net too wide' (Hong Kong Standard, 1 June 1995). After a tense, hour-long debate on 31 May 1995, Legislators passed Mr. Ho's motion in tight vote.

The flexing of the Legislative Council's political muscle in resisting the government's proposals on itemised charges and higher medical fees did not take place in a vacuum.   Upon the release of the Provisional Hospital Authority Report and the Primary Health Care Report in 1989 and 1990 respectively, some political parties and grassroot bodies advocated that more resources should be allocated to the public health care system instead (United Democrats of Hong Kong, 1990; Lee, 1990). During the Legislative Council's debate in response to the consultation document *Towards Better Health*, the then United Democrats of Hong Kong, the largest political party, justified the maintenance of the low-fee policy on the ground of considering health care as a social welfare service, and their view was also supported by many other 'pro-welfare' political parties and individual Legislators.

[The] charges for health care services should not be based on operating costs, nor should itemised charging be adopted...[Since] healthcare is a social welfare service, the Government should take full responsibility for looking after the health of the general public and should in no way introduce the principle that patients should bear a greater burden of healthcare costs. (Hong Kong Legislative Council, 13 October 1993)

Thus, the government's attempts to place restrictions on social rights to health care were resisted by the public and politicians. Before the introduction of indirectly elected seats in the Legislative Council in 1985, the making of public policies in Hong Kong was strongly shaped by the alliance between the bureaucrats and the capitalists (see Chapters 4 & 5). Between 1985 and 1991, the government was faced for the first time by a group of elected legislators who were sometimes critical of government proposals and pressed their opposition to the point of voting against the government (Miners, 1994). Six years later in 1991, the Legislative Council had members who were directly elected by universal suffrage for the first time. While in 1995, all members of the Legislative Council were either elected by universal suffrage, or elected from so-called functional constituencies. The latter category is comprised of special interest groups which are afforded the right to have an elected representative, such as for example, doctors, lawyers, engineers and so on. As a result of the changes in the political structure of Hong Kong, conflicts between political parties and those between political parties and the government have become a common feature in the debates on the development of social welfare and social services (Chow, 1994).

Although the government is faced with more critical and active examination of its proposals, it cannot be said that it is prepared to accept major amendments to its policies or resolutions passed by the Legislative Council. Irrespective of strong political pressure and resistance, the government still insists on maintaining the principle of formalising itemised charges and standardising the differences of fees between different public hospitals. To persuade the public to accept the practice of charging for specific items, the government has adopted two measures. First, probably in view of political pressure exerted by the politicians, the

Hospital Authority has abolished charges for several items, 'including replacement joints, spinal implants and special accessories required for blood transfusion' (Hospital Authority, 1995b). The fact is that not all itemised charges are scrapped as demanded by Mr. Ho's motion passed by the Legislative Council. As advances in medical science have made a constant stream of new equipment and items available to doctors, the Authority may, at any time, charge for newly available items not funded by the government. Second, the government proposes to allow patients with a family income up to a certain limit to receive medical subsidies or exemptions for specific items. Hence, more relaxed fee-waiving measures are employed to legitimate the formalisation and standardisation of these charges (see next sub-section for more detailed discussion). It is hard to predict whether these two measures could help to reduce political pressure against the government's policy on itemised medical fees. But it is obvious that itemised charges as well as higher user fees would continue to be a hot political issue partly in view of the further development of democracy and partly in view of the citizens' decade-wide experience with low-fees policy.

Fee-waiving Measures

Fee-waiving is an important component of the safety-net approach that is used to show the government's promise of 'no turn away' policy: no one is denied adequate medical treatment through lack of means. However, this is also used to legitimate the reduction in government subsidy to the non-target groups. Certain groups are recommended in *Towards Better Health* to be given a full or partial waiver without going through means-testing procedures, they are: (a) public assistance (now known as comprehensive social security assistance) recipients; (b) disability allowance recipients; (c) persons aged 70 years and above in receipt of old age allowance and (d) unemployed chronically ill patients. Group (a) would be immediately given a full waiver as is the current practice, while the other groups would be granted a partial waiver at a certain percentage of the fees paid by non-targeted groups (Hong Kong Government, 1993a:para.4.15).

Under this proposed arrangement, the non-target groups would have no choice but to be means-tested if fee waiving were sought. Besides, if the Hospital Authority could succeed in charging higher fees, the partial-waiver groups may need to apply for fee waiving. These two factors would increase the likelihood of a rise in number for means test usually characterised by stigma and inconvenience. The fact is that even though the current practice is to charge only low fees, 78 per cent and 13 per cent of the inpatient fees in psychiatric and non-psychiatric hospitals were waived in 1991/92 (Hong Kong Government, 1993a:para.1.20).

As regards charges for specific medical items, the current Secretary for Health and Welfare proposed to allow families with an income of up to HK$16,000 a month to receive partial or full medical subsidies (Eastern Express, 1 June 1995). As household rather than personal income would be used to determine patients' ability to pay, the 'family responsibility' to care for the welfare of its members would be reproduced.   Besides, patients of old age might feel bad to have their own family went through the means-testing process which is not amenable to promoting a sense of dignity for old people themselves.

Moreover, the government has decided to expand the role played by a charity fund named the Samaritan Fund to provide assistance to financially needy patients to meet the cost of specific 'private-purchase' items. A grant of HK$20 million will be provided by the government to the Fund which is made up of donations from charitable trusts, organisations and the wider community (Hong Kong Government, 1995b:119).   Charity organisations are to be asked to provide an extra HK$15 million for the Fund on top of the promised government's grant so that some 800 patients or three times the number of existing recipients will benefit (Hong Kong Standard, 2 November 1995).

This shows that charges for 'private-purchase' items will not be abolished and that global budget for health care will not be used to finance these specific items.   Instead charity funds and charity organisations would be asked to offer a helping hand. If the Samaritan Fund could not effectively meet the increase in applications for financial assistance, first priority would be given to emergency cases. Those patients requiring specific medical items for cold or elective surgery would then be deprived of the opportunity to improve their health status. This also implies that those who could afford to meet the cost of 'private-purchase' items would have more convenient access to elective surgery or procedures.

In the 1990s, a safety-net system to offer financial help to the needy to meet these itemised charges will then be linked to the spirit of charity and ability to pay rather than social rights. Such a practice is consistent with the government's intention to reduce the citizens' social rights to health care. In relation to the total hospital budget, the sums of charitable funds involved are marginal.   Their ideological significance is greater: the

Hospital Authority would continue to use funds raised through charitable sources that should otherwise be totally met out of general revenue, and the inadequacy of charitable funds would be used to legitimate itemised charges for 'private-purchase' items that may increase alongside further technological improvement in medicine.

The Shared Care Approach: Redirecting Patients' Demands to the Private Sector

Rather than further extending the time frame and passively waiting for the public acceptance of the so-called 'percentage subsidy approach' and the standardisation of itemised charges, another important step has been taken to reduce patients' demands for highly-subsidised medicine in an indirect way. This section will discuss the shared care approach adopted by the Hospital Authority to achieve such a purpose.

Establishing an Interface between Specialists and Primary Care Doctors

In an era characterised by the prevalence of chronic illness, the Hospital Authority has identified six priority chronic disease groups for attention. They are cancer, cerebrovascular disease, ischaemic heart disease, end stage renal failure, chronic lung disease and diabetes mellitus (Hospital Authority, 1994; 1995a). Within the six priority disease groups, a shared care approach has been recently developed to better manage the chronic conditions of patients with diabetes or hypertension. The stated purpose of the approach is to establish an interface between the specialists and the primary care doctors to provide optimal and continuous care to the patients (Hospital Authority, 1995a:31). To establish such an interface, these patients attending the Hospital Authority's specialist outpatient units are to be jointly cared by the Authority's specialists and primary care doctors.   Shared care programmes are characterised by establishing communication and referrals between these two parties via the use of common clinical protocols and structured referral system (Hospital Authority, ibid:31).

Recent changes in health policy in the UK have also emphasised the importance of applying the shared care approach to certain groups of chronic patients by involving hospital consultants and general practitioners (Goldberg and Jackson, 1992; Bennett, et al., 1994). Such an arrangement is considered to be of particular importance for those with chronic, long-term conditions who require continuity of follow-up and may require to cross from primary care to specialist care and vice versa. If communications are efficient and referrals are effective, this approach could help to deliver appropriate care suitable for the level of patients' need, and could free valuable hospital services and beds as a result of the transfer of patients' care into the community. However, shared care in the UK has, to some extent, shifted the cost of prescribing expensive drugs from the hospitals to the general practitioners (Orme, 1991).

Hong Kong is a different health care environment from the UK. Hong Kong people do not have registration with a single primary care doctor as in the UK. As a result, it is usual for Hong Kong patients to seek consultations or treatments from several primary care doctors. In developing shared care programmes, patients in Hong Kong have to assume a more central role and to feedback the information from several primary care doctors through a patient-held record (McGhee, 1995).

Redirecting Patients' Demands for Public Medicine

Factors Accounting for Boosting Patients' Demands for Follow-up Care by General Practitioners in the Private Sector   The public general clinics provide service on a first-come-first-serve and quota basis. That means, patients attending these clinics still have to confront many considerable barriers to primary medical care. To avoid these barriers, patients usually prefer to attend private practitioners providing primary medical care as a market commodity. The adoption of shared care would not do away all these undesirable barriers to public general clinics. This is an important factor in accounting for the likelihood of patients' attending private practitioners in the case of shared care.

Patients cannot self-initiate attendance at public specialist clinics without a doctor's referral. Because of the inadequacy of these services in meeting rising public demand, it usually takes patients nearly three months for a first-time attendance to a specialist clinic. The factors of long queue and inconvenience could serve to 'encourage' public patients to attend private specialists instead. However, specialists charge higher fees than the general practitioners. For example, in a survey on private consultation fees in 1992, it was found that general practitioners charged from HK$80 to HK$300 for each consultation, while the range of fees for each consultation was from HK$150 to HK$600 (Hong Kong Government,

1993a:9). So, the pricing factor could be a serious barrier in discouraging working-class patients from using private specialist services.

Until the adoption of the shared care approach, the health care system of Hong Kong was characterised by one-way referral from the private sector rather than two-way referral between the public and private sectors. Besides, patients discharged from public hospitals may not have had the confidence to attend general practitioners in the private sector for follow-up or chronic care. The implementation of shared care programmes allows the Authority's specialists to refer their patients to general practitioners in the private sector.   Such a practice could persuade the diabetes or hypertension patients to attend general practitioners rather than specialists. No doubt, those who have limited choice but to seek treatment or follow-up services provided at public specialist clinics would still suffer from the problems of long queues and inconveniences.

Moreover, the Hospital Authority has taken active measures to promote follow-up or chronic care managed by general practitioners in the private sector (Hospital Authority, 1994:30). For example, currently four Hospital Authority's Diabetic Centres are organising educational sessions for general practitioners (Hospital Authority, 1995a:31). In addition, regular discussion and evaluation of shared care arrangements between specialists and primary care doctors could help to boost public confidence for the latter.   Backed by specialists' support and training, general practitioners are more ready to follow up diabetic, hypertensive or other chronic patients.   This represents a good business opportunity for primary care doctors in the private sector especially in view of the long-term care needed by chronic patients.

Implications   The diabetic shared care programmes will be rolled out to all eight hospital clusters in 1995/96. Each hospital cluster will soon develop a hypertension shared care programme with local primary care doctors to better manage stable and uncomplicated hypertensive patients currently followed up in the Authority's specialist outpatient clinics. The next step involves more structured arrangements between the Authority's specialists and primary care doctors, and extension to other chronic diseases (Hospital Authority, 1995a:31&38). A rapid development of shared care programmes may actually signify a trend towards greater involvement of private general practitioners in following-up the Authority's specialist outpatient clinics. Further, making use of primary care facilities and resources in the private sector may also legitimate a much slower development of new general outpatient clinics in the public sector.

The development of shared care programmes and the consequent establishment of a two-way referral system between the public and private sectors are expected by the Authority to have the effect of reducing the hospital admission rate and specialist clinic attendance for patients in the programmes by 10 per cent (Hospital Authority, ibid:40). This could help to make better use of the available health care resources. The fact is that hospital care is very expensive, and the average cost of medical care provided in public specialist clinic is three times higher than that provided in public general clinics (Hong Kong Government, 1993a). However, such a result would largely be made possible by involving private practitioners rather than general outpatient clinics in the public sector. In the UK, the case of cost shifting of expensive drugs from hospitals to general practitioners is not borne by patients themselves. However, in Hong Kong, the case of cost-shifting in shared care programmes is likely to be shifting from public financing to private financing since patients have to pay out-of-pocket for attendance at private clinics.

The rapid development of shared care programmes without meeting apparent political pressure has to be understood in relation to the government's promise of maintaining its low-fees policy in primary care. The reduction of patients' demands for highly-subsidised outpatient services are not realised by directly reducing the level of state subsidy, but by shifting part of the workload originally taken up by the Authority's specialist outpatient clinics to private clinics. As long as the main concern of the public and the politicians is on opposing higher user fees, patients' demands for highly subsidised health care can be reduced in a more subtle way. Indeed, within the context of Hong Kong, the predominant role already played by the health care market in primary care has provided the infrastructure for the redirecting of patients' demands from the public sector to the private sector.

Conclusion

Confronting the problem of reducing or containing patients' access to highly subsidised public medicine, the state has to deal with a complex set of political issues. Within the context of Hong Kong citizens' long term experience of low-fees policy in health care, the government's desire to reform the pricing structure of public medicine is anything but easy.   In spite of this, it looks apparent that the reform of health care pricing policy is still on the political agenda. Confronting increasing demand for public medicine, the Hospital Authority has employed the shared care approach to divert demand by inducing patients to finance their follow-up or chronic care in the private health care market. Whether this would significantly reduce demand for health care provided in specialist outpatient clinics remains to be seen; but it implies that other less politically contentious means or approaches may be used to reduce demand for highly subsidised medicine in an indirect way and to reaffirm the importance of relying on oneself and the family for welfare.

7 Semi-Private Beds: Enhancing Competition and Choice?

Introduction

Alongside efforts made by the government to persuade Hong Kong's citizens to accept higher fees and to standardise itemised charges for specific medical materials or accessories, emphasis is also placed on increasing choice in the public sector. The idea of choice sounds attractive to the public since the only choice that is available to public patients is their freedom to choose which general outpatient clinic (within a particular region) to attend (Hong Kong Government, 1993a:para.3.13). Another so-called 'choice' available to all patients is the choice between public and private health care. Certainly, those who cannot afford to pay are left with no choice but to go public. As regards public hospital care, patients cannot choose which hospital they want. Nor can they freely choose their own doctors or timing of hospitalisation unlike the situation in private sector health care. In the case of accident and emergency, patients are transported to the nearest public hospital for treatment. While in the case of elective or cold surgeries, patients are most likely admitted to their regional hospital (Chapter 5).

In the context of Hong Kong, the government proclaims offering public patients a choice of semi-private beds of higher cost recovery potential as a real and affordable choice. Two hospitals began to introduce semi-private beds on a pilot scheme basis at the end of 1994. This type of bed was first introduced to Ruttonjee Hospital on 20 July 1994 and Tsan Yuk Hospital on 11 October 1994 (Ming Pao, 16 May 1994). The pilot projects are implemented to determine the demand from the public on actual experience before a decision is made to decide 'how best to extend it to more public hospitals' (Hong Kong Government, 1995b:119). It is estimated in *Towards Better Health* (para.4.13) that 'some 2,000 beds could initially be made available for semi-privaterooms'. This is not a small figure at all as this is about ten per cent of beds available in public hospitals.

179

In addition, competition has also become a keyword of health care reform in Hong Kong. *Towards Better Health* (para. 4.16) emphasises that the level of fees charged for semi-private beds could serve as a benchmark for the private sector and thus facilitate healthy competition with private hospitals. The discussion in Chapter 5 has already shown that the public and private sectors exist as almost two separate independent entities: neither competition nor co-operation is created between the two sectors. So the 'choice' element of semi-private beds and the promotion of competition at the inter-sector level are important areas for analysing health care reform in Hong Kong.

The chapter examines whether the setting up of the Hospital Authority in Hong Kong is amenable to enhancing competition between hospitals, and whether the introduction of semi-private beds will promote choice and competition both on intra- and inter-sector levels.

The Case of Hong Kong: Corporatisation without Competition?

Enhancing Integration of Public Hospital Services

The Hong Kong Hospital Authority was formally established with the enactment of Hospital Authority Ordinance in 1990 and took over the control and management of public hospitals in 1991. The Hospital Authority was chosen to tackle the major problems of public hospital care, like over-centralisation, inflexibility, low staff morale, long waiting lists, overcrowded conditions, poor co-ordination between ex-government and ex-subvented hospitals, etc. (Scott, 1985; Provisional Hospital Authority, 1989; Hospital Authority, 1994). However, the Ordinance does not require the separation of providers from purchasers of care through the creation of the internal market like that implemented in the UK. The fact is that the corporatisation exercise would have been an opportunity for the introduction of competition between public provider units on an intra-sector level (i.e. between public hospitals). While there have been talks about the Authority's headquarters assuming the role of health care purchasers, nothing concrete has emerged (Hospital Authority, 1994). In spite of the introduction of greater administrative and financial flexibility into the system of public hospital care, the health care delivery mechanism organised by the Hospital Authority is still characterised by the public integrated model rather than the public contract model (Chapter 2). Also, there has not been any fundamental change in the financing arrangement between the hospitals and the Authority's head office: budgets are allocated to individual hospitals according to historic cost basis and new projects, if there are any (Yuen, 1994). In the public sector, money does not follow the patients, and there is no need for public hospitals to compete with one another for survival as a consequence of the lack of provider competition.

Prior to the establishment of the Hospital Authority, public hospitals were divided into two types: government and subvented hospitals (Chapters 4 and 5). By incorporating these two types of public hospitals under the management umbrella of the Hospital Authority, and by bringing the remuneration and fringe benefits package of subvented hospital staff in line with that of their government counterparts, the government believed that better integration of public hospitals and medical resources could be resulted. In particular, the corporatisation exercise was believed to be of particular importance to help raise the occupancy rate of subvented hospitals and reduce overcrowding of some government regional hospitals (Scott, 1985; Provisional Hospital Authority, 1989). So, it easily leads to the impression that integration rather than competition was to be strengthened. Moreover, the corporatisation of public hospital services has brought an end to the government's exploitation of the relatively much less attractive fringe benefits and promotion prospect of ex-subvented hospital staff (Chapter 5). That is, the government can no longer exploit the differences between former government and subvented hospitals since the establishment of the Hospital Authority: the government has to spend much more for the same throughput of services compared to the pre-Hospital Authority's era.

Non-expansion of Private Paybeds

As public hospital care is highly subsidised, there exists an inherent disincentive for private hospitals to compete with public hospitals for patients, thereby resulting in a seemingly 'dual monopoly' with each sector serving different types of patients (see Chapter 5). It is in fact almost impossible for private hospitals to compete for patients with their counterparts in the public sector because the former cannot afford to provide health care without even realising the cost of provision.

The establishment of the Hospital Authority may result in more fee-paying private patients via the expansion of private paybeds. If this practice were further strengthened, inter-sector competition between private and public hospitals would be enhanced. However, the number of private paybeds (1st and 2nd class) available in the Hospital Authority is just about 2 per cent of the total number of public hospital beds (Wong, 1998). Because of the non-expansion of private paybeds, these beds are still largely used as a fringe benefit provided to senior civil servants or senior staff of the Hospital Authority (see Chapter 5). During the interview, the ex-Secretary for Health and Welfare explained to me that:

> [t]he hospital beds in the private sector only cater for some 18 per cent of the population with 10 per cent of all hospital beds. Nevertheless, it has a special role to play in meeting the needs of those patients who could afford to pay the economic fees. The further expansion of private paybeds [in public hospitals] could mean, if we are not careful enough, the collapse of the private sector. That's bad. It is bad because it will not make the most of the resources available in the private sector and may frustrate the doctors if there will be only one avenue [the public sector] for them to provide hospital care. (Interview)

Thus, it seems that the government wants to retain the role played by the private sector and to avoid a further increase in direct competition with the private sector via the expansion of private paybeds provided in public hospitals. But as will be discussed later, the provision of semi-private rather than private beds may help promote inter-sector competition in Hong Kong.

Non-expansion of Opportunities for Consultants' Private Practice in Public Hospitals

The Hospital Authority enjoys greater flexibility in dealing with personnel matters such as salary scales, hiring and firing and the use of part-time staff. The Authority may also allow senior doctors or consultants to undertake private practice in public hospitals. However, in the context of Hong Kong, the idea of allowing non-teaching public hospital consultants to have private practice had not ever been raised in any official documents until the Scott Report was published in 1985. It was observed that experienced doctors and consultants preferred to set up their own business in the private health care market in order to make much bigger profit (Ng, 1990). The idea of private practice might be used as a concession to reduce the consultants' resistance to the setting up of the Hospital

Authority, or it might be used to prevent the further drainage of experienced staff from the public to the private sector in Hong Kong.

The Scott Report proposed that revenue from private practice should be divided, on an agreed basis, between the hospital and the doctors concerned, and that the level of direct financial benefit to the individual doctor should be restricted to around 25 per cent of the basic salary (Scott, 1985:para.9.20). In the past, only senior doctors or consultants employed under university terms could enjoy some rights of private practice. However, they did not personally receive any direct financial benefit for providing private services in teaching hospitals: the fees charged being divided between the university and the government. Although they attended private patients, hospital consultants working in non-teaching hospitals did not receive any additional remuneration nor did they retain any portion of the fee so charged in their unit or department for service development or research activities (Scott, 1985:para.9.4.2). Up till now, however, all these practices remain the same, and private practice has been confined to those consultants employed under university terms (Yuen, 1994), which result in the non-expansion of opportunities for private practice in public hospitals.

If private practice is further encouraged, the number of paybeds will become much larger, and the use of paybeds will not be largely restricted to senior civil servants and Hospital Authority employees. In addition to the government's wishes to retain the role played by private hospitals in meeting the needs and/or demands of private patients, the medical profession itself is also divided as to the proposal of private practice in public hospitals. The current President of the British Medical Association (Hong Kong Branch), openly specified three dangers of allowing private practice for consultants working in public hospitals in an authoritative directory circulated and used within the medical and dental profession (Law, 1993). First, the consultants' attention would be more diverted to their private patients. Second, the consultants would have no incentive to shorten the hospital waiting list as this would reduce the pool of private patients. Third, the consultants would delegate the care of public patients to junior doctors resulting in increasing the workload of the latter but without giving them any financial reimbursement for the extra work done.

Even though the Hong Kong Medical Association represents the interest of the entire medical profession and plays a very important role in health policy making, it may not be supportive to the proposal of private practice in public hospitals since this may undermine the interests of private practitioners who constitute the majority of the medical profession. In view of retaining their private patients and in view of safeguarding their financial interest, it is conceivable that private practitioners will continue to resist the proposal of private practice. Rather than expanding opportunities for private practice, a scheme entitled 'Flexible Employment Terms' was launched in July 1993, allowing private practitioners in four specialities to work either as full-time medical officers on a short-term basis, or as part-timers (Yuen, 1994). This measure is used to supplement the medical expertise of public hospitals since the majority of the medical profession are private practitioners. Nevertheless, private practitioners have not yet been given admission privileges to facilities in public hospitals for their private patients.

It can be seen from the above discussion that the corporatisation of public hospitals in Hong Kong has not, up till now at least, led to the expansion of private paybeds nor opportunities for consultants' private practice. If all these are realised, competition between health care providers on both intra-sector and inter-sector levels will no doubt be induced. Such an analysis provides the background and context for examining the introduction of the product of semi-private bed and the kind of competition and effects it will bring about in Hong Kong.

B-class Beds: Characteristics and Features

The idea of semi-private beds was firstly introduced in the 1985 Scott Report. This report regarded private beds (both first and second class) provided in public hospitals as A-class and public ward beds as C-class (para.11.5.2); and recommended semi-private beds as B-class beds of which the standard was somewhere between A-class and C-class beds. The major areas for improvement were in terms of space, privacy and amenities. The report emphasised that the standard of B-class bed should be comparable to that of private beds in the 'dormitories' available in private hospitals. In 1985, more than 60 per cent of hospital beds were provided in the dormitories of private hospitals (para.11.18). Regarding medical treatment, the report suggested that B-class beds should not seek any significant differentiation in medical treatment from that available in public wards. However, this report agreed that patients in B-class beds would tend to have their medical treatment supervision handled directly by more senior medical staff (para.11.5.1). The private ward patients in public hospitals have indeed long enjoyed this kind of privilege despite the fact that nothing has been specified in policy terms.

The Provisional Hospital Authority supported such an idea (1989:para. 12.6). But a bit unlike the Scott Report, it strongly emphasised that the standard of medical treatment should be the same in all classes of wards (para.12.6.3). The consultation document *Towards Better Health* further reaffirmed this point and emphasised that an important differentiation should be made between 'hotel' services and medical care. The consultation document clarifies that patients occupying B-class beds should not enjoy 'preferential treatment over general ward patients either in terms of choice of doctors or priority for elective surgery'. In other words, no queue jumping would take place for those patients using these beds.

During the interview, the ex-Secretary for Health and Welfare told me that 'semi-private beds can be provided in different classes, say, B1, B2, B3...etc., according to the different levels of amenities and accommodation provided'. According to the actual experience of the pilot projects on semi-private beds in two selected hospitals, they enjoy the freedom to determine the level of amenities for these beds. For example, in Tsun Yuk hospital, two types of semi-private beds of different levels of fees are provided: two-bed rooms and single-bed rooms. Thus it can be seen that hospitals can flexibly modify the pricing of and the amenities provided in semi-private beds.

With respect to the level of fees, the Scott Report recommended a significant cost recovery from B-class beds. That is, B-class beds are of much higher cost-recovery potential than public ward beds. The Provisional Hospital Authority proposed two different charging practices for B-class beds. The first option follows the principle of marginal cost. '[B-class] beds should be subsidised to the same extent as beds in public wards, and the patients would pay the additional cost between the B-class and public wards' (para.12.6.4). This means that users of semi-private beds have to pay 100 per cent for additional facilities and amenities provided, while they can enjoy the same level of subsidy for the rest of medical care as public-ward patients do. The second option looks very much alike the recommendation of the Scott Report: '...setting the fee as a percentage of total cost but at a higher percentage of recovery than that for the public wards' (Scott, 1985:para.12.6.5). This means that the production cost of hospital care is averaged out, and the semi-private-ward patients have to pay much more or get less government subsidy. The consultation document finally recommended the second option, and the flat rate fee charged could be set at 40 per cent or 60 per cent of the operating cost per bed day, with the rest of the cost being subsidised by the government. In short, upon the successful implementation of B-class beds, public hospitals would have three types of bed of varying standard and price.

B-class Beds: Core Product and Enhanced Benefits

A hospital care product consists of two major components: a core product satisfying basic health care needs, and a set of enhanced benefits which may or may not be relevant for maintaining or restoring health (Ten Have, 1995). The core product refers to medical treatment and procedures meeting the medical needs of patients. For example, a woman in labour wants the hospital to assist her to have a safe and easy delivery. As regards enhanced benefits, it has two different types: medical and non-medical. Choice of experienced doctors and priority for elective surgery are examples of enhanced medical benefits. Public patients may suffer from being deprived of such enhanced medical benefits that are of direct or indirect relevance for satisfying health care need. For example, they may queue up for a long time for elective surgery to have their health status improved. Usually, the medical profession and the urgency of medical need determine how long the public patients have to wait for a surgery. If patients want to jump the queue and enjoy enhanced medical benefits, they may choose to consume private medicine or use private beds provided in public hospitals provided that they are willing and able to pay economic fees. As a result of the consumption of enhanced medical benefits, private patients can have their medical needs met more quickly than their counterparts in the public sector. In this case, unnecessary suffering often experienced by those patients who cannot afford to go private can be avoided.

The non-medical aspect of enhanced benefits is concerned with facilities and amenities not relevant for maintaining or restoring health, but are purchased to satisfy individual preferences, demands or wants. A better standard of amenities will be surely of benefit to patients especially in view of the fact that confinement to hospital bed is not usually regarded as a pleasure.

The experimentation of B-class beds can show that the government wants to make it possible for public patients to use additional or enhanced amenities. That is, additional hotel services or amenities should no longer be only restricted to senior civil servants or senior employees of the Hospital Authority. As emphasised by all the relevant reports and consultation documents, B-class beds are provided to meet additional users' wants in hotel facilities and services rather than to enable the patients to enjoy extra medical benefits. Such an emphasis is made to justify the implementation of B-class beds that their users would not have any priority over public-ward patients.

Product and User Differentiation

The experimentation with B-class beds signifies the government's attempts at product and user differentiation. In the past, with the exception of private-ward patients, public patients had no chance to get extra benefits even for those who could afford to do so. So, the B-class bed is a new product that can enable public patients to enjoy additional benefits. In this way, public hospitals could provide different levels of inpatient services that are clinically equivalent but have different amenities. Within the public health care system, product differentiation is in fact not a new concept as could be evidenced by the provision of private wards and public wards. But this will further expand upon the widespread implementation of B-class beds.

Product differentiation does not strictly or directly imply the exercise of price discrimination, for different products can be charged at the same price. However, the intention underlying the provision of B-class beds is to cater for the middle income groups who cannot afford to stay in private hospitals or in private wards of public hospitals but would be willing to pay a higher fee for better amenities (Scott, 1985). The middle-income group has therefore been singled out as a particular segment among the users of public hospital care. Therefore, the product differentiation strategy adopted is also one that can lead to the further differentiation of users of public medical services. Three types of user segment could then be identified, namely, users of private, semi-private and public wards respectively.

Theoretically, any public patients are free to choose which type of bed they want to use. Practically speaking, however, because of the lack of provision of private beds (including first and second class) in public hospitals, they are, in most cases, used as a privilege offered by either the government or the Hospital Authority. Public patients may choose to use

B-class beds. However, they have to satisfy the basic condition of paying more for this since substantial user charges would be placed on patients using upgraded ward facilities. That is, alongside product and user differentiation, the pricing structure of public medical services will also be reformed towards the direction of higher cost recovery.

B-class Beds: Attracting Private or Public Patients?

B-class Beds as an Inter-sector Interface Product

As discussed before, the product of B-class beds is primarily targeted to attract the middle-income group to use additional amenities made available in public hospitals.   The enhanced benefits of hospital care provided in private hospitals usually cover both medical and non-medical benefits, while those provided by semi-private beds are said to be, in policy terms, confined to non-medical aspect only. As far as the level and scope of enhanced benefits are concerned, private hospital care is a much better choice.   However, since charges in private hospitals are set to recover the total bed cost and cover profit and private medical professional fees, patients who can afford to pay more for amenities but who cannot afford the full private hospital charges may prefer to use the product of B-class bed. Pricing is then an important factor in shaping patients' demand for semi-private beds provided in public hospitals.

Compared to the price of private hospital care, the price of B-class beds is competitive in two ways. First, although patients have to pay a higher fee for using this product, they would still be partially subsidised by the government, say, 40 to 60 per cent as recommended in *Towards Better Health*. Private hospitals and private practitioners may choose to cross-subsidise the less well off patients by charging the more well-off patients higher fees and charges. Such a possibility cannot be totally ruled out; however, it is very unlikely that such a practice would become a general rule for it would most probably attract lots of less well-off patients and consequently add strains on full cost recovery or profit-making.

Second, private hospital care is pegged to each individual case. If a patient has to go through major or sophisticated surgery involving complex treatment and advanced medical technology, he or she has to pay a very expensive price out-of-pocket unless covered by adequate medical insurance or employers' fringe benefits. If B-class beds are linked to the concept of pegging fees to actual cost of each case, it may prove to be very expensive in certain cases. In actual charging practice, however, the operating cost of all acute hospital beds is averaged rather than calculated case by case. In other words, B-class bed patients would just be charged a higher flat rate fee. Certainly, if they want to employ their own nurse or caretaker, they have to pay an extra economic fee.

The long queue for public medical services is an important factor encouraging patients to go private (see Chapter 2). The ex-Secretary for Health and Welfare said that '[About] 10 per cent of those in private hospitals are earning HK$4,000 a month. They're on the breadline' (Ball, 1993). It can be imagined that to obtain earlier access to medical services by going private, these patients on the breadline would use most if not all of their savings or seek loan from their relatives, friends or whatever sources. With respect to elective or cold surgeries, if patients consider the time factor or early treatment to be of utmost importance,   the competitiveness of private medicine can be maintained.

However, in the case of accident and emergency, the difference that enhanced medical benefits offered by private hospitals can make would be much   reduced because the time factor could be discarded under such circumstances. According to official statistics, more than 25 per cent of public patients are admitted through the Accident and Emergency Departments (Census and Statistics Department, 1993).   This type of patient may choose to use semi-private beds but without being forced to join the long queues for public medical services. So, in this case, B-class beds would probably have a better chance to compete for patients and the competition pressure put on private hospitals would be greater. Moreover, in respect of maternity cases, the time factor is also relatively insignificant, since giving birth to a baby is not considered as an elective surgery that can be delayed.   In fact, one of the hospitals which was chosen to implement the pilot project of semi-private beds is a maternity hospital (i.e. Tsan Yuk Hospital).

From the above analysis, it can be seen that the factor of pricing may function effectively to attract some private patients to go public and use B-class beds instead particularly those patients who can avoid the long queues for public medical services. *Towards Better Health* (para.4.16) states that:

[s]emi-private rooms also facilitate healthy competition with private hospitals...It is possible that the level of fees charged for semi-private rooms

would serve as a benchmark for the private sector. These developments may, in the long run, attract patients away from the public system, thus lessening the burden on the public sector.

It is clear from this quote that the government wants to introduce competition between the public and private sectors via the introduction of B-class beds. If B-class beds prove to be competitive enough, they can then serve to establish an interface between the two sectors with respect to the competition for patients. The government anticipates that the private sector may then, in the long run, make the price of their health care products more competitive in order to attract more patients. The lowering of the price of private medical care sounds attractive to the public since it has long been criticised as very expensive even when compared with the US (Ball, 1993).

Deadweight Effects

One argument that comes forward in response to the creation of this inter-sector interface product is that of the 'deadweight' effect (Pirie and Butler, 1988). *Towards Better Health* (para.4.17) mentions that 'semi-private rooms may create a reverse flow of patients [from private hospitals] into public hospitals, thereby straining the [public health care] system further'. The effect is described as 'deadweight' because government might subsidise those already in private medicine.   Giving these patients government subsidy would cost the government a dear price to generate competition on the one hand, and reduce the amount of public subsidy available for meeting the needs of public patients staying in public wards on the other hand. The more competitive the semi-private beds, the more patients will be drawn away from private hospitals, and the higher the degree of deadweight effects will be generated as a result. The increasing consumption of B-class beds following a reverse flow of patients into public hospitals will turn out to contribute to an increased financial burden on the Hospital Authority in spite of the fact that it can charge these patients higher user fees. Some of the policy makers and politicians I interviewed discarded such a possibility, however.   The following quotations can well illustrate this.

We think not because in the private sector you can choose your doctor. But we can't choose doctor in public hospitals. But it will attract more public patients to use such beds. The relationship between doctors and patients will be one of the deterrent factors which will prevent people from using the public sector if they have the money. (Ex-Secretary for Health and Welfare, Interview)

Compared to private medicine, our choice is different, since public patients cannot choose their doctor and the timing of hospitalisation. Thus, a reverse flow of patients from the private sector is unlikely. (Chief Executive of the Hospital Authority, Interview)

The provision of B-class beds would not attract private patients since they do not have choices of doctors and timing of which they could enjoy in the private sector. Remember the only improvement is only concerned with hotel service only. Because private hospitals offer a choice of doctor and render faster treatment, most of their patients would stick with the private sector. (A Legislator elected from the Medical and Health Care Functional Constituency, Interview)

I don't think so. The reason is that the product of B-class bed is different from the products offered in the private sector. Public patients could not choose their own doctors, and schedule their admission. (An appointed Legislator, Interview)

From these quotations, it can be seen that the ideas of these policy makers and politicians are very similar to the differentiation made between medical and non-medical benefits. They tend to believe that the provision of enhanced medical benefits is an important factor preventing a reverse flow of patients from the private sector from taking place. But their belief is somewhat contradictory with what was described in the consultation document as healthy competition between the private and public sectors. As stated by the consultation document, the price or level of fees of the B-class bed is also an important factor attracting patients to use it. Upon a widespread introduction of B-class beds, there is no way for the private sector to be totally immunised from engaging in competition - whether healthy or unhealthy - with the public sector. So, it is very difficult, if not impossible, to keep competition going but without generating deadweight effects at the same time. The question is therefore more concerned with the degree of deadweight effects generated rather than whether they will take place or not. However, from a political point of view, the discarding of the possibility of 'unhealthy' competition by some politicians can serve to legitimate the decision of policy makers in implementing B-class beds.

As can be shown from the following quotations, three interviewees were aware of price as an important factor to attract private patients to use B-class beds.

> In fact, the product of B-class bed is different from that offered in the private sector. But the factor of price will cause some kind of competition between the public and private sectors. (A member of the Health and Medical Development Advisory Committee, Interview)

> As there is still a heavy subsidy for B-class beds from the government, some of the users of private health care will be attracted to use them. I think there should be a system to attract patients from the public wards rather than from the private hospitals. (A directly elected Legislator, Interview)

> B-class beds have certain attraction as the patients are more certain about the fees which are fixed at a flat rate. While in the private sector, it is not so. So, the implementation of B-class beds might encourage private patients to use public medical services as a result, and thus the government has to give more subsidies. (A Legislator elected from the Medical and Health Care Functional Constituency, Interview)

The competition generated on the inter-sector level is amenable to the creation of deadweight effects. To some likely users of private medicine, paying less for hospital care may be an incentive for them to choose B-class beds especially if they can avoid the long-queues in cases like emergencies and giving birth to a child. The generation of a deadweight effect is caused by the flow of patients from the private sector to take advantage of government subsidy when using B-class beds within the public sector. As an inter-sector interface product, B-class beds could generate a deadweight effect that could outweigh the cost recovered from patients by charging higher user fees.

The generation of a deadweight effect implies that a particular segment of middle-income patients will not use medical care as a commodity in the private health care market. Competition for patients in the market can either be price- or quality-based; but the products are still provided as commodities. Inter-sector competition is facilitated not by introducing a new commodity but by a subsidised product with enhanced amenities made available in the public sector. In theory, the public sector can compete with the private sector by expanding the provision of private beds as a commodity but without generating a deadweight effect. Nevertheless, it is inconsistent with the wish of the government to retain the role played by private hospitals (see above discussion).

B-class Beds as an Intra-sector Interface Product

Towards Better Health (para.4.16) states that the introduction of B-class beds is 'conducive to...diverting public subsidy from those who are willing and able to pay more for greater personal comfort to those in financial need'. As discussed above, inter-sector competition is closely associated with the generation of a deadweight effect. So, this quote should not be understood in relation to the concept of inter-sector competition. Rather, it refers to attempts made to attract those patients who would most likely use public wards if semi-private wards were not made available in public hospitals. Viewed by the government, B-class beds will, therefore, provide a good measure to reduce the overload of public hospital care as interpreted by over-subsidising those patients who can afford to pay more but not to the extent of going private. That is, this will help to reform the pricing structure of public medical care according to patients' ability to pay (see Chapter 6), and make the system of public medical subsidy a discriminatory rather than a non-discriminatory one by the provision of such an innovative product.

To attract such a particular segment of patients from public-ward users would generate no competition with private hospitals. Semi-private wards may, however, 'compete' with public wards for patients not in terms of price, but in terms of better amenities. B-class beds can then be considered as an intra-sector interface product in public hospital care both in terms of the standard of hotel services and the level of fees or government subsidy. To determine whether the product of B-class bed consumed at a particular moment is an inter-sector or intra-sector interface product will depend on whether a deadweight effect is generated or not. Indeed, the Health and Welfare Branch and the Hospital Authority would like to persuade the public to believe that the provision of B-class bed will help reduce the overload of public hospitals and raise more revenue for the needy but without subsidising the private patients at the same time.

Administrative Flexibility and Financial Incentive

As discussed in Chapters 2 and 5, there is little incentive for a government department to increase charges if all the extra revenue goes directly to the Government Treasury. However, as a public body, the Hospital Authority enjoys a greater degree of administrative flexibility in providing health care and is allowed to retain 50 per cent of whatever extra income it receives (Provisional Hospital Authority, 1989; Hong Kong Government, 1993a). Furthermore, each public hospital can retain part of the extra income generated for research or development purposes. In the event of inadequate funding from the government, public hospitals may tend to raise funds from providing more B-class beds of higher cost-recovery potential. The Hospital Authority and its hospitals may thus fully make use of their administrative flexibility and autonomy enshrined in the 1990 Hospital Authority Ordinance to adjust either the number or the level of fees of semi-private beds.

As stated in the 1993 consultation document (para.4.13), the actual provision of semi-private wards would not be determined by quota but 'assessed against prevailing demand'. The Scott Report (para.11.5.5) made it clear that 'the decision on "B" class pricing is a policy decision first and a marketing decision subsequently'. In other words, patients' demand on semi-private wards would be employed to determine the number of beds made available as semi-private ones. So, the number of semi-private beds can be more than the initial estimated figure of 2,000 if there is found to be a higher demand. An appointed Legislator told me that:

[a]s far as I know, no fixed percentage of B-beds was proposed. It might be varied from hospital to hospital according to luxury/privacy offered, as deemed suitable for the district. For example, the demand for B-beds may be higher in Hong Kong Island than Kowloon. That's why each hospital determines the percentage for itself, according to its own demand. (Interview)

Towards Better Health (para.4.17) states that '[the] market mechanism will indicate the appropriate level of fees and number of beds to be made available'. This implies that public hospitals may reduce the level of fees in order to attract more patients using these beds, or increase the level of fees in case of over-demand. There exists quite a big difference with regard to the price of semi-private beds: HK$600 per day in Ruttonjee Hospital, the two-bed rooms at HK$800 per day and single rooms at HK$1,200 per day in Tsan Yuk Hospital. Flexibly adjusting the level of fees or the number of beds according to market signals is an innovative measure that has not ever been adopted in public hospital care. All this shows that the Hospital Authority and its hospitals can use their own autonomy and flexibility to enhance the competitiveness of the product of semi-private beds.

B-class Beds: The Nature of Choice

This section discusses the nature of choice that will be made available as a result of the introduction of B-class beds. The stigmatisation effect created will also be discussed.

B-Class Beds as a Choice

Towards Better Health states that the introduction of B-class beds represents 'a real choice...made available to those who demand something better than general ward accommodation but for whom top range hospital care may be too expensive' (para.4.16). The government has associated the idea of choice with B-class beds, but not with patient choice of doctors, or proxy users' choice of provider units. As can be seen from *Towards Better Health*, the idea of choice is linked to a higher percentage of cost recovery. So, patients cannot take advantage of this unless they can afford to do so. All of the policy makers and politicians (including the 'pro-welfare' ones) I interviewed also agreed that a choice of better amenities should be provided to the users of public hospital care, and that higher fees should be charged. The following quotations illustrate this point.

> Under the public hospital system, there is virtually very little [choice]. Most private beds are used by senior civil servants, and the ordinary patients couldn't have the choice...I think people should have their own choices over the amenities if they are willing to pay more. (The ex-Secretary for Health and Welfare, Interview)

There is a need for B-class beds as the well-off patients would like to have more privacy and better facilities. And such a provision can also offer more choices for the patients. (An appointed Legislator, Interview)

As long as the public is willing to pay more for better amenities, the product should be provided in public hospitals. Choice should be given to those who could afford better quality services. But the improvement should be confined to the non-medical dimension. (A directly elected Legislator, Interview)

Reform of health financing must be considered in relation to health care delivery. The B-class bed is an additional product and a choice that allows pricing to be used. (Chief Executive of the Hospital Authority, Interview)

Those who are willing to pay more will receive hotel services, and they do so by choice. Public concern is likely to be less even if the degree of cost recovery for B beds are higher...Consumer choice should be linked up with quality enhancement. (A member of the Health and Medical Development Advisory Committee, Interview)

It can be seen that a choice provided by the public health care system was considered to be very desirable. These quotations also defined the boundary and features of choice to be offered. That is, the scope of choice should be restricted to hotel services rather than other enhanced medical benefits, and that patients should pay a price choosing to use semi-private beds. Among all the quotations, the one made by the Chief Executive of the Hospital Authority is most specific about the relationship between choice, pricing and health care delivery. To the Chief Executive of the Authority, the B-class bed is but an idea that could be linked to health care financing and choice at the same time.   He further elaborated the idea of choice as follows:

[n]o one would be compelled to use the B-class bed. It is all by choice, or by self-selection. I think self-selection is particularly attractive because it not only minimises administrative costs, it also expands the choices available to our users. This mechanism gives them an incentive to reveal their willingness to pay for better amenities...The self-selection approach to health care will be realised as a result of the introduction of B-class beds, or amenity beds, if you like. (Interview)

This quote echoes what has been said in *Towards Better Health*: 'It is administratively simple to implement...Moreover, no one will be compelled to opt for a semi-private room' (paras.4.16 and 4.17). Since there is no need for the relatively well off patients to go through any means-testing procedures, it is not only administratively simple but also financially inexpensive.

All the politicians and policy makers I interviewed strongly favoured the implementation of a pilot scheme of B-class beds so as to give middle-income patients more choice and generate more income to improve the service quality of public health care. They appreciated the positive effects created by the provision of another choice of semi-private wards as long as public ward patients would not be the losers. The politicians would like to see that the introduction of B-class beds is a win-win solution both to the better-off patients and the public-ward patients. While the policy makers as represented by the ex-Secretary for Health and Welfare and the Chief Executive of the Hospital Authority have continued to reaffirm the public that the semi-private wards would be a win-win solution. Overall, political resistance to the introduction of B-class beds as a new choice to public patients is far less than that encountered in the implementation of the percentage-subsidy approach discussed in the last chapter.

The B-class Bed as a Choice?

First, in the context of Hong Kong, the demand for B-class beds is initiated or led by patients themselves as long as they can afford to pay higher user fees. However, this is narrowly restricted to the choice and consumption of an alternative or interface product, rather than being expanded to include the selection of doctors or hospitals

Second, B-class beds are to be introduced in public rather than private hospitals. In other words, such an innovative product or such a choice is to be confined to hospitals wholly publicly owned, and privately owned hospitals will not be able to afford to provide a similar product.

Third, the product of B-class bed is a choice augmented with hotel services. Whenever patients choose to use B-class beds, it is certain that the non-medical benefits that patients derive will be somewhere between public wards and private wards provided in public hospitals. It is relatively easy for the users to judge the quality of amenities or hotel services. Restricted choice available in public hospitals would then be related to something that is more certain.

Fourth, a choice made available by introducing B-class beds is concerned with both quality and money: paying more for better level of amenities. The nature of choice is then developed around the idea of cost sharing of which patient choice has to be backed with the ability to pay. Simply, those unable to afford to pay more cannot enjoy such a 'real and affordable' choice. As discussed above, the government is willing to meet rising public expectation as long as patients are ready to pay more for better amenities. So, the area in which choice is to be expanded is related to its potential for cost recovery. Any decoupling between 'choice' and 'the ability to pay' would most probably be viewed by the government of Hong Kong as being inconsistent with its purposes in reforming the health care system. That is, if some of the public wards were upgraded without asking patients to pay more, and the choice were expanded to include the selection of doctors or hospitals, the government's purposes to reduce social rights to health care and to set higher user fees discussed in the last chapter would have been undermined. Regarding money as a passport to a choice would have the effect of encouraging the public to believe that the making of a better choice without paying a financial price is not a feasible alternative in Hong Kong.

Stigmatisation and Choice

The introduction of B-class beds would create within the public hospital sector a significant private subsystem. Hong Kong has already established a two-tiered system in hospital care both on inter-sector level (i.e. public versus private hospitals) and intra-sector level (i.e. private wards versus public wards). The expansion of B-class beds would make the two-tiered system more evident on the intra-sector level as the differences of amenities would become more evident to public patients. The implication of social stigma generated cannot be overlooked then.

In view of the low-expectation and low-quality care provided at public outpatient clinics, and in view of the fact that a much larger proportion of outpatient care is provided in the private sector, it is almost unavoidable for patients to experience a sense of social stigma during the consumption of public outpatient care. As regards outpatient service, patients may avoid the social stigma from affixing to them by employing the exit strategy, i.e. going private. Nevertheless, with respect to inpatient service, the exit strategy is not a feasible one to a very large proportion of public patients. With the introduction of B-class beds, there is no need for public patients to go private, and to pay an economic fee to improve the quality of hospital care. To facilitate public patients' access to better amenities at an 'affordable' price would generate a stigmatisation effect: an even much stronger social stigma is likely to be attached to the users of third class wards in public hospitals.

Without the implementation of B-class beds, it is very likely that the public-ward patients will experience less stigma. Basically, there are two reasons for this. First, most of the hospital care is provided in public wards in public hospitals. Second, private beds are mostly provided as fringe benefits to senior civil servants and Hospital Authority's employees. With a widespread introduction of B-class beds, these two factors would be changed accordingly. First, the proportion of hospital care provided in public wards in public hospitals will be reduced. Second, backed with their ability to pay, public patients can have access to hospital beds with quality amenities and facilities. A stronger social stigma is likely to be attached to the users of public wards in public hospitals. Some public patients may then be 'encouraged' to make use of B-class beds to avoid stigmatisation. This would create a vicious cycle of further reinforcing the stigmatisation effect if more and more patients choose to use B-class beds. A sense of stigma imposed on public-ward patients would therefore serve as a push factor that can increase the attractiveness of B-class beds. An important point is that public patients have to pay a financial price for using B-class beds to get rid of the stigma. Those who cannot afford to pay more would be left with no choice but to experience a stronger social stigma. So, the assertion made by the government that patients who are unable or unwilling to pay more will not be affected by the B-class bed policy is largely a myth.

Prospects for Implementing the B-Class Beds

Nevertheless, the prospects for introducing B-class beds are not yet promising, particularly in view of the private hospitals' opposition in terms of their calling on the Hospital Authority to scrap private and semi-private beds. The Private Hospital Association – which was formed for the first time in the medical history of Hong Kong – called on the government to limit access to public hospital services to the most needy and those above the safety net should be charged a fee similar to that charged in private hospitals. The proposal was to bring patients back to the private sector and to draw a line between so-called 'free welfare' and charged services provided in public hospitals.

The Association's promotion of the safety-net approach is seemingly consistent with the government's desire to persuade all citizens that they should have fewer social rights to publicly-funded health care as they may perceive or believe.   However, as far as the implementation of semi-private beds is concerned, the Association's standpoint is quite different from that of the government and the Hospital Authority.   Since the establishment of the Hospital Authority, the market share of inpatient service in terms of patient days provided by private hospitals has been reduced from about 10 per cent in 1991 to 7.9 per cent in 1994 (Hospital Authority, 1993; 1995a).   The Association's worry is that following the full implementation of semi-private beds in public hospitals, more private patients would go public, and the market share of private hospitals' provision of inpatient service would be further reduced.

In a meeting with Secretary for Health and Welfare Katherine Fok Lo Shiu-ching, the Preparatory Committee members of the Private Hospital Association complained that B-class beds had siphoned patients away from private hospitals and endangered their business if not their survival (Hong Kong Standard, 7 June 1996).   As a result of strong pressure exercised by the Association, the planned expansion of the pilot project of B-class beds into other public hospitals came to a halt, and the project could only be maintained at the 1995/96 level (Sing Tao Daily, 22 April 1996). The power of the private health care providers has thus become a major barrier to the introduction of semi-private beds in public hospitals. Unless the government and the Hospital Authority can convince the private hospitals that their interest would not be sacrificed, a widespread introduction of semi-private beds in public hospitals will no doubt invite their strong opposition (Wong, 1996; 1999).

Conclusion

The Hospital Authority has reintegrated former government and subvented hospitals but without promoting intra-sector competition by separating providers and purchasers of health care.   Instead, since the Authority was set up, the government has to commit more financial resources for standardising the remuneration package and thus it can no longer exploit the much less attractive terms of employment provided by ex-subvented hospitals.   Moreover, because of various ideological and political reasons, the Hospital Authority has not been able to generate extra revenue or competition with private hospitals by increasing the number of paybeds or allowing hospital consultants to have the right to private practice in public hospitals.

The above discussion has shown that semi-private beds are an innovation especially in terms of their dual characteristics: serving as an interface product between public-ward beds and private beds in public hospitals, and that between public hospital care and private hospital care. It appears that the government as well as the Hospital Authority would like to see the provision of semi-private beds as largely an intra-sector interface product primarily attracting public-ward rather than private-hospital-sector patients to use them.

The idea of choice tried out and to be further developed has reflected the government's attempt to meet the rising public expectation according to the patients' ability to pay. Ideologically, it is consistent with the safety-net approach discussed in the last chapter to reduce social rights to highly subsidised medical care. Since the introduction of semi-private beds is presented and perceived by many politicians as a win-win solution, it has become less politically contentious than the so-called 'percentage-subsidy' approach discussed in the last chapter.

It is very tempting for the Authority as well as the government to make it a policy to provide B-class beds in public hospitals, which are of higher cost-recovery potential than public-ward beds. Nevertheless, the private health care providers have become the most important barrier to the introduction of B-class beds as they take it as a threat to their business interest in the inpatient service market. What is clear is that we cannot afford to underestimate the power of the private sector in shaping health care policy in Hong Kong.

8 Health Insurance and Financing

Introduction

Ever since the release of the Scott Report in 1985, health insurance as a means to finance health care has become a hot issue among bureaucrats and politicians in Hong Kong. Several months after the establishment of the Hospital Authority in December 1990, the Health and Welfare Branch formed the Medical Insurance Study Group, chaired by its former Secretary, to examine different major types of medical schemes found in other developed countries and to make recommendations suitable for Hong Kong. The Medical Insurance Study Group considered eight schemes that were suggested by different group members as relevant to Hong Kong. As a whole, all these schemes can be re-categorised into two major types: social insurance-based schemes and voluntary health insurance schemes. These two broad approaches to promoting health insurance formed the two options for public consultation in *Towards Better Health* published in 1993. Finally, the former approach was dropped, and the latter one was proposed as an important mechanism to regulate and stimulate private health insurance in Hong Kong.

This chapter discusses the regulatory framework within which private health insurance and the semi-private bed scheme can be mutually reinforced. This chapter is divided into three major sections. The first examines the reasons why social insurance as an approach to financing health care was not considered appropriate in the context of Hong Kong. The second examines the nature of state regulation applied to facilitating the growth of private health. Finally, the third critically discusses the nature of choice and competition promoted upon the implementation of the co-ordinated voluntary insurance approach.

Constraints upon Implementing the Social Insurance Approach

There are both structural and technical constraints in implementing the social insurance approach in Hong Kong. Technical constraints can be solved if the government and the society at large are committed to the establishment of social insurance in financing and delivering health care. I will argue that underlying the technical constraints are the powerful structural constraints which have played an important role in suffocating the development of social insurance in the field of health care. In the following discussion, the different constraints are to be critically examined.

Compulsory Public Health Insurance Perceived as an Hypothecated Health Tax

In the eyes of the government, compulsory public health insurance constitutes hypothecation of revenue which goes against established government financial principles and practice (Wong, 1999). The implementation of social insurance in health care is perceived as a threat to the practice of financial principles enjoyed by the government and its bureaucrats. If an hypothecated health tax were implemented, health funding would no longer come out of the general pool of taxes collected by the government. Governments in other countries also often dislike hypothecated taxes dedicated to a particular field as it reduces their freedom and flexibility in budgeting (Holliday, 1992). A member of the Health and Medical Development Advisory Committee also echoed this point as follows:

> [h]ypothecated tax is a possibility. But the public may request the hypothecation of revenue for other social services as well. The raising of a health tax will set a bad example which in the long run will disturb the flexibility enjoyed by the government in distributing financial resources among different programmes. Personally, I do not favour this possible alternative. (Interview)

The point is that the hypothecated health tax would not only be clearly identified in government accounts, but would also appear as a separate line entry on individuals' tax demands and statements. This could succeed in increasing the public's ability to express a clear preference with regard to health spending, and would mean a threat to the autonomy of the government in allocating financial resources to health care enveloped under the general category of annual public expenditure. In addition, the social insurance approach also implies rising taxation. The ex-Secretary for the Health and Welfare Branch put it in a straightforward way that:

> [c]ompulsory public health insurance equals a tax increase...There are very few taxpayers in Hong Kong. Those who contribute insurance money will be likely those who pay tax. The elderly and the chronically ill are unable to contribute...The employers would not favour the compulsory [insurance] scheme...It will be a great financial burden on the taxpayers and the economic structure. (Interview)

The consultation document *Towards Better Health* strongly states that:

> [i]f employers were required to insure all their workers...it would represent an open-ended commitment to employers which could fracture the market. Any additional requirement to cover the workers' families and children would further add to cost. (para.37)

Put another way, compulsory public health insurance represents a tax increase which is perceived as a threat to the low-tax policy long regarded as the cornerstone of the success of the Hong Kong economy. An appointed Legislator emphasised that:

> [s]ocial insurance will increase the cost of production for the employer which will adversely affect their competitiveness...As the low-tax policy has to be maintained, it seems to be unacceptable that the much less favoured social insurance approach should be implemented in the context of Hong Kong. (Interview)

So, to the government itself, the implementation of compulsory public health insurance represents a threat both to its freedom to allocate resources and to its commitment to maintain the low-tax policy in Hong Kong (see Chapter 6).

In Need of an Infrastructure for Implementing the Social Insurance Approach?

Towards Better Health remarks that 'The start-up cost of a public insurance scheme involving some 5.75 million people is enormous' (para.4.27). So, the government regards it as being very expensive to set up the infrastructure to run a centralised health insurance for all the people in Hong Kong. A member of the Health and Medical Development Advisory Committee emphasised that:

> I do not favour the central or compulsory public health insurance scheme as Hong Kong does not have such kind of infrastructure, say, for the CPF [Central Provident Fund].   And the administration cost for running a programme for about six million people is really expensive. (Interview)

The question of whether a CPF should be established in Hong Kong to enable workers to secure better retirement protection has been debated ever since 1967.   Instead of proposing the setting up of a CPF, a consultation document released in October 1992 came up with a proposal for a compulsory private provident fund entitled the 'Retirement Protection Scheme' (RPS) which would be organised on a decentralised basis (Government Secretariat, 1992). In fact, the recommendation of the 1992 consultation document was similar to a business and professional group's proposal which opposed 'the concept of a central provident fund or other mandatory centrally administered scheme' (Business and Professionals Federation of Hong Kong, 1991:2). The public consultation, however, ended with strong public opposition, especially that from the grassroot organisations, worrying about the financial guarantee of the scheme should the private financial institutions become bankrupt (Mok, 1994). Many other politicians I interviewed also reflected the opinion that Hong Kong lacks the infrastructure to set up and run a public health insurance scheme for health care unless the central provident fund can be implemented. From the following quotations, it can be seen that the first priority was given to the setting up of a CPF which has a long history of debates in the policy circles.

> If central provident fund can be established, it will provide the infrastructure for setting up the compulsory public health insurance scheme. It can save much administration cost. (A directly elected member, Interview)

The compulsory public health insurance scheme can be considered if the CPF scheme is implemented. Priority should be given to CPF first. (A Legislator elected from the Labour Functional Constituency, Interview)

The CPF is more urgent. Its implementation can establish the basis for implementing the public health insurance scheme. I think compulsory health insurance is very unlikely to be implemented if the basic infrastructure is not well established. (A directly elected Legislator, Interview)

We strive for two goals: first, central provident fund, and second, central health insurance...After setting up the CPF, it is more efficient to administer the central health insurance package as the basic infrastructure has already been set up. Or the two schemes can share the same infrastructure, and thus more cost-efficient...As far as I know, all political parties support the CPF scheme, but not the central medical insurance scheme. The Liberal Party is especially against the idea of compulsory medical insurance. (A directly elected Legislator, Interview)

To some politicians, although the public health insurance scheme is accorded a second priority to central provident fund, the question of setting up the infrastructure is more a technical question which can be solved if central provident fund can be established in Hong Kong. However, as most of the attention of the politicians was drawn to the setting up of a centralised CPF rather than a decentralised RPS, and as the support for compulsory public health insurance scheme was not as widespread as that for CPF, the government could make the most of this situation to turn down the social insurance approach to health care. It does not mean that with the setting up of the CPF, the compulsory insurance approach to health care would immediately follow. What seems to be apparent is that the lack of a centralised infrastructure or a compulsory contributory scheme for a good cause can be effectively used by the government to legitimate its decision not to implement the social insurance approach to health care.

A Transitional Approach to Compulsory Public Health Insurance?

The debates over the choice between private insurance and social insurance included the possibility of gradually progressing from the former to the latter. A member of the Health and Medical Development Advisory Committee explained during the interview that:

[i]f more and more people buy insurance on a voluntary basis, the change to a central and compulsory one could be made easier. But at present, as only about 10 per cent of Hong Kong people have medical insurance, it is not the right time to set up a centralised system. (Interview)

The former Secretary of Health and Welfare Branch also expressed the same kind of opinion as below:

[y]ou know, although the number of people buying medical insurance is increasing at a rate of 40 per cent per annum, there are only about 14 per cent of Hong Kong people who have private health insurance...Personally, I am not against the social insurance approach, but it is not the right timing to do so. If there are more and more people buy their own [health] insurance, the government may consider transforming the private insurance system into a public one. In fact, we shouldn't deny this possibility. (Interview)

However, would the 'transition thesis' be a possibility or just a false hope that is used to diversify the public pressure imposed upon the government for a more equitable health care financing system in Hong Kong? It is difficult to foresee in the Hong Kong context whether private health insurance will become more and more popular and whether its growing importance will be interlocked with the established interests of the medical profession and private hospitals to put a barrier to certain state policies. If all this became possible, it would tremendously constrain the progression from a private to a public insurance system. What is clear is that the government does not have a plan for such a so-called 'transition' from a private insurance system to a public insurance system. It might therefore be figured as a mere possibility used to justify the implementation of the regulated voluntary insurance scheme.

Compulsory Public Health Insurance is Cost-inflationary?

Towards Better Health highlights that compulsory public health insurance providing 'universal and comprehensive coverage will lead to overutilisation...and therefore cost escalations' (para.4.27). A member of the Health and Medical Development Advisory Committee also expressed the same worry: 'If we encourage the implementation of compulsory medical insurance, cost escalation might become fiercer. Only those pressure groups, in particular Meeting Point, would favour such an idea' (Interview). A directly elected member however held a different viewpoint. He said, 'Competition between the providers will help, in the long run, to reduce the price' (Interview).

A Legislator elected from the Medical and Health Care Functional Constituency stated that:

[t]he major barrier for the implementation of a compulsory medical insurance scheme comes from the government itself...There is a possibility that the implementation of an insurance scheme might induce abuse. But abuses can be kept under control, say, to control the behaviour of the providers. (Interview)

Indeed, the assumption underlying those methods of capping provider reimbursement employed in social insurance-based system is that providers, not patients, are the main generators of demand for costly medical care services, for example, hospitalisations, high-tech procedures, expensive drugs and so on. Cost-containment incentives have been developed and further modified or expanded for these important medical care 'consumers' (Donaldson and Gerard, 1993). If Hong Kong can establish the Canadian kind of system with only one single purchaser, the system is well placed to exert a powerful control on health care costs. Firstly, the public administration of insurance funds minimises overhead costs. Secondly, the central insurer is in a much better position vested with stronger bargaining power to negotiate with health care providers, so that the government keeps tight control over fee and cost increases (Abel-Smith, 1994; Marmor, 1995).

Alongside the portrayal of the cost escalation tendency of health care in general and that of a public insurance system in particular is the government's emphasis placed on efficiency and cost-effectiveness. *Towards Better Health* reminds the public the importance of paying special regard to the 'financial implications for service providers, consumers and third party financiers...collectively when charting the course of reform' (para.3.19). The consultation document has tried to persuade the public to believe that the social insurance approach is not consistent with the objective of cost containment, or would not give 'the community and individual users good value for money' (para.3.17). The government's placing a mistrust on the social insurance approach to containing health care cost has added further weight to the argument that the 'transition thesis' is used to legitimate the implementation of the co-ordinated voluntary insurance approach than as a framework to establish a social insurance system for health care in the long run.

Compulsory Public Health Insurance is Contrary to the Philosophy of Positive Non-intervention?

Private health care is almost left unregulated in Hong Kong (see Chapters 2 and 5).   In applying the social insurance approach to health care financing, the government has to take up an active role in negotiating with health care providers, both public and private (if the scheme is designed to integrate both sectors), regarding their levels of service, fees and charges, plans for development and use of resources.   All this is at odds with the government's policy of 'positive non-intervention' in private health care. It is indeed one thing to control what one is providing, and it is another to interfere with market forces governing what one intends to purchase. From the viewpoint of the medical profession, any regulation of medical fees and charges is considered as measures taken to undermine their economic autonomy (Fung, 1991; So, 1991).   Unlike their counterparts in the US, the private medical practitioners of Hong Kong have long enjoyed a very high degree of economic autonomy with little intervention from the government.   Both historically and psychologically speaking, the local medical profession is very unprepared to have their economic autonomy undermined in this way.   Their fierce opposition to regulatory measures applied to their use of resources and their level of fees and charges can, no doubt, be anticipated.

The lessons from other social insurance-based systems is that countless political struggles and seemingly endless negotiations between the three parties, namely, the government, the medical profession and the health insurance industry, are the basic rather than unusual features (Helms, 1993).   As discussed in Chapters 3 to 5, the medical profession, as a body, is a In addition to keeping the 'positive non-intervention' policy in health care, the government is aware of the great political constraints and costs involved in dealing with the medical profession especially if it has to be involved in funding private doctors.   Taking all this into consideration, the goal of simplicity to administer emphasised by *Towards Better Health* may be interpreted as a rationale for keeping minimal government intervention in private health care and avoiding to create direct confrontation or conflicts with the medical profession especially in relation to their economic autonomy in pricing their services.

If the social insurance system incorporates both the public and private sectors, users of private health care could receive government subsidy. In fact, upon the implementation of this scheme, a clear distinction made between public and private sectors might be rendered meaningless as the providers would receive payment from the central insurer (Fung, 1992). Although the government emphasises that an interface should be established between the public and private systems, the purpose is not to dissolve the dual health care system and set up a 'monopolistic' system via the social insurance approach but to encourage more co-operation between the two systems, for example, in the use of advanced medical equipment (Hong Kong Government, 1993a:para.2.15). The maintenance of the existing dual system of health care is considered by the government as an important measure to make room for the market to prosper and to cater for the wants and demands of the consumers on the one hand, and on the other, to demonstrate its political commitment to its 'positive non-intervention' policy.

Compulsory Public Health Insurance as 'Collectivism' and 'Welfarism'?

The consultation document *Towards Better Health* strongly stated that 'the compulsory insurance approach is based very much on the idea of "collectivism" which some developed countries have tried and sought to abandon' (para.4.27). An appointed member also strongly felt that 'Hong Kong people do not like to see an increase in the tax rate and an introduction of "welfarism" representing the centralisation of welfare' (Interview). The integration of the public and private sectors and an increase of 'hypothecated tax' following the introduction of social insurance are perceived by both the government and the capitalists as 'undesirable' moves towards 'collectivism' and 'welfarism'.

So, the attack on the social insurance approach has its ideological roots: the application of the social insurance approach to health care financing and delivery is contrary to the wishes of the state to reduce citizens' social rights to health care in Hong Kong (Chapter 6). Confronting a greater pressure upon the government for expanding the development of social services and social welfare, Sir David Wilson (1989:para.50), the ex-governor of Hong Kong, in his speech to the Legislative Council, claimed that:

[w]e do not intend to provide a western-style welfare state. To do so risks encouraging a mentality of dependency that is alien to the Hong Kong way of life.   Instead, we concentrate much of our efforts, and of our available resources, on the young people of Hong Kong, who represent our future, and on those who cannot fend for themselves.

It can be seen that the significance of the Hong Kong way of life (Hong Kong's mode of capitalism) is emphasised by means of labelling the western-style welfare state as a dangerous thing that is perceived to be susceptible to encouraging a mentality of dependency upon the state for the sake of improving individual welfare (Chiu and Wong, 1998). To avoid such a 'welfare-state tragedy', the government's welfare strategy in concentrating available resources on those who can contribute to the economy of society and to those who are least able to help themselves is justified by its own welfare philosophy.   Indeed, the philosophy of investment logic and welfare residualism is made evident from this quote. In many official documents, the government emphasises that old people have become the major users of public health care. In view of the change of demographic environment, the continuing provision of heavily subsidised public health care has largely served the purpose of maintaining the 'non-working' or 'economically inactive' population rather than facilitating the young (the 'economically active') to get appropriate treatment, who can contribute to the economy. The government may fear that available public resources might be wrongly concentrated on those who do not represent the future of Hong Kong. Because of this, it is no wonder that the goal of cost containment in public health care has been considered very important nowadays.

Moreover, stepping into the 1990s, the Social Welfare White Paper re-emphasises that:

[t]he challenge for Hong Kong is to improve services without creating the sort of dependency culture that has emerged in some developed industrialised societies, a phenomenon that removes the incentive to work and undermines the productive engine of the economy. (Hong Kong Government, 1991:para.5)

This has re-emphasised that the improvement of social service has to be closely monitored so that a dependency culture will not be created in Hong Kong. According to the residualist welfare philosophy of the government, to set up a public 'monopolistic system' funded by social insurance would encourage people to rely on insurer(s) for their health care needs, and to put more pressure on the government or the employer to contribute more to the health tax which may in the long run 'undermine the productive engine of the economy'.

The Politics of the Social Insurance Approach to Pensions However, what is really surprising is that five months after the publication of *Towards Better Health*, the Hong Kong government itself announced its intention to apply a social insurance approach to pensions on December 15, 1993. This is because only about one year previously (October 1992), the consultation document on RPS released by the government recommended that 'the future [RPS] system be decentralised, comprising individual retirement protection schemes run by banks, trustees, insurance companies or employers themselves, as in the case at present' (Government Secretariat, 1992:4). As a result, the consultation document clearly declared that the government 'does not support a universal pension system' (ibid:6). In July 1994, the Government Secretariat published a consultative paper on Old Age Pension Scheme (OPS). The OPS is different from the RPS or the CPF on two major points. First, OPS provides immediate benefits upon implementation. A RPS or CPF will take at least thirty years to yield meaningful benefits for the retired workers. Second, OPS is not employment-related, and provides retirement protection for all eligible elderly citizens including housewives, the disabled and the current elderly population. Since a RPS or CPF is employment-related, it will only cover those who have regular jobs and regular contributions for a long period of time, and therefore, leaves the majority of the population unprotected.

The social insurance approach to pensions is run on a pay-as-you-go system: current collected income has to pay for pensions to people at certain age irrespective of their past contribution record. This is not considered as an equitable approach according to the principles of desert and merit which have been long cherished by the business world in Hong Kong. Similarly, public comprehensive health insurance is inherently close to a full pay-as-you-go system: insurance collected 'goes out quickly to cover bills of members of the risk pool' (Glaser, 1991:23). The government's sudden shift of its attitude on retirement policy was out of public expectation. It was also inconsistent with the criticisms put forward by the consultation document *Towards Better Health* on the social insurance approach to health care financing and delivery.

Such a sudden change of attitude towards the social insurance approach to pensions has to be understood in relation to the political context of Hong Kong and the change of governorship from David Wilson to Chris Patten in 1992. China's commitment to the preservation of human rights and civil liberties in Hong Kong was completely destroyed after the Tianmen Square massacre taking place in 1989 (Scott, 1995). Aside from the enactment of a Bill of Rights, which Chinese officials promptly implied would be repealed after 1997 (South China Morning Post, June 4, 1991), constitutional reform was announced by Chris Patten in October 1992 and was used by the Hong Kong government as a means to establish a more democratic political institution for protecting human rights in the future Special Administrative Region on the one hand, and to gain its legitimacy before the transfer of Hong Kong's sovereignty to China on 1 July 1997 on the other hand.

China saw Mr. Patten's proposal as an insult. Lu Ping, the Director of the State Council's Hong Kong and Macau Office, said that the Governor's proposal committed three violations: firstly, violating the Sino-British Joint Declaration made in 1984; secondly, failing to meet the requirements of the Basic Law; and thirdly, turning down the agreements previously reached by the British and Chinese governments concerning the 1995 election (Tai Kun Pao, 24 October 1993). Not only the Chinese government but also the conservative business interests, like the Business and Professional Federation, the General Chamber of Commerce and the Chinese Chamber of Commerce came out strongly against Patten's political blueprint (Ching, 1993). The conservative and yet powerful business interests considered that Chris Patten's reform would end their political domination and threaten both their political and economic interests (Scott, 1995). It was within such a context that the government badly needed the support of the general public in order to balance the force of the Chinese government and capitalists. An OPS rather than a CPF, which could immediately bring benefits to old people upon implementation, was manipulated by Chris Patten to release the tension between the government and the working class in the area of social services and enlisted their support on the political reform. By diverting the public's attention to the debate on a seemingly good package of OPS, the government partly reduced its immediate pressure in the transitional period.

Nevertheless, the government took a half-hearted attitude for pushing the OPS from the start. As emphasised in the consultative paper, the implementation of the OPS would be subjected to the 'general public acceptance; and discussion with the Chinese Government' (Government Secretariat, 1994:1). The OPS proposal received great support from the working class. The Hong Kong Workers Alliance's survey found that nearly 80 per cent of respondents were willing to contribute to the OPS. Moreover, a grassroot federation called 'Alliance for Fighting for a Retirement Scheme for All', which was formed by thirty-three organisations, held a demonstration to show their support to the scheme (Ming Pao, 31 October 1994). Like the case of constitutional reform, the OPS was strongly opposed by capitalists and the Chinese government. The capitalists feared that the OPS was a starting point for the development of 'welfarism' in Hong Kong, and that the scheme would 'run into huge deficits and involve enormous costs from the community' (South China Morning Post, 21 April 1994). The Chinese government also shared the same views of the conservative business interests in Hong Kong. The New China News Agency made it clear that retirement and welfare were two separate issues. This meant that only those who were working needed a retirement scheme, and those who were of the labour market and those who did not contribute to their own pension schemes, should continue to apply for public assistance (Ming Pao, 18 July 1994). In other words, the Chinese government openly opposed a universal pension scheme. Moreover, the three most influential political organisations, the Meeting Point, the Democratic Alliance and the Liberal Party reached a compromise for pushing the government to carry out a CPF rather than an OPS. Thus, Hong Kong still lacked a strong working class political party for defending their own rights.

Noting that the Chinese government did not support the OPS, and noting that the British economic and trade interests would suffer if London continued its 'confrontation' approach (South China Morning Post, 1 October 1994), the government of Hong Kong changed its attitude. The OPS was finally dropped and replaced by a Mandatory Provident Fund Scheme (MPF) which is very much similar to the RPS proposed in 1992. It looks apparent that the OPS served the political needs of the government since it represented a 'no-loss' or even a 'sure-win' scenario. On the one hand, it could help to gain general public support, and from the working class in particular, which was used to balance the joint opposition of the Chinese government and capitalists against Chris Patten's constitutional reform. If the OPS could be implemented, the Hong Kong government could gain one more point for its legitimacy. On the other hand, if the

OPS were turned down, the responsibility for expanding welfare to the citizens of Hong Kong could be shifted to other parties, and the Chinese government in particular, since the factor of China's attitude was identified in the consultative paper as being critical to the implementation of the OPS. At the time the OPS was announced, it was used to enlist public support to the state so as to back itself at the time of confrontation with the Chinese government on the issue of election to the Legislative Council. After the constitutional crisis was over, the OPS was suppressed and finally withdrawn to please the Chinese government and capitalists. Because of the very strong political consideration of a social insurance approach to pensions, rather than a real concern for further improving the welfare of old people, social welfare in Hong Kong finally comes to a standstill.

Implications for a Social Insurance Approach to Health Care As soon as the political objectives of the OPS were achieved, the scheme was withdrawn, and the debate over a pension scheme for the citizens of Hong Kong is back to square one. The coming out of the recently proposed MPF organised on a decentralised basis represents no breakthrough at all or almost a dead end to the application of a more equitable centralised approach to the retirement policy that has been debated for 28 years since the late 1960s. If the OPS could be implemented, the use of a social insurance approach to the financing and organisation of welfare could be given a better chance for development in Hong Kong. Such a scenario could provide a fertile ground for the application of the social insurance approach to health care as well.

Another important point is that a social insurance approach to pensions or health care was considered as a fundamental change to the welfare system of Hong Kong beyond 1997. This was regarded as a politically sensitive issue, and everything beyond 1997 had to seek the full support of the Chinese government. The above discussion has shown that the Chinese government did not buy the social insurance approach to pensions for fearing that it would jeopardise Hong Kong's economy. The fact is that the Chinese government had joined with capitalists to oppose the OPS. It seems that China will do nothing to harm Hong Kong's economy as Hong Kong can act as the 'economic dynamo for southern China' (Scott, 1995:207). Shortly before the Sino-British Joint Liaison Group opened its fifth round of expert talks in Beijing on 28 November 1995, the Chinese team leader Chen Zou'er lambasted Britain over the government's welfare expenditure in the past five years, and warned that 'Hong Kong is heading for economic disaster with its escalating welfare spending' (Hong Kong Standard, 29 November 1995). This further shows that China wants to constrain Hong Kong's fiscal measures so that the possibility of welfare state in the future Special Administrative Region is almost killed. In short, since China is keen to maintain the Hong Kong's mode of capitalism after 1997, it is entirely understandable that it prefers the co-ordinated voluntary insurance approach to the social insurance approach regarded or labelled as a move towards 'collectivism' and 'welfarism'.

Private Health Insurance and State Regulation

Co-ordinated Voluntary Insurance: Nature and Context of Regulation

The co-ordinated voluntary insurance scheme was considered by the government as an ideal approach to promoting health insurance in Hong Kong. Government intervention in the health care market has long been kept to a minimum, therefore, the proposed introduction of this scheme can be regarded as a milestone of state intervention in regulating the health insurance market. Before examining the nature and context of such regulation, the fundamental features of this voluntary insurance will firstly be described.

Fundamental Features of the Scheme The main purpose of a public designated body proposed to be set up by the government is to examine insurance plans submitted by health insurers, and 'approval would only be given if a plan meets certain criteria for adequacy of coverage and appropriateness of premium' (Hong Kong Government, 1993a:para.4.18). The criterion of cost containment - whether on provider-side or consumer-side or both - may also be included (Health and Welfare Branch, 1991:14). However, no one would be forced to take out insurance, and no insurer would be required to submit all their health insurance plans for approval by the designated body. It is emphasised that only those plans involving the use of public facilities, say, B-class beds, whether or not in conjunction with private sector facilities, have to be approved by the designated body before they are marketed to the public. Plans involving only private sector facilities would be exempt, although the insurers may also submit such plans for the designated body's approval (para.4.19). The ex-Secretary of Health and Welfare Branch explained that:

> [i]t's wrong in a Hong Kong spirit to control the marketplace. But we do want to exercise some degree of voluntary control, voluntary, and we mean it. To come to us with a plan so that we can say this plan would provide x amount of service and the premium should not be more than y. The plan will be compulsory only when it covers the public hospital sector...At the moment, 14 per cent of people buy insurance. But they don't know what they are buying. A stamped approval from a designated body would give them a kind of quality assurance. (Interview)

Her explanation stated above almost repeated what was mentioned in the consultation document *Towards Better Health*. She just wanted to emphasise that the approach is voluntary rather than compulsory in nature and that approval given by the designated body would serve as a kind of quality assurance for buyers.

Four different parties were suggested to compose the designated body: government bureaucrats, the insurance industry, the medical profession and consumer interests. However, would such a composition of members be susceptible to creating conflicts between the different parties, especially between the medical profession and the insurance industry? What are the nature and context of such regulation?

Regulation of Voluntary Insurance: Nature and Context The regulation of voluntary insurance does not imply any systematic planning or monitoring of all or a significant proportion of health care activities and resources in Hong Kong. It is up to the market actors, i.e. the insurers, to market their health insurance plans, both in terms of deciding the scope of coverage and the amount of premium. The regulator, i.e. the designated body, just sets the rules and procedures. The regulator's main instruments are rules which serve to approve health insurance plans or advise the insurers to modify their insurance plans if approval is to be sought from the designated body. The task of the regulatory body would be to regulate general contract conditions and standards. Besides the major task of approving of submitted health insurance plans, the designated body would leave to the insurance industry, the providers, and the insurance holders or patients to decide what insurance arrangements to be made, and what services to provide, how and by whom.

Therefore, the designated body, in nature, would not serve complex functions like the centralised insurer or sickness funds in some social insurance-based systems do. It does not mean that the government bureaucrats would not get in some troubles with the other three parties in the designated body. But it is likely that the troubles would not be as big as those confronted by the centralised insurer or sickness funds. Also, the government or the designated body would not involve itself in making serious, long-lasting and recurrent negotiations between the medical profession and the insurance industry over all the financing and reimbursement matters as exemplified in some social insurance systems in developed nations.

It is likely that the parties involved in the designated body, especially the medical profession and the insurance industry would try hard to advance their own interests and conflicts may take place as a result. Alongside the expansion of health insurance since the late 1980s, more and more conflicts taking place between these two parties. For example, in response to some of the insurance companies which had started the practice of enlisting their doctors, the Hong Kong Medical Association (HKMA) (1991:2) asserted that:

> [t]here should not be any list of doctors issued by the insurance companies. Any list should be compiled by the employer or HKMA...Contracts should be made between the employer and the doctors. The insurance companies should only act as funding agencies to receive bills from doctors and reimburse doctors. The middleman, whether in the form of insurance company, medical benefit consultant or medical administrative service company, was undesirable.

The medical profession is afraid that insurance companies will have more say on the fee schedule of medical services and will undermine their economic autonomy as a consequence if the latter is given the right to enlist their own doctors (Fung, 1991). Because of the concerted efforts made by private doctors and the HKMA, the Hong Kong Medical Council finally resolved that insurance companies be prohibited from the enlisting of doctors. Such a decision made by the Council was based on the belief that a list initiated and built up by insurance companies and published for reference to the insured is a violation against the restriction on doctor advertising (Yuen, 1994b).

However, the 'win-lose' scenario could not fully explain the complex relationship between these two parties. Under many situations, a 'win-win' scenario for these two parties is possible. For example, in a survey undertaken by the Hong Kong Medical Association in 1992, more than three quarters (76%) of the respondent members of the Association favoured the promotion of private insurance as a means to finance health care, although some respondents still emphasised that 'Citizens and medical profession should be protected from profiteering and manipulation by medical insurers' (Hong Kong Medical Association, 1992:12). Private practitioners like to see a constant growth of private health insurance in Hong Kong because the insured patients' demand for private medicine may be boosted as a consequence of the reduction of financial barrier. In fact, at the point of departure, the proposed approach to promoting private health insurance did not result in any complaints from the medical profession and the health insurance industry.

During our interview, the Chief Executive of the Hospital Authority said: 'about 30 per cent of insured patients use general beds of public hospitals, since their premium is so low. It seems that Hong Kong people just have limited knowledge about medical insurance'. So, the under-regulation of health insurance in Hong Kong has been a good reason for the government to start off with some intervention in this field. However, the government could have promoted private health insurance via the giving of tax concessions rather than through the establishment of a regulatory mechanism. A member of the Health and Medical Development Advisory Committee explained as follows:

> [p]ersonally, I encourage the government to give tax concessions to those who buy medical insurance. But I believe that the government would not favour such an idea as the Finance Branch firmly believes that the taxation system should be kept as simple as possible. (Interview)

To the government itself, the co-ordinated voluntary insurance scheme fits well with its parameters in reforming health care. Firstly, the scheme is simple to administer and can be set up with low costs. The implementation of the scheme would just involve the setting up of an office to register and regulate the health insurance plans. Compared with the setting up of a social insurance scheme, the start-up costs for the scheme would be much lower. In addition, the scheme is simple to administer without getting the government directly involved in negotiating arrangements for paying health care providers if both public and private sectors are incorporated under a social insurance system.

Secondly, the government is of the view that 'in the absence of widespread use of medical insurance, private hospitals are expensive and may be inaccessible to many...[and] the aim of reform should be to improve accessibility to both the public and private sectors' (Hong Kong Government, 1993a:paras.3.9&3.11). So, from the government's point of view, accessibility to both public (mainly referring to B-class beds) and private health care can be enhanced with the promotion of private health insurance. However, to enhance patients' access to private medicine primarily involves unfair choices as the decisions about the use of health care resources in the private sector are conditioned by patients' ability to pay or to afford an insurance policy. The use of progressive rather than regressive methods for determining patients' financial contributions to health care is indeed more consistent with the purpose of enhancing working-class patients' access to health care (Aday, 1994).

Thirdly, the duality of the health care system can be maintained, and is thus less disrupting to the health care system as a whole in the eyes of the government, especially with respect to retaining the role played by the private sector (Chapter 7). In addition, the consultation document *Towards Better Health* reassures the citizens of Hong Kong that 'For those who could not or did not wish to take out insurance, heavily subsidised public services would still be available' (para.4.20). This is indeed a restatement of the government's guarantee that no one would be prevented from obtaining adequate medical treatment through lack of means. The promise to maintain a heavily subsidised public health care system has thus served to legitimate the government's decision to promote private health insurance.

A Regulated Insurance System and the Demand for Health Insurance

The health insurance market in Hong Kong can be divided into two distinct sub-markets: the corporate market and the non-corporate market. In the former case, employers purchase insurance schemes for their employees; while in the latter case, people buy health insurance on an individual basis. Compared with the corporate market, the non-corporate market is relatively insignificant (Yuen, 1994b): most of the health insurance schemes are purchased on a corporate rather than an individual basis. There are four reasons accounting for the relatively low percentage of population in Hong Kong which takes out non-corporate medical schemes. Firstly, since private health insurance which comprehensively covers private medicine is very expensive, not many people can afford it. Secondly, there has been a proliferation of employer-sponsored medical schemes which usually cover the young, well salaried and better-educated employees (Hedley et al., 1990; Census and Statistics Department, 1993). If well-paid employees are provided with health insurance as fringe benefits, their personal or non-corporate demand for health insurance is consequently reduced. Thirdly, those without health insurance may pay out-of-pocket if private health care is sought in the event of illness. Such a strategy can reduce a monetary loss in the form of monthly or quarterly premium. A study in 1987 indicated that less than 5 per cent of the population in Hong Kong were covered by private health insurance and only 21 per cent of those who went to private hospitals carried private health insurance (Yuen, 1988a and 1988b). The percentage of inpatients going private with private health insurance cover could have increased substantially in recent years as it was estimated that 12 per cent of the population in Hong Kong were covered by medical insurance (Hong Kong Government, 1993a). But it is reasonable to believe that there remains quite a considerable proportion of patients who have to pay out-of-pocket for seeking treatment and hospitalisation in the private sector. The fact is that in the case of jumping the public queue for early treatment or elective surgery, even low income groups who could not afford to purchase private health insurance had gone private (see Chapter 7). Finally, the public hospital care system serves as an insurance against financial risks in the event of hospitalisation. The term 'insurance' used here has nothing to do with the actuarial concept of private insurance or is not so much a technical description of a system based on the assessment of risk, but is used in a way to suggest 'protection' for the general public.

Although employers are not required by law to provide health insurance to employees, it is common for the large (200 or more employees) and medium (100 - 200 employees) size corporations to offer medical benefits as fringe benefits in order to attract and retain employees, especially those of higher ranks. The employers may either self-insure or purchase medical schemes. The corporations' preference for insurance in hospital care coverage is not difficult to understand because of the need to insure against the high costs of hospitalisation once incurred (Downey, 1993). It is the traditional function of health insurance to share risks among the insured members. However, as comprehensive coverage for hospitalisation is expensive, this has even prevented some of the large and medium size corporations from offering low-rank or even mid-level employees a hospitalisation scheme. Compared with these corporations, small-size companies (less than 100 employees) in general provide very few hospitalisation benefits to their employees (Yuen, 1994b). Moreover, insurance policies for larger corporations are normally sold at a lower price, while those for small and medium size companies - which however form the mainstay of the economy of Hong Kong - are more expensive. Indeed, 'bulk' purchase and sales make possible a substantial reduction of expenses in marketing, billing, processing and other administrative overhead costs (Fein, 1989). In return, the larger group rates can be reduced greatly. It is within such a context that many companies in Hong Kong - especially those of small and medium-size - do not find health insurance attractive. The point is that these companies may self-insure themselves in the provision of outpatient services to their employees, and rely on the public hospital care system to provide hospital care to their employees.

Relationship between Regulated Health Insurance and B-class Beds A directly elected Legislator said that: 'There exists certain relationship between medical insurance and B-class beds. The premium for Class B beds' insurance will be much lower' (Interview). A member of the Health and Medical Development Advisory Committee further elaborated that:

> [t]he encouragement of medical insurance should be accompanied with the introduction of B-class beds as private medicine is very expensive. The premium for enough coverage for private medicine is very high, say, several hundred dollars each month, depending on the age of the insured. With the implementation of B-class beds, the premium could be lowered. The general companies would not like to contribute so much for its employees for the consumption of private medicine. Thus, B-class beds together with the stamped approval of insurance schemes could encourage more companies and individuals to purchase medical insurance...Most of the companies in Hong Kong are small or medium enterprises. Public hospital care [B-class beds] can penetrate into this market niche. (Interview)

The relationship between B-class beds and regulated health insurance is mutually reinforcing. As discussed in the previous chapter, the fees of B-class beds are charged on the basis of a daily-standardised charge. To the insurer, this is a sound mechanism to control overcharging or price discrimination practice on the side of providers.   In addition, unlike private beds provided in public and private hospitals, semi-private beds are subsidised by the government considerably.   Because of these two factors, the insurer could offer health insurance plans covering the B-class bed at a much attractive price.   That is, the provision of B-class beds could lower the insurance premium and thus encourage employers and individuals to purchase health insurance. Backed with the twin package of the provision of B-class beds and regulated insurance plans purchased at lower prices, health insurance can penetrate into small size companies on the one hand, and facilitate large and medium size companies to extend the provision of hospitalisation benefits to mid-level or even to low-rank employees on the other hand.

On the other side of the coin, those patients with insurance cover including B-class beds will most likely seek hospitalisation in a B-class bed rather than a public-ward bed of a public hospital.   It is because the insurer rather than the patient will be largely responsible for the costs incurred by using the B-class bed. Since the link between demand and payment is indirect if patients are covered by private health insurance, it is not surprising that the demand is higher than when people have to pay out-of-pocket all by themselves.   Thus, an increase in 'B-class bed' insurance would have the effect of increasing the use of B-class beds.   Alternatively, patients may use a private hospital, subject to co-payment of any excess cost by them.   Since private hospital care is very expensive, the chance for the insured person (taking out insurance mainly targeted at the possible use of B-class beds) to use a private hospital is relatively slight.   However, patients may take the alternative of private medicine if they do not want to wait for a long time for cold surgery.

A Co-ordinated Voluntary Insurance Scheme: Creating Choice and Competition?

The government believes that with the setting up of a designated body for approving health insurance plans, both choice and competition would be enhanced. The argument is that both the effects of choice and competition are restricted, and benefit the relatively well off population only.

Choice and Competition: Government Viewpoints

Towards Better Health emphasises that the regulatory framework set up by the designated body would facilitate private insurance companies to 'compete with each other in greater openness and transparency to users' (para. 4.18). It is believed that greater competition between health insurance plans approved by the designated body would help drive down the insurance premium and would ultimately benefit the consumers. Another kind of competition will be generated between registered and non-registered plans. A member of the Health and Medical Development Advisory Committee explained that:

> [c]ompetition between registered plans versus non-registered plans will be created. In order to gain the trust of the consumers, the insurance companies may end up submitting most of their insurance plans to the designated body. This will make the insurance plans more open and transparent to the public. (Interview)

In short, two different kinds of competition will be created, and they are competition between different registered plans, and competition between registered and non-registered plans. The first kind of competition is believed to be consistent with the neo-liberals' belief in the use of market forces in driving down the insurance premium; while the second kind of competition may result in promoting the popularity of registered plans and in enhancing people's trust on the designated body. Competition is thus viewed by the policy makers as being amenable to generating two desirable effects: promoting health insurance and benefiting the consumers at the same time.

To the policy makers, there are also two kinds of choice available to the public upon the promotion of health insurance plans. First, the consumers would have a choice over different types of insurance plan, both registered and non-registered. Second, the public would have a choice to go private or have an access to a new choice of semi-private beds provided in public hospitals if they are financially protected by an insurance plan. To the government, if more and more people are insured by private health insurance, the demand for heavily subsidised public-ward beds would be reduced, and thus 'the burden of financing healthcare would be more evenly distributed between Government and those who are better able to look after themselves' (para.4.20). Thus, the expansion of choice in health care via the implementation of voluntary insurance and B-class beds is presented by the government as a 'win-win' solution - being beneficial to those patients with means and those without.

A Critique of Competition

It cannot be denied that the two kinds of competition described above may be created with the setting up of a designated body. If approved plans could ensure adequate coverage and reasonable premiums, this may induce further competition between registered and non-registered plans, and in the long run may help to promote the image of the designated body in registering or approving plans. However, the designated body may receive complaints from insured persons with regard to the adequacy of coverage and the level of co-payment after actual utilisation. The problem of patients' complaints will be much less serious with those registered plans involving only the use of public facilities since the way that B-class beds charged can effectively get rid of the price discrimination practice evident in the private sector (Downey, 1993; Hay, 1992). The picture will be different if registered plans cover the use of private medicine. Since the insurers in Hong Kong do not have the right to enlist their own doctors to provide comprehensive health care, they cannot exercise control over the fee-charging behaviour of doctors. The continued predominant practice of the fee-for-service approach among doctors in the private sector would be likely to induce provider abuses and may therefore increase the level of co-payment responsible by the insured patients. If patients' complaints cannot be effectively handled, the 'authority' of the designated plan in registering plans involving the use of private hospitals will be undermined.

Moreover, private insurance plans are risk-rated, which means that the level of premium reflects the relative likelihood of the insured person to claim for insurance benefits, and those who are more likely to be heavy users of medical care have to pay a higher premium or are even excluded from joining any private schemes (Fein, 1989). To insurance companies, the best way to ensure profit making is to select the 'good risks' and to exclude the 'bad risks' (Luft and Miller, 1988). So, competition between insurance plans may help to make the premiums more competitive for the 'good risks', while the insurance companies would use whatever methods to discourage the 'bad risks', like elderly and sick applicants, so as to keep costs down. In other words, the 'desirable' effects generated by competition will be made possible at the expense of the 'bad risks'. The relatively 'bad risks' may even have to pay a higher premium in order to make premiums attractive to the 'good risks'.

This raises an important question: who will benefit from the type of competition created by the regulated approach? Most probably, this will benefit the 'good risks' only. If competition is to benefit the less well off and the sick as well, the government may decide to use a social insurance approach designed to induce provider-side or purchaser-side competition or both. The Canadian system representing a centralised social insurance system can enhance provider-side competition; while the sickness funds approach adopted by Germany can enhance both provider-side and purchase-side competitions since people may choose their own sickness fund serving as their health care purchaser (Appleby, 1992). The adoption of the regulated voluntary insurance approach may just end up benefiting a very small group of people whose medical needs are not as great as those of 'bad risks'.

Notwithstanding the careful use of cost containment measures, the promotion of private health insurance schemes would unavoidably lead to an increase in health care expenditure. The reason is that private insurance is not so conducive to efficient use of resources (Folland, Goodman and Stano, 1993). In the context of Hong Kong, because of competition for buyers, it was estimated that around 20 per cent to 40 per cent of the premiums collected were used on advertising, marketing, commission, administration and other paper work. Another 15 per cent to 20 per cent of the premiums were for profit making. As a result, only a portion of the insurance premiums was directly spent on financing health care consumption (Wong, 1990). Therefore, although private health insurance can serve to pool risks and minimise individuals' expenses on health care at the point of consumption, it plays a considerable role to increase health care expenditure on an overall basis. The case of the US can well illustrate the cost-escalating tendency of private health insurance. Thus the government's argument that the use of market competition will in the long run drive down the prices of private health insurance plans is thrown in serious doubt.

A Critique of Choice

From the above sub-section, it can be seen that the bad risks will not benefit from the competition induced unless they are employees in companies which purchase private health insurance on a corporate basis. The high-risk groups and the working class are likely to be deprived of the choice to pick up private health insurance. Inequalities of choice for an enhanced access to better health care will be further widened. A failure for the high risk groups to purchase any insurance plans may be due to some other factors other than their own purchasing power backed by their income or private wage, for example, age, job nature, health status, past record of illness and other related factors. The insurance companies welcome the working class to purchase an insurance plan provided that they are regarded as low risks or good risks. The main reason for their failure to get one is their low income which makes a monthly contribution of several hundred dollars unaffordable. To the high-risk individuals of working class background, a choice for private insurance plan is mostly a dream rather than a possibility.

In most cases, if health insurance is provided as a fringe benefit, the exchange value of the labour of the employee has to be taken into consideration. From a corporate point of view, the exchange value of the employee is a very important factor in determining the fringe benefit package. Those who are viewed as having higher exchange value measured in terms of rank and salary are those employees that the employers would most likely to retain and attract and vice versa. In addition to low-paid employees, part-time workers, the underemployed, people working in dangerous occupations, and highly mobile employees like construction workers are very often, if not always, excluded from benefiting from medical insurance benefits provided by employers. All these groups with great needs for financial protection cannot get even a modest plan to minimise the financial risks associated with ill-health and accidents. To ensure profit making, the corporate decision to provide medical fringe benefit to the employees responds to their exchange value rather than to their needs.

If health insurance is linked to employment, the insured employees will usually lose their benefits upon retirement, and it is very difficult for them to extend their insurance policy as a result of a change of employment status. In the context of Hong Kong, all major private insurance companies marketing health insurance plans, like Blue Cross, Cigna and Carlingford Insurance, charge the age group 61-65 four times more than those aged 40 or below. A physical examination report is required from the attending doctor of the insurance company for any applicant over age 60 or who is currently under medical treatment (such expenses have to be borne by the potential insurance buyers). Therefore, even though a retired person is allowed to continue his or her insurance policy with coverage equivalent to that provided by the previous employer, he or she has to pay higher premiums because of his or her age, and because of the change of the nature of insurance plan purchased on an individual rather than a corporate basis. According to my survey in 1993, there exists no insurance plan in Hong Kong which covers age 66 and above even for those who have enrolled in a plan earlier. If this practice has not been changed yet, age 66 will become an absolute dividing line beyond which individuals can no longer benefit any more from private insurance plans - even for those who can back their choice with enough purchasing power.

Theoretically, those patients with insurance plans can have three choices: going private, using B-class beds, and using public-ward beds. The final choice is unlikely since there is no need to insure against the financial risk of using a public-ward bed unless fees are significantly increased. Going private is a very expensive option; while using B-class beds is a comparatively less expensive option (Chapter 7). Thus, it is reasonable to believe that if individuals' and corporations' opting for a private insurance plan is mainly a consequence of the introduction of B-class beds, the regulation approach would increase the likelihood of being kept in the public sector rather than going private. However, being kept in public hospital but using better amenities has a different meaning. Firstly, the consumption of B-class beds represents an option to go for better 'hotel' facilities, somewhere between going public and going private; or it may be named as going semi-private within the public sector. Secondly, the consumption of B-class beds within the public sector is an option for those who can afford to pay out-of-pocket, or for those who are insured against the financial risks of such a consumption. To those who cannot afford to pay out-of-pocket, or without having an insurance plan for using a B-class bed will have no choice but to use a public-ward bed; or in the traditional sense of being kept in the public sector without having a choice to go private.

The implementation of the co-ordinated voluntary insurance approach will not change the market mechanism through which freedom to choose is pursued and achieved are private ownership and rewards. In a 'market-led' approach, unless one is insured by his or her employer, choice for those who cannot afford to pay for a commodity would contract as choices follow ability to pay (Johnson, 1995). The emphasis placed on private and occupational welfare or the private wage in financing health care is very similar to the industrial achievement-performance model.   This model 'holds that social needs must be met on the basis of merit, work performance and productivity' (Titmuss, 1974:31). The working class and those who are out of the employment market are usually deprived of a choice to pick up a health insurance plan; or in other words, they would be left with no choice but to use public-ward beds.   Therefore, if there is any successful promotion of private health insurance following the implementation of the registration of health insurance plans, it will be underpinned by an ideological force emphasising self-reliance and merit and a belief that private health insurance enhances personal choices in health care.   A further acceptance of these neo-liberal beliefs in health care will fit in with the government's purpose in expanding the role of private financing.

Prospects for State Regulation in Private Health Insurance

The government wants to promote the use of private health insurance as a means to finance both private medicine and the new product of B-class beds provided in public hospitals.   As discussed above, the regulation approach and the provision of B-class beds is mutually reinforcing.   If the image and 'authority' of the body designated to regulate private insurance can be strengthened, and if the demand for private financing of health care in Hong Kong can be stimulated as a consequence, the private financing of health care in Hong Kong can be further enhanced.   Within the context of increasing privatisation of social services in Hong Kong (Chiu and Yu, 1992), it is reasonable to believe that the promotion of private health insurance will also serve to privatise health care in terms of financing medical consumption in two ways.   Firstly, the widespread use of private health insurance can encourage more people to go private. Secondly, if the opting for health insurance plans is stimulated by the lower premiums as a result of the coverage of B-class beds, it will increase the likelihood of using B-class beds which have a high cost-recovery potential.   Such an increasing role of individual/corporate or private financing of hospital care fits well with the government's emphasis on reducing subsidies on patients' medical consumption.

However, as the implementation of B-class bed scheme is still in the pilot stage, and as the scheme is closely related to the state's approach to the promotion of private health insurance, the prospect for setting up a designated body for the health insurance industry is still uncertain. Both private health care providers and health insurers would like to see the promotion of private health insurance. The major area that these two parties disagree with is the anticipated impact of the implementation of the B-class bed. Even without the implementation of B-class beds, the government may consider applying its proposed approach as a first step to regulating health insurance. But the government's recognition of the under-regulation of private health insurance is one thing, and its commitment to enforcing some more progressive state regulation in this industry is another thing. It seems that the scheme of B-class bed not only serves as a legitimation for state regulation in health insurance, but also as a necessary condition for implementing its proposed regulation approach. So, the prospects for state regulation in private health insurance would much depend on the progress of the experimentation of B-class beds in public hospitals.

Conclusion

An examination of the nature of the regulation approach has shown that it is unlikely to expand the benefits of choice and competition to the wider public. The promotion of private health insurance will not benefit the high-risk group and the working class. Individuals' access to an insurance plan will depend on their own purchasing power or their own exchange value viewed by their employers.

Along with the desire of the state to promote private health insurance, the taxation-based system of public health care is to be maintained, and health insurance is regarded as a supplementary rather than an alternative way to financing public hospital care. Health insurance is taken as a means to promote private financing of health care rather than being viewed as a mechanism to integrate the financing and provision functions of health care in Hong Kong. However, the logic for implementing the desired regulation approach of the state is not that straightforward. It is, after all, tied up with the interest of the private health care providers and the delicate balance between the private and public sectors in health care. It does not mean that the state will easily give up its idea to further promote private health insurance. But the ideal plan cannot proceed as smoothly as the state expected at first place particularly confronting the unsettled condition of the scheme of B-class beds.   Because of this uncertainty, the use or expansion of private health insurance in Hong Kong is still largely dependent on the market force and the employers' provision of health insurance on the one hand, and on the extent to which the rationing of health care, and hospitalisation in particular, is applied to public patients on the other.

9 Promoting Informal Health Care

Introduction

Informal health care provided in the form of unpaid labour has long been an important part of the health care system. In actual practice, informal health care refers to informal diagnosis and treatment of acute illness, actions implemented to nurse the sick or manage the symptoms of chronic illness or disability, and also daily 'routines' and measures used to promote health maintenance and prevent diseases; it includes both aspects of care-for-others and self-care (Graham, 1984; Stacey, 1988). Graham (1991) suggests that unpaid informal care is usually done within a home-based setting and governed by the bonds of kinship. The majority of informal care provided in the UK has been found to be provided by family members (Walker, 1982). In the US, Doty (1986) reports that about 75 per cent of functionally disabled older people are cared for solely by family members, and that women provide the vast majority of this unpaid labour. Within the context of Hong Kong, older people who are in need of care are also mainly cared for by family members, particularly their immediate female kin whereas care provided by other relatives, friends and neighbours constitutes a very small proportion of informal care (Working Group on Research for International Year of the Family, 1994; Ngan and Kwok, 1992 & 1993; Chow, 1988). The family has been the main provider of long-term health and social support to its dependent members, and dwarfs the role played by the formal health and social care systems (Brody and Brody, 1989).

The role played by the family and the community in providing 'better health care to individuals' (Working Party on Primary Health Care, 1990:para.9.45) has been explicitly identified in official documents in the 1990s. Phases like 'community carers system' (Hospital Authority, 1994:5), 'informal caring network' (Hospital Authority, 1995a:12), 'community as carers' (Hong Kong Government, 1995b:para.5.30), 'community as partners in health' (Hospital Authority, 1998:10) have emerged in official documents. Establishing a closer interface between the formal health care system and the community carer system has become a major concern of health care reform in Hong Kong nowadays.

Another important development in the 1990s is the state's active promotion of Chinese medicine as evidenced by the publication of four official reports on the promotion of Chinese medicine and the status of Chinese medicine practitioners in the 1990s (Working Party on Chinese Medicine, 1991, 1994; Preparatory Committee on Chinese Medicine, 1997a, 1997b). Chinese medicine has long been and is still an integral part of Hong Kong Chinese culture, and is widely used by the public despite the continuing dominance of Western medicine. The consumption of Chinese medicine is home-based and domestic labour-intensive in nature, and is heavily reliant on informal care. Thus, the government's interest in the role and further development of Chinese medicine as an alternative system of health care and treatment has significant implications for expanding the role of informal health care, both in terms of self-care and family care.

This chapter argues that, already the predominant provider of health care, the informal sector is set to expand via two important strategies implemented by the state: promotion of community health care and Chinese medicine respectively. The community health care strategy is an explicit one to incorporate the informal sector, in particular the family, to provide a pool of carers participating in the care of the chronically sick, older people and other dependent members, whereas the promotion of Chinese medicine, a quasi-formal form of health care, is an implicit one to promote informal health care, both in terms of self-care and family care. The argument is that within the political environment of emphasising cost-containment in health care, the implementation of community health care and the further promotion of Chinese medicine are of strategic importance in providing a material and ideological context for reducing public demand on highly subsidised health care, in resourcing formal health care, and in reinforcing family care and self-reliance ideology.

Expanding the Role of the Community Carers' System: Policy Objectives of the Government

Older People and the Chronically Ill as Two Major User Groups of Health Care

The Health and Welfare Branch and the Hospital Authority have identified two major issues confronting the Hong Kong's health care system nowadays: the disproportionate increase of the population of older people and the prevalence of chronic illness. Firstly, the population aged 65 or above will be increased at a rate of 22 per cent between 1994 and 2000, compared with 3 per cent of the overall population within the same period (Hospital Authority, 1995a:4). The population of older people is expected to rise from 11.6 per cent (0.71 million) in 2001 to 12.3 per cent (0.79 million) in 2011 (Hong Kong Government, 1993a: para.2.3). Secondly, the major causes of mortality and morbidity have now been dominated by the prevalence of chronic illnesses (Hospital Authority, 1995a:4). Accordingly, older people and the chronically ill have been identified as the heavy users of public medical services. In most official documents, however, these two groups of patients are considered to be significantly overlapping with each other. For example, it is stated in the 1995 Rehabilitation White Paper that '[w]ith...an ageing population, the morbidity pattern in Hong Kong has shifted towards chronic diseases. Many of them are disabling in nature and these patients will require long term rehabilitation care' (Hong Kong Government, 1995b:para.5.1).

Older people occupy on average 40 per cent of bed-days in public hospitals and comprise 21 per cent of patients at the specialist clinics of the Hospital Authority, and constitute an estimated 30 per cent of patients at the general outpatient clinics of the Department of Health (Hong Kong Government, 1993a:para.2.5; Working Group on Care for the Elderly, 1994:paras.251 and 257; Liu and Wong, 1997). The ex-Secretary for the Health and Welfare Branch portrayed older people as the major users of expensive medicine by stating that:

[i]n the past, our population was relatively young. However, nowadays, you know, our population has become older. That means, young people are getting fewer and fewer in number; whereas elderly people are getting more and more. It's our duty to provide adequate health care to the elderly. But at the moment, they are heavy users of our public health care system...The trend

of ageing is a very important factor in affecting the use of our valuable health care resources. (Interview)

There have been no official figures concerning the use of public health care facilities by the chronically ill. However, the Hospital Authority has identified the major causes of hospital admissions as being coincident with the leading causes of death in Hong Kong. It was reported that the number of patients treated in public hospitals for colonic cancers in 1992 was increased by 162 per cent as compared to 1982. Corresponding figures for ischaemic heart disease and blood diseases increased by 110 per cent and 92 per cent respectively (Hospital Authority, 1994:29). In fact, the top three killers which almost account for 60 per cent of all the causes of mortality are chronic diseases: malignant neoplasm, heart diseases and cerebrovascular diseases. Infectious and parasitic diseases for which the acute care approach is more suitable have become relatively fewer in number, accounting about 3 per cent of the total annual deaths of Hong Kong (Census and Statistics Department, 1995:38). Chronic illnesses may appear at any age, although most people experience them in their old age. Most of the chronic illnesses are incurable, and their chronic symptoms or residual disability may, however, be effectively managed if there is an adequate provision of health and social care support.

Older people can be very healthy and productive until they grow very old (Sidell, 1995). Preventive health care services are certainly of great use to the general population of older people. While for those who have chronic illness(es), rehabilitative and long-term care services are especially important. According to a local survey, it has been found that out of the 1,172 persons aged 55 or above, 53.5 per cent have joint chronic problems, while 82.7 per cent of them have one or more type of chronic diseases (Chi and Lee, 1989). However, having chronic illness(es) may not as a consequence significantly undermine the self-care capability of older people. Their conditions can be very stable although continuing care is needed (Radley, 1994). Generally speaking, the majority of older people, including those who have chronic illness(es), are capable of coping with personal care such as eating, bathing, toileting, dressing and walking (Chi and Lee, 1989; Chow, 1988). To be old, or to be chronically ill, is not necessarily dependent, nor consequently consumptive of hospital care resources.

The demographic projection of the population of older people and the prevalence of chronic illnesses are not sufficient causes for increasing medical care expenditures. There are three other equally important causes of increases in health care spending. Firstly, the intensity of medical care could increase as a result of the number and complexity of procedures performed by the health professionals (Wolfe, 1993). Secondly, the cost of a given amount of medical care rises more rapidly than the general inflation rates (Folland, Goodman and Stano, 1993). Thirdly, the medical profession has a bias towards expensive acute care which is highly specialised and high-tech, and doctors most often determine what is needed because of the information and power asymmetry between them and patients (Chapter 4). To the surprise of the general public, the Hospital Authority (1995a:24) also criticised its bias towards high-tech acute care by stating that 'the organisation of health care provision have traditionally been one along professional grouping of providers according to their training and specialisation, and leaned heavily towards acute, high technology, hospital care'. Because of the undesirable prevalent culture within the formal health care environment, health care resources are much more allocated to acute hospital care, which leads to the under-development of ambulatory and community health care, and other long-term care services. For example, as far as the public health care utilisation of older people is concerned, hospital care is a far more major component than primary health services since the former constitutes 97.4 per cent of public health care spending on the elderly (Central Policy Unit, 1993). The advances in expensive high-tech medical treatment and procedures, high salary or compensation for increasingly specialised health care providers, and the provider-driven-demand are also potential factors for escalating health care costs.

Purposes of Expanding the Role of the Community Carer System

Paradoxically, the heavy users of public medicine are subjects to be blamed and 'cared' for at the same time. But as will be discussed below, this paradox is underpinned by the same concern of the government in aiming at cost containment in health care. The Working Party on Primary Health Care (1990:para.9.32) recommended the promotion of 'community participation, in particular the family and neighbours', and the provision of 'training and professional support and personnel at all levels, including volunteers and care-givers involved in providing health care for the elderly'. Emphasising the role played by the family and neighbours for the (social) care of older people is commonplace in government documents.

However, it is the first time for an official document to specify the need to expand their role in providing *health care* for older people. The Hospital Authority (1995a:12) also emphasises that 'carers in the community such as family members, other care-givers, self-help groups, and community organisations...form the informal caring network in the community which participates in the process of rehabilitation, maintaining and improving health'. Not only the role of the informal caring network is recognised, but also intimate collaboration with 'welfare agencies, family members and community carers' is considered essential to provide continuous and holistic care to patients (Hospital Authority, 1995a:5). It seems that the importance of the informal sector in health care has been recognised by both policy makers and health care providers to supplement the work of 'formal' health care. So, what are the purposes behind the expanding role of the informal health care system, especially in view of the challenges of an ageing population and the prevalence of chronic illness?

Firstly, cost containment is a paramount objective underlying the improvement of primary health care and the setting up of the Hospital Authority. As stated in the Primary Health Care Report, investment in primary health care is subscribed to the principle of cost containment and the use of resources in the most efficient and effective manner. It is expected that through encouraging primary health care and community participation, excessive demand on expensive hospital services can be reduced (Working Party on Primary Health Care, 1990:paras.4.10&4.11). By involving the community in the provision of health care, cost containment is thought to be realised by promoting self-reliance and reducing dependence on formal health care (ibid:para.4.11). In addition, the Hospital Authority stresses that faced with the escalating cost of health care, cost-containment has become a national priority in many developed countries, and that Hong Kong is no exception (Hospital Authority, 1994:86). The strategy adopted by the Hospital Authority to contain health care cost is by effective management of health care resources and closer collaboration with other formal health care providers, like private practitioners (Chapter 7), and carers in the community (Hospital Authority, 1994:86; 1995a:5). Hence the informal health care sector has been identified as playing an important part in the blueprint of cost containment in (formal) health care.

Secondly, a related goal to cost containment is to reduce the rate of hospitalisation of those requiring long-term care. The Primary Health Care Report stated that 'the issues of keeping patients out of hospitals and encouraging ambulatory care are particularly relevant to the elderly' (Working Party on Primary Health Care, 1990:para.9.21). It further adds that the progressive increase in the population of older people aggravates the demand for health services as they are perceived to be high-risk population in experiencing illnesses. Taking into consideration the need to reduce their dependence on hospital care, the Working Party strongly recommended that 'the elderly should be one of the most important target groups for receiving primary health care' and that 'family, the government and the elderly themselves' should be responsible for meeting their growing and changing needs (ibid:paras.9.27&9.29). It is emphasised that such a strategy is cost-effective having regard to older people's demand on the more expensive hospital care (ibid:para.9.27). The Working Group on the Care of the Elderly has recognised that some elderly patients may not need long-term hospitalisation (1994:para.85). By reducing unnecessary hospitalisation of patients, hospitals can concentrate their resources on the treatment of the acutely ill (ibid:para.88). Thus, the hospital setting is not regarded as an appropriate 'workplace' for meeting the health care needs of elderly patients both with respect to the use of health care resources and their long-term needs. It is also within this context that the informal caring network in the community including family members, volunteers, neighbours, and voluntary welfare organisations is promoted and expanded.

Thirdly, the promotion of community participation is pursued with a view to preventing or deferring the need for long-term institutional care (Working Party on Primary Health Care, 1990:9.32.b; Working Group on Care for the Elderly, 1994:para.85). The policy is to provide a system of primary care integrated with community involvement where prevention and rehabilitative care are based primarily in the local community and most important at home. The goal is to keep the elderly and chronically ill patients within the community and especially at home as long as possible. In the eyes of the policy makers, home-based prevention and rehabilitation is a much cheaper alternative compared to institutionalisation. Such a goal is consistent with the community care approach adopted in 1979. The aim of the community care approach is to enable older people to live in the community for as long as possible, and to provide residential places for those who for health or other reasons, can no longer live with their families on their own (Hong Kong Government, 1979). The Hong Kong government believes that 'community care is a better system of service delivery and it is cost-effective...[and] better "value for money"'" (Working Group on Care for the Elderly, 1994:para.89).

From the above, it can be seen that the purposes of preventing or deferring the need for hospitalisation and long-term institutional care, and to keep patients within the community as long as possible are in agreement with the paramount purpose of cost containment. These three goals are not necessarily bad if the needs of older people and the chronically ill can be well addressed at the same time. But cost containment in Hong Kong has been narrowly defined by the policy makers as attempts made to containing the growth rate of the health care cost in the public sector. However, cost containment can also refer to the costs that patients and their caregivers have to pay, an almost neglected concept in health care (Henke, 1992). Transport, waiting time, care burden, and opportunity cost in caregiving process are concepts on which cost containment could focus. This approach, however, is not included in the debate of cost containment within the circle of policy makers in Hong Kong.

Social Construction of the Informal Sector with respect to Community Health Care

Before examining the strategy adopted by the state in expanding the role of informal carers, this section discusses the social construction of informal health care by the government itself. Four distinct but interrelated views on the informal sector as defined or identified in official documents released in the 1990s will be discussed. These views form the basis on which the role of the informal sector is to be further expanded in the current health care reforms.

The Informal Sector as an Important Part of the Community Carer System

Firstly, the informal sector has been portrayed as community carers participating in the process of providing health care to patients and dependants, including rehabilitation and health maintenance. They are also regarded as health care 'providers' in an informal sense in contrast with formal health care provided by paid medical professionals or allied health professionals working in health care settings. Informal carers are responsible for providing care; whereas health care providers are assigned with the tasks of producing health care services meeting medical or nursing needs of patients. The Chief Executive of the Hospital Authority explained that:

> [t]he community has two important roles in the provision of health care: as consumers and carers...Community or informal carers refer to a diversity of carers, including family members, relatives, self-help groups, voluntary community organisations and also welfare agencies providing residential or long-stay services. They all play an important role in the treatment process...In particular, families support patients during illness and assist in the medical rehabilitation process. (Interview)

According to the conception of the Hospital Authority, community or informal carers refer to a diversity of carers, both paid and unpaid. Formal carers working in a non-health care setting, like welfare agencies, are considered as paid carers providing social care or personal care rather than formal health care; while informal carers or the informal sector provide informal health care. So, the network of community or informal carers has been defined in a broader sense, just excluding the formal health care providers with qualified or professional training, both in public and private sectors. The informal sector is portrayed as an important part of the community carers system, and as an important part in the whole process of continual and holistic care, which is expected to provide the supportive environment for patients, for example, psycho-social and economic support, assistance in daily living and patients' health maintenance and improvement (Hospital Authority, 1995a:12). It appears that the informal sector is expected to provide a broad category of care; its contribution is counted not only in terms of unpaid caring labour but also economic support.

The Informal Sector as Community Resources

The 1995-1996 annual plan of the Hospital Authority (1995a:24) states that 'There is also general neglect on the need to involve and empower community carers in the treatment process, which leaves the valuable community resources in offering continuous care to the patient untapped'. Community carers are viewed as community resources which would be left untapped if they are not involved in the treatment or rehabilitation process. The Chief Executive of the Hospital Authority emphasised that:

I think we have to establish a closer interface between the health care providers and the community carers system. The community carers, like the patients' families, can provide valuable resources for the benefits of our patients in the treatment and rehabilitation process. In the past, our approach to health care was too hospital-oriented, we had left many valuable community resources untapped. We have now adopted a more out-reaching approach and make sure that the resources available from the community can be better utilised. (Interview)

So, the community, and in particular the family has been portrayed as a pool of resources that could be tapped or mobilised to add extra resources for the benefits of patients. The Hospital Authority (1995a:25) emphasises that 'resources are always limited...and maximisation of the benefits of available resources' are urgently required. Unlike internal resources, financial, physical and manpower - which can be freely utilised by the Hospital Authority in the production of medical care, the resources available from community carers are not owned by formal health care institutions. Instead, the 'ownership' of this type of resources belongs to community carers themselves. In other words, such resources are 'external' to health care providers, and could only be mobilised rather than used or distributed according to the command of health planners or the hospital management. In mobilising the resources from the informal sector, an important task of the Hospital Authority is to heighten the awareness of informal carers to enhance and supplement the care given in public hospitals (Hospital Authority, 1994:56).

The White Paper on Rehabilitation also emphasises that if community resources are to be used, promotion of a caring attitude among the family members and the community is deemed desirable (Hong Kong Government, 1995b:para.5.5). Community resources are not as available and flexibly employed as organisational resources. To the policy makers and providers, community carers can be motivated to contribute more to the pool of resources through the promotion of a caring attitude so as to meet the specific needs of patients. The better the sense of caring attitude, the more the community resources would be available for mobilisation and use.

Although the contribution of community carers is voluntary rather than compulsory, it is emphasised that they should be involved in the delivery of health care so as to make an input of resources into the services provided (Working Party on Primary Health Care, 1990:para.4.11). Hence, community carers are deemed to be 'obliged' to contribute personal efforts and to be involved in the process of treatment and rehabilitation, particularly in relation to the provision of care on a continual basis. Besides, a successful mobilisation or enhancement of carers' involvement in the health care process can enlarge the pool of community resources. In addition to the promotion of a caring attitude emphasising moral obligation or volunteerism, other strategies employed can include education and training, provision of supporting services to patients and their carers, and community health care services. All this will be discussed in another major section. In short, the informal sector is viewed as a significant source of externally available resources which can be better mobilised or enhanced to make an extra input into the services produced by formal health care providers. Without the support or back up of community resources, the continuity of care will be disrupted as formal health care providers may not have enough resources to provide appropriate services.

The Informal Sector as a Pool of Unpaid Caring Labour

This comes to the third point that the contribution of community carers is, at least, implicitly viewed as being free to or uncompensated by health care providers or institutions. On the contrary, formal health care is not free, and providers have to be compensated with salaries. The resources contributed by the informal sector qualified by the feature of free or unpaid caring labour which, if compensated, would no doubt significantly dwarf the budget available for producing health care in the formal sector. The caring labour of community carers has not become a market commodity. It is typically contributed on an unpaid basis at home or in the community.

Nevertheless, nothing is free. In addition to the direct costs for caring of the sick or the dependent - the additional expenditure on medical appliances, drugs, transport, etc. - there are the costs of lost opportunities for earning. The direct and indirect costs of caring will be discussed in further detail in the section discussing the strains of informal carers. What is clear is that the seemingly free caring labour is contributed at a price by informal carers. The mobilisation or enhancement of unpaid caring labour may in fact ultimately shift the cost in the use of community resources to the informal sector.

The Informal Sector as an Ideal Context for Self-care

Policy makers and providers view self-care as one of the important components of informal care. The Hospital Authority (1995a:48) emphasises that 'for medical care to be effective, patients need to understand the nature of their illness and comply with treatment protocols. They may be required to change their life style to promote and maintain health'. Thus, the focus of self care is placed on individual responsibility to seek treatment from health professionals and comply with the medical treatment protocols. As Stacey (1988) reminds us patients are also health workers actively engaged in their own care. Informal health care can be something done by the individual or to the individual. The labour-intensive character of health services, particularly in meeting the increased demand for chronic illness management, has been a good rationale for formal health care providers to emphasise self-care as resources.

However, as informal health care is largely limited by the state to the provision of care to dependent or chronic patients who would otherwise need long-term institutional care, self-care has been placed within a community or family context. That is, self-care and care contributed by informal carers are viewed as being mutually complementary to each other. For example, while emphasising the self-care potential of psychiatric or ex-mental patients, the Hospital Authority realises that it has to 'render valuable advice and support to family members and carers in the community for [these] patients, to ensure compliance to treatment and prevent relapse and re-admissions'. (Hospital Authority, 1994:47). Besides, the Working Party on Primary Health Care (1990: para.3.8&4.10) recommends that 'self-care which places in the family' should be incorporated as an important level of care provided in the health care system of Hong Kong, and that 'individuals and their families have a decided role in taking care of their health needs'. While the extent of self care is recognised as an essential level of care, the policy emphasis is more on care for the elderly and dependent patients instead of care-for-self, especially in view of their heavy 'demands' on expensive hospital care. The community or the family context is assumed to be the best workplace for facilitating self-care and to make the latter an important resource in the treatment or rehabilitation process.

Community Health Care Strategy: Rose Garden for Patients and their Carers?

In 1994, the Hospital Authority firstly announced that its vision to the year 2000 is to establish a seamless health care system through collaboration with other health care providers and carers in the community, so as to ensure continuity of care provided to patients (Hospital Authority, 1994:4). To realise such a vision, services provided by the Hospital Authority are re-categorised into four different types: acute care, extended care (long stay or rehabilitation), ambulatory care (out-patient or day basis) and community care. It is clear that the first three types are not new at all, but the fourth type of health care seems to be a 'new' concept which did not come out until 1994. According to the definition of the Hospital Authority (1995a:17), community care is 'mostly outreaching in nature supporting patients or their care-givers at home or in the community setting'. Hence, although community care as a type of health service is a new term, its concept is not so new. Existing services such as community nursing service and domiciliary occupational therapy also belong to this type of health care. However, new services are also developed along this line: community-based geriatric assessment teams, community-based psychogeriatric teams and community-based psychiatric teams. The out-reach services provided by these teams are believed to have the effect to involve and support community carers to take better care for both elderly and ex-mentally ill patients in the community context (Hospital Authority, 1995a:41). The Department of Health has also begun to run elderly health centres since 1993. Unlike the community-based teams organised by the Hospital Authority, which mainly supplement the rehabilitation care of patients and better monitor the pre-admission and post-discharge programmes for patients, the elderly health centres emphasise prevention and early detection of disease among older people.

Community care and ambulatory care have been identified as two major components of the community health care strategy which was originally proposed in the Primary Health Care Report released in 1990. Another major component of this strategy includes community support services provided by the Social Welfare Department, subvented non-governmental organisations and the Hospital Authority; they include multi-services centres, day care centres, home help, respite services, patient resources centres and social security measures.

Another major emphasis of the community health care strategy is on the setting up of comprehensive pre-discharge planning programmes for elderly and chronically ill patients to better cater for their diverse needs in medical rehabilitation and long-term care. Indeed, pre-discharge planning in Hong Kong is poorly developed. According to Woo's survey, only 26 per cent of her respondent elderly patients were given advanced notice of discharge (Woo, 1994). The Working Group on Care for the Elderly (1994:para.283) believes that '[l]ack of proper pre-discharge planning often resulted in unnecessary hospital admissions and affected the quality of life for elderly people'. The Working Group recommended the setting up of comprehensive pre-discharge planning programmes in public hospitals to cover all elderly patients in all clinical specialities instead of being limited to the speciality of geriatric medicine (ibid:para.286).

As concerned with the medical rehabilitation of the chronically ill, there was not any pre-discharge planning programmes for them before 1994. As at the end of April 1995, there are only two newly appointed rehabilitation consultants responsible for the co-ordination and development of medical rehabilitation services for patients suffering from various chronic illnesses - one in Kowloon Hospital and one in Tung Wah Hospital (Hong Kong Government, 1995b:para.5.9). Since the majority of hospital admissions has chronic symptoms or consequences, the appointment of two rehabilitation consultants is undoubtedly very far away from being adequate to meet the needs of the chronic patients in this area.

The context of Hong Kong has also made it complicated and difficult to properly manage pre-discharge planning. Firstly, the lack of a GP support system makes it difficult to ensure continual care (Chapters 5 and 6). Medical follow-up of discharged patients is mainly provided by outpatient clinics in public hospitals, which is a major factor in aggravating the waiting list problem. If discharged patients go to general outpatient clinics run by the Department of Health, doctors may not have details of their previous admission(s) (Hospital Authority, 1995a). Likewise, separate sources of authority and funding for the various health and social welfare organisations are not conducive to the most efficient and co-ordinated management of the pre-discharge planning and post-discharge care.

It is beyond doubt that comprehensive pre-discharge planning is important in enhancing long-term care and reducing hospital re-admissions. However, it just constitutes one of the factors in realising these desirable goals; other important factors include attending the needs of carers, and provision of community services support, community-based nursing care, management of medication, and subsequent ambulatory care to patients (Williams and Fritton, 1988). So, the nature of the discharge problem is not only concerned with the planning of discharge, the crux of the problem is usually the lack of necessary follow-up services and long-term care provided to both patients and their carers.

Community Care and Ambulatory Care: A Critical Discussion

As far as the involvement of and support to community carers are concerned, the setting up of three different types of community-based teams in the 1990s is an innovation. Such an approach is considered to have the potential to bridge the gap between hospital treatment and ambulatory care (Working Group on Care for the Elderly, 1994:para.88). However, all the three types of 'community-based' teams are in nature hospital-based and led by either a consultant or senior doctor. These teams also provide inpatient, day patient and outpatient services, but most importantly they are assigned with the specific task to reach out to community residential settings or patients' homes to provide medical care and education or training to community carers. A total of 5 geriatric assessment teams have been established in 1995, and a total of 8 teams will be established to cover the whole territory before 1998. Nonetheless, in actual practice, these geriatric teams focus most of their efforts on out-reaching hostels, residential homes, and care-and-attention homes for the elderly. The formal or community carers working in non-health setting are provided with support and training in the management of symptoms and illness for the elderly. The Hospital Authority aims to achieve a 10 per cent reduction in the unplanned hospital re-admission rate and specialist outpatient attendance rate in these residential settings. (Hospital Authority, 1995a:41). Again, the psychogeriatric teams and psychiatric teams mostly limit their outreach efforts to residential settings for the elderly, and half-way houses and sheltered workshops for the ex-mentally ill respectively. Thus, those elderly and ex-mentally ill patients living in 'collective households' rather than domestic households; and those paid community carers rather than unpaid family carers could benefit more from this out-reaching approach.

The bias of the out-reaching approach towards collective households and paid community carers may be explained by the relative cost-efficiency and the 'demonstrable' results achieved in the community rather than home-based setting. Under the pressure of cost-containment, it seems unlikely that the out-reaching bias will be corrected in the near future. In other words, family carers responsible for taking care of their sick members will be mostly deprived of the benefits generated by the 'innovative' out-reaching approach.

The first elderly health centre was opened at the Nam Sham Estate, a public-housing estate, in Shum Shui Po in May 1994. Mr. Chris Patten, the current Governor of Hong Kong, announced in 1992 that a total of seven elderly health centres will be established (Working Group on Care for the Elderly People, 1994:para.273). The main services provided by elderly health centres are concerned with health promotion, health screening and health education among the general elderly population. Health promotion and early detection of diseases for old people are desirable goals. This could also help prevent unnecessary hospitalisation and long-term institutionalisation. However, the targets of the elderly health centres are limited to those age 65 or above. From a prevention point of view, the effectiveness of health prevention or promotion programmes may be better achieved if the age can be reduced to 50 (Hong Kong Council of Social Service, 1995). The underlying reason for such a policy and practice may finally be tied up with the government's desire to control the amount of resources devoted to this area. It is certain that if those aged between 50 to 64 are also included, more elderly health centres have to be established to cater the needs of a larger population. Moreover, the functions of elderly health centres have not been expanded to include rehabilitation services and other continuing care for elderly patients discharged from hospitals. If these functions were also included, the rehabilitation and continual health care needs of discharged elderly patients and their family carers may be better satisfied.

The continuity of health care has long been a serious problem in Hong Kong. After hospital discharge, patients may wait for more than 3 months for seeing a specialist for the first time (Hospital Authority, 1995a). The doctor who offers treatment during the acute phase of the illness usually supervises the medical rehabilitation activities of an elderly or a chronic patient. But as commented in the 1992 Green Paper on Rehabilitation that doctors prefer to 'devote most of their time and interest to acute care', and as a result, the diverse needs of patients suffering from various chronic illnesses are not properly met (Hong Kong Government, 1992:para.5.9).

The Primary Health Care Report and the consultation document *Towards Better Health* recommended the promotion of family medicine through closer collaboration with the private sector. However, it did not recommend a family medicine GP system set up in Hong Kong. The fear of the government is that improving the quality of ambulatory care services would attract more patients from the private sector (Hong Kong Government, 1993a). The joint management of certain chronic patient groups by public and private practitioners discussed in Chapter 6 is also a clear evidence of retaining the market sector serving as the predominant provider in primary care. Those patients who could not afford to pay for 'quality' ambulatory care provided in the private sector would continue to suffer various inconveniences incurred by going public (Chapters 2 and 6).

Community nursing services and domiciliary occupational therapy are the other two main types of service categorised under the heading of 'community care'. They are only available to discharged patients from hospitals. The majority of service users are old people. Usually, domiciliary occupational therapy gives advice to those persons with physical or mental handicap. Although these two services have a much longer history than out-reach services described above, Chi and Lee (1989), in their survey, found that their use by old people was terribly low: only 0.7 per cent used community nursing service and even none of their respondents used domiciliary occupational therapy. In her recent survey of old people discharged from hospital in 1993, Woo (1994) confirmed the same result: only 3 per cent used community nursing service and none of her survey's respondents used domiciliary occupational therapy.

The Hospital Authority (1995a:29) emphasises that 'true continuity of care can only be achieved through a seamless health care arrangement with primary health and community carers'. Although the role of primary health care has recently been recognised in Hong Kong, it is just regarded as a level of care to complement hospital-based services like the case of many other developed countries (WHO, 1987; Malcolm, 1994). Hospitals as organisational entities still dominate the provision and direction of health care, including acute care and community health care, in Hong Kong. Within this context, it is very unlikely for primary health care to develop into an organisational entity and make referrals to secondary or tertiary care for patients. Having regard to the realities of the power structure biased towards hospital care and specialist medicine, the shift of resources from acute care to primary health care and long term health care is thrown in doubt.

As a whole, the Hospital Authority and the Department of Health have given due attention to community care as a type of health service. However, the functions of elderly health centres are much limited, and could not be developed into an organisational entity to provide generalist, holistic, continuing and comprehensive health care to old people. The newly developed out-reach services mainly provide medical care and continuing health surveillance for those living in collective households or residential settings. Those elderly and ex-mentally ill patients and their family carers living in domestic households are largely deprived of the benefits of such an 'innovation'. As will be shown in the next sub-section, the limited provision of non-hospital care to those patients with a family is not a new phenomenon. It appears that the 'innovations' of community care continue to sustain such a phenomenon.

A Critical Examination of Community Support Services

'Traditional' Community Support Services   Apart from community care and ambulatory care, community support services perform an important source of support for elderly and chronic patients to be cared for or rehabilitated in the community. The main kinds of services include multi-service centres, day care centres, home help, respite service, and the newly developed patients resources centre.

Multi-service centres for older people first came into operation in 1977. The centres intend to be operated on an integrated basis whereby services provided include home help, counselling, social activities, laundry, bathing, canteen facilities and community education. There were 18 multi-service centres in 1993. It was planned to establish a total of 14 additional multi-service centres for older people by 1997. However, up to September 1997, only nine more centres, were established (Hong Kong SAR Government, 1997:125). Such an undertaking is indeed well behind schedule and fails to fully satisfy the needs of older people.

Day care centres for the elderly are another community support service implemented ever since the late 1970s. Its main purpose is to provide personal care and limited nursing services for elderly people, who are still mobile but in declining health and lack family members to look after them on a full-time basis (Social Welfare Department, 1993). The current services provision is even worse than the multi-services centre. There are only 12 day care centres but the demand is 31. Chan et al. (1993) criticises that day care centres are not complementary to family care. For example, their opening hours cannot fit in with the demand of the working class families, and they find it very difficult to escort their elderly members to day care centres during the day time. Therefore, those who are much in need are often unable to benefit from this type of service.

Moreover, the provision of respite service is kept to a bare minimum. This service was first introduced in 1989. It provides temporary residential care for elderly people or people with a disability for not more than two weeks so as to provide short-term relief to the families (Hong Kong Government, 1995b). As concerned with respite service for the elderly, there are at present only 13 places available for all family carers to compete in Hong Kong.

The Hospital Authority (1995a:48) emphasises that a home help is often required by individual patients to cope with illness. The home help service is a unified service, providing meals, personal care, escort, laundry and home management services. Although home helps are not confined to old people, about 80 per cent of the users belong to the elderly group (Working Group on Care for the Elderly, 1994). As at September 1997, the government fails to provide a total of eight additional home-help teams to cater the needs of the community (Hong Kong SAR Government, 1997:124).

The lack of transport and escort services for the frail elderly and the chronically ill to receive community health care is another important issue to be dealt with. According to Chi and Lee (1989), some 40 per cent of their elderly respondents had difficulties in visiting a doctor because of the lack of escort or transport facilities. Woo (1994) has found that 75 per cent of her elderly respondents recently discharged from the hospital could not attend the outpatient clinics for medical follow-up without relying on relatives or friends to accompany them. According to the Working Group on Research for International Year of the Family (1994), 89.6 per cent and 85.5 per cent of the female respondent carers have to escort the elderly to obtain medical treatment and social welfare services respectively. While a survey on the needs of chronic patients also reflects that transport or escort allowance is widely supported by the respondents (Chan et al., 1992:22). The Working Party on Primary Health Care (1990:para.9.39) was aware of this problem, but felt that support from informal carers would be more appropriate. There are probably two reasons for turning down the idea of enhancing the transport and/or escort arrangements for the needy: first is the consideration of the financial implication of the service or arrangements; second is the promotion of patients' reliance on their relatives or friends to provide the escort service.

Chi and Lee (1989) found that the usage of community support service was very low: only 1.8 per cent of the respondents used multi-service centre, 1.1 per cent used home help service, and 0.3 per cent used day care centre. Woo (1994) also found in her study that there was only 1 per cent of discharged respondent patients using home help service. It is also found that chronically ill patients discharged from hospitals have to rely almost on their own personal or family resources as community support services for the chronically ill is not designed as an integral part of patient care (Chan et al., 1992:21). Because of insufficient resources input from the government, the provision of the above services are all in large shortfalls. As a result, priority is given to those without family support. In a study conducted in 1988 by Chow on the elderly on waiting lists for care and attention homes, he found that community support services were mostly received by respondents who live alone' (Chow, 1992). Although the majority of elderly and chronic patients live with their family, it does not imply that their need for community support service is necessarily less. Chow (1988) also found in his study that more than half of the carers in his samples wanted home help services in order to release their caring burden.

In spite of the laudable goal of providing support to patients and their carers, Woo (1994:219) concluded from her study that very few discharged patients received formal social support, the majority of support being provided by the informal sector. Another local study concerning cancer patients receiving chemotherapy also found that the majority of care and support received by the respondents were provided by their family especially their spouse and parents (Ma et al., 1990). Community support services are not available to all carers in need of help, and most of them are apparently left to care alone under the current service provision. This phenomenon is very much consistent with what is happening now in the delivery of out-reach services provided by the Hospital Authority. The caring responsibility shouldered by family carers is further reinforced by the policy practice of the government through giving priority to those patients living alone or in collective households. As Moroney (1980:2) ironically criticised, 'families face a penalty if they care and a reward when they cease caring'.

Patient Resource Centres as an Innovation: Further Shifting the Caring Burden to the Family? Vested with the purpose of enhancing and supporting the role of patients, their families and the community as carers, eight patient resource centres are established in eight major hospitals. The main functions of these patient resource centres are to conduct educational and training talks for patients and their families, and to facilitate the formation of self-help groups for those patients and their families who have to confront similar problems in the management of chronic illness and symptoms.

In the eyes of the Hospital Authority (1994:55), the patient resource centre has provided a basis on which patients and their carers can be mutually involved in the acquisition of 'knowledge and skills on how to promote health, and how to adjust and cope with impairment and disability, and how to maintain and improve health status'. The Authority further emphasises that its approach to education and training for patients and their carers is essentially different from the traditional moral approach with respect to positively empower carers in several ways: helping them to identify patients' need; inculcating them knowledge and understanding for patients to maintain and improve health; providing them knowledge on specific chronic illness or disability and some basic skills to do health monitoring or surveillance work (1995a:35; 1994:56). It is expected that through enhancing the quality of informal health care, a continuity of care for patients can be better ensured. There is no doubt that family carers should be better supported with training and education. Nevertheless, within the context of vastly inadequate community health care or tangible services provided to informal carers, and the emphasis of further expanding their role in health care, family carers would likely be morally pushed to offer more.

Moreover, the patient resource centre facilitates the formation of and provides basic support to self-help groups. These groups are characterised by patients sharing common sufferings with which conventional allopathic medicine has little to offer. The group provides a context for patients and carers to compare themselves with similar others, to obtain specific information about medical issues, to search for self-identify and build up mutual support (Taylor et al., 1988; Lock, 1986). Broadly speaking, two levels of support can be enhanced: inter-patients level and inter-carers level. On the one hand, the mutual support that patients and carers get from the self-help group may fulfil their needs for affiliation and self-efficacy. On the other hand, they may provide tangible support to one another especially at time of crisis. The Chief Executive of the Hospital Authority also emphasised the advantages of self-help groups as follows:

> [o]ur patient resource centres have provided good support and information to patients' groups. They [the members] can help each other.   They also organise programmes and outings by themselves. If we HA, as a public body, wants to use the open area of the commercial or shopping complex for an exhibition or a mass programme, we have to pay the market rate. But if our patients' group makes an application, they can get it with a good discount or even free of charge. (Interview)

Thus, the Hospital Authority views self-help groups as a focal point to draw community support and resources. On the one hand, the functions of self-help groups in enhancing psycho-social support cannot be denied. On the other hand, as self-help is enhanced within a family and community context, the Hospital Authority can make use of these groups to tap more resources from patients, their families and the wider community.   The Authority's support given to self-help groups is mainly confined to education and some co-ordination. Other tangible support is kept to a minimum. Besides, self-help group members (including patients and their families) are provided with no transport allowance, and free rehabus (rehabilitation bus) service is only available for special outings. Most often than not, the hospital is quite far away from where they live, and transport cost is a real burden to many patients and their families. If self-help groups are not well supported with more tangible services, for example, transport allowance, free or highly subsidised escort service, and more comprehensive rehabilitation services, the financial, escorting and other caring burdens of patients and their family carers might be increased rather than reduced.

Social Security: a Real Support to Patients and their Family Carers? In Hong Kong, the Social Security Allowance Scheme (SSAS), formerly known as Special Needs Allowance Scheme before October 1992, is a kind of social security measure employed by the government to encourage the families to look after their disabled or elderly members (Patten, 1993). The SSAS consists of two kinds of allowance: normal disability allowance and higher disability allowance. The normal disability allowance is payable to those severely physically disabled certified by a public doctor having 100 per cent loss of earning capacity as defined by the First

Schedule of the Employees' Compensation Ordinance (Kwok and Yeung, 1993). The higher disability allowance is twice the rate of normal disability allowance, and is payable to those who are eligible to normal disability allowance and who require constant attendance from others in their daily life (e.g. dementia, double incontinence). The eligibility criterion for SSAS is indeed very harsh. People suffering from severe physical disabilities do not necessarily suffer long term loss of 100 per cent earning capacity if they could receive successful rehabilitation. In other words, if the recipients of normal or higher disability allowance could regain some per cent of earning capacity, they would no longer be eligible for an allowance.

In 1992, the normal disability allowance rate was about 14.3 per cent (and the higher disability allowance rate was thus about 28.3 per cent) of the monthly income of manufacturing worker (Census and Statistics Department, 1992). Such a low rate does not sufficiently take into account of the special needs arising from severe disability, for example, in the use of extra-ordinary expenditure on rehabilitation aids, prosthesis and orthosis, mobility and orientation assistance, physiotherapy, occupational therapy, and long term medication. People with disabilities and being eligible for the Comprehensive Social Security Assistance (CSSA, formerly known as Public Assistance Scheme before October 1992) will be given special subsidies covering a wide range of items, including alternative transport costs, rehabilitation aids, and exemption from hospital and out-patient clinic charges (they are, however, administratively inflexible and impose inconvenience and stigma on the recipients). Given the diverse needs of the disabled and the rising costs of special need items, people with disabilities whose family income is above the CSSA level (which is same as the rate of disability allowance) have been under growing financial hardship to meet their special needs. In fact, the normal or higher disability allowance is so low that there is a lack of incentive for the family members to quit their full-time job to care for their disabled or elderly members.

There has not been yet any allowance scheme specifically designed for the chronically ill. Chronically ill patients are not entitled to normal or disability allowance unless they are medically certified as having 100 per cent loss of earning capacity. There are two reasons for excluding chronic illness as the criterion for public assistance. First is the government's fear of crushing the work ethics of Hong Kong people (Chapter 5); and second is the financial implication of chronic illness allowance. However, most persons with chronic illness face financial problems and many are discriminated against and stigmatised in the labour market (Gerhardt, 1990). Employers are usually reluctant to hire workers with a chronic illness who have to take regular leave for medical follow-up.   If the chronically ill are left with no choice but to continue to work to make a living, their health conditions may be worsened. For example, it is found that the pneumoconiotics would have their health rapidly deteriorated if they take up a full-time job (Hong Kong Workers' Health Centre, 1993; Pneumoconiosis Mutual Aid Association, 1994).   Since chronic illness seriously affects the ability of patients to earn a decent income, it was reported from a survey that about 63.6 per cent of the chronically ill respondents had severe financial difficulty (Chan et al., 1992).

Like disabled patients, the chronically ill have to spend a considerable amount on necessary medical expenses which are not recognised in current financial assistance schemes. The study of Yeung and Tam (1993) found that 93.8 per cent of the respondents met their medical bills with their own or family resources without getting any government allowance. About 20 per cent (18.8%) of the respondents even resorted to loans to cope with the extra medical expenditure. Unless the government expands the scope of disability allowance to cover the chronic patients, and unless the government significantly increases the rate of disability allowance, the families and the patients would be left alone to cope with the additional medical expenditure incurred all on their own.   In spite of the government's emphasis to confront the challenges of chronic illness, the chronically ill and their families are still much marginalised by the social security system of Hong Kong. The chronically ill have to lose all their earning capacity, or their family income has to be spent down to a level eligible for CSSA before they could get any government assistance. The social security approach to chronic illness is just minimal or remedial since it does not take into account the recurrent extra medical expenditure of the chronically ill, which is essential to maintain life and to exercise better control over the illness. The social security system of Hong Kong is too remedial to supplement informal health care.

Portrayal of Family Responsibility in Health Care

After critically examining the community health care strategy in detail, it can be seen that promises as to the spectrum of services or support to enhance informal care, and facilitate long-term care especially to chronically-ill and elderly patients remain vaguely defined and inadequately developed. Not much tangible support is specifically provided to informal carers to deal with their caring burden and stress, physical, social and financial.

The Working Party on Primary Health Care (1990:para.9.1) states that the majority of rehabilitative services for patients 'should preferably be provided in the home environment rather than in institutions', and further adds that 'this is particularly relevant in a Chinese community like Hong Kong where the family remains the major support unit'. Because of the recognition of the role of the family in health care, the Working Party (ibid:para.9.45) is optimistic that there is plenty of scope for innovative approaches to mobilise the family to provide better health care to patients requiring rehabilitative care.

By emphasising family responsibility, the majority of community resources will continue to be tapped from the family. In other words, the family-caring network can be and should be further expanded to cater the health care needs of dependent family members who otherwise would require expensive hospital care or long-term infirmary care. However, such a trend in the health and rehabilitation fields is 'unhealthy' in the sense that the family as a 'natural' caring unit would become something taken-for-granted and its caring burden would be overlooked. This point will be discussed in further detail later.

Promotion of Chinese Medicine: Furthering Self-reliance

The above discussion has shown that the discourse of informal health care focuses on the family's role in taking care of its dependent or chronically ill members. The implementation of the community health care strategy also appears to largely depend on the family to provide informal health care and finance additional medical expenditure incurred by the dependent. This section will argue that the promotion of Chinese medicine is also strongly reliant on the family's provision of informal care and financing of expenses incurred in the use of Chinese medicine not yet and will not be subsidised by the government.

Promoting the Status of Chinese Medicine Practitioners

However, for socio-historical reasons, the practice of Chinese medicine in Hong Kong has not been subjected to control as a professional discipline in terms of registration and qualification (Chapters 3 to 5). Nowadays, Hong Kong has about 7,000 Chinese medicine practitioners, and some 1,600 retail herbal shops (Preparatory Committee on Chinese Medicine, 1997a). There are many different forms of Chinese medicine, including herbal medicine, bone-setting and acupuncture. A recent survey on Chinese medicine practitioners has revealed that nearly 90 per cent (89%) of practitioners in Hong Kong are herbalists (Wong et al., 1993b).

Surveys done in the 1970s and 1990s indicated that the public are more confident in Chinese medicine than in Hong Kong's Chinese medicine practitioners (Lee, 1980; Wong et al., 1993b). The absence of a licensure system may be an important factor in reducing the trust of the public in Chinese medicine practitioners, for the public cannot be certain whether a practitioner of Chinese medicine is qualified or not. Compared to the Western-medicine counterparts, Chinese medicine practitioners are put in a much more subordinate position, and the latter have no say at all in health care policy in Hong Kong (Chapter 3). The medical profession has enjoyed structural superiority over other para-medical professions and alternative health care providers, including the practitioners of Chinese medicine (Lee, 1982).

To facilitate the further development of Chinese medicine, the Working Party on Chinese Medicine (1994), which was chaired by the then Deputy Secretary for Health and Welfare and composed of academics, doctors and representatives of relevant government branches and departments, recommended the registration of Chinese medicine practitioners. A preparatory committee has now been set up, advising on legislation providing a statutory framework for the registration of Chinese medicine practitioners. The legislation is aimed at providing for the establishment of a statutory body to replace the preparatory committee upon its enactment. The preparatory work for setting up the registration framework and the final registration of Chinese medicine practitioners has involved many difficult tasks for the opinion of Chinese medicine practitioners is divided rather than united as concerned with the criteria for registration (Working Party on Chinese Medicine, 1992: para.2.27). It is anticipated that the legislation for the establishment of the Traditional Chinese Medicine Council will be introduced in the 1998/99 legislative session, and from year 2,000 onwards, the registration of Chinese medicine practitioners will be implemented (Preparatory Committee on Chinese Medicine, 1997b).

Registration Set-up as a 'Natural' Response to Political Pressure and Patients' Interest? The change of government's attitude or policy towards the registration of Chinese medicine practitioners can be considered drastic, for before the 1990s the government adopted a conditional tolerance approach to Chinese medicine (Chapters 3 to 5). Chinese medicine practitioners are free to organise associations by themselves in improving their own welfare and the standard of their practice. As in 1992, there were 13 of these associations (Working Party on Chinese Medicine, 1991:para.2.18). However, all these associations have their own admission criteria and there are no agreed regulatory measures against misconduct by members. Chinese medicine practitioners join these associations on a voluntary basis. The organisations of Chinese medicine practitioners have mutual contacts; but they have not yet come together in some overall representative body in fighting for their own interests or in exerting joint political pressure on the government to recognise their professional status. A recent survey conducted in 1991 revealed that 86 per cent of the respondents (Chinese medicine practitioners) were in favour of some form of registration for themselves (Wong et al., 1993b). But this was just an indication of the personal opinion of individual Chinese medicine practitioners. As far as the issue of registration is concerned, the support of Chinese medicine practitioners is important. However, because of the lack of joint political pressure exerted by Chinese medicine practitioners, the individual rather than collective voice for registration among the practitioners is not a sufficient factor to explain the government's attempt to establish a registration mechanism for Chinese medicine practitioners.

The Report on Chinese Medicine 1994 states that 'many people considered that regulation of TCM [Traditional Chinese Medicine] practitioners is vital to safeguard consumer interests' (para.4.2). So, is the registration mechanism a natural outcome of safeguarding patients' interest? There are two reasons for suspecting such an explanation. First is the factor of patients' perceptions on the use of Chinese medicine. Many local surveys have demonstrated widespread belief within the public that Chinese herbal medicine produces fewer side effects (Lee and Cheung, 1989; Wong et al., 1993a; Lam et al., 1994). There has been little public demand or pressure to control herbal medicine. As a result, the public pressure on ensuring the safety of Chinese medicine could not be strong enough to push the government to regulate or register Chinese medicine practitioners. Moreover, among the 2,000 Chinese medicinal materials available in Hong Kong, there are only about '50 herbs which have a narrow safety margin and should be regarded as "potent" or "toxic"' (Working Party on Chinese Medicine, 1994: para.5.3). What is important is that Chinese and Western medicines are different in nature. Most Chinese medicines are used in compound prescriptions, and the toxicity of medicinal materials can be neutralised with appropriate preparation and in suitable combination. The efficacy for treatment can even be enhanced with the use of 'toxic' herbs. Nevertheless, because available 'toxic' herbs are few in number, the government may even ban the sale of these herbs totally, and patients' safety can be consequently ensured without going through the more difficult task of setting up a registration mechanism.

Thus, the decision to establish a mechanism for the registration of Chinese medicine practitioners should not be understood as a 'natural' response of the state to the disunited pressure of the Chinese medicine practitioners nor the public demand for ensuring Chinese medicine safety.

The commitment to the development of Chinese medicine is stated in Article 138 of the Basic Law that '[t]he government of the Hong Kong Special Administrative Region shall, on its own, formulate policies to develop Western and traditional Chinese medicine and to improve medical and health services'. China is in fact one of the few countries where there is an integration of Chinese and Western medicine at both outpatient and inpatient levels, and where there are legal provisions for the registration of both Chinese and Western medicine practitioners (Wong and Chiu, 1997). So, the resumption of China's sovereignty over Hong Kong has provided a politically favourable context for the development of Chinese medicine.

The promotion of the status of Chinese medicine practitioners may be understood as an indication of the state's exercising of its autonomy in expanding the role of Chinese medicine and Chinese medicine practitioners in the health care system now dominated by high-tech Western medicine. In his study of the establishment of the British NHS, Klein (1989) points out that it was the decision of government to establish a NHS which transformed the power of the doctors by creating mutual dependence. Martin (1994) has also convincingly argued that the state has been as important, if not more so, as the doctors in the development of post-war British health policy. The discussion of Chapter 3 has shown that the government of Hong Kong played an important role for the structural power assumed by the medical profession and the marginalisation of Chinese medicine and Chinese medicine practitioners. So, the government may also exercise its own autonomy in promoting the use of Chinese medicine according to the explicit and implicit objectives it wants to achieve. As will be discussed later in this Chapter, the promotion of the status of Chinese medicine practitioners has to be understood in relation to the ideological and material implications for the consumption of Chinese medicine.

Undermining the Structural Power of the Medical Profession? With the implementation of the registration system, the public are able to distinguish between those with training or qualification and those without. As a result, registered Chinese medicine practitioners may gain more trust in the community. Moreover, the registration system will further augment some of the advantages perceived by patients in seeing a Chinese medicine practitioner. Local surveys have revealed that the relationship between patients and Chinese medicine practitioners are more egalitarian in the sense that patients have greater access to information and explanations about the etiology and treatment of illness (Lee, 1980; Wong et al., 1993b). Similarities between Chinese medicine practitioners and their patients in their concepts of health and disease causation may be an important factor in facilitating doctor-patient communication. The fact is that traditional health beliefs about the 'hot/cold' and 'poisonous/wet' concept were found to be strong among public outpatient service users (89%), and the general public (86%) (Hedley et al., 1990). However, it is common for Western medicine doctors to ignore the traditional ideas of etiology, or with little regard given to the traditional health beliefs of their patients (Koo, 1989). The coming registration of Chinese medicine practitioners may thus help enhance the status of Chinese medicine practitioners and increase public confidence in their status and practice.

Although the coming registration of Chinese medicine practitioners represents an important milestone in the development of Chinese medicine, the structural power enjoyed by the medical profession is not directly threatened. The most important point is that Chinese medicine has not been incorporated within the official health care system nor the hospital care system. Chinese medicine practitioners would continue to be confined to the market sector and the 'primary' health care system like their present situation. The medical profession still obtains greater power to control the society's health affairs. A Legislator elected from the Medical and Health Care Functional Constituency emphasised that:

> [t]he medical profession has a duty to ensure the best of health care is being delivered to patients. It is with this in mind that I have been trying to push for a proper registry of Chinese medicine practitioners and a structured control of Chinese medicine. (Interview)

The medical profession has been trying to bring the issue of Chinese medicine under its control and to convey to the public that it has an predominant say over the social organisation of health care in Hong Kong. Moreover, financial support of the government is given almost entirely to Western medicine rather than Chinese medicine consumption, Chinese medical education and research. First of all, the government has not incorporated Chinese medicine into the official health care system (including both hospital and primary health care), nor subsidise people's consumption of Chinese medicine. It seems that the government wants to adopt a more 'cost-effective' approach to promoting the development of Chinese medicine without generating political pressure on the government to provide publicly-subsidised Chinese medicine.

Further, even with the registration of Chinese medicine practitioners, they cannot call themselves doctors as can their counterparts qualified to provide Western medicine. The medical profession will probably continue to gain from the state the right to assert dominance in institutional medicine and health affairs. On the contrary, Chinese medicine practitioners will continue to be excluded from the health care policy-making circle, and they are restricted with respect to their power to regulate the technical content of their work.

It is difficult to foresee whether the economic interests of the medical profession will be significantly threatened following the registration and regulation of Chinese medicine practitioners; but as long as the state and the medical profession are politically and/or financially resistant to the idea of integrating Western and Chinese medicine in the formal health care system, the medical profession will continue to enjoy structural and political power over their Chinese medicine counterparts confined to the periphery of formal medicine.

Promoting the Use of Chinese Medicine

Health Education on Chinese Medicine As mentioned above, Hong Kong people are more confident with Chinese medicine than Chinese medicine practitioners. Probably in view of this, the government adopts the health education approach in promoting the safer use of Chinese medicine. Instead of banning the sale of potent or toxic Chinese medicinal materials, the Preparatory Committee on Chinese Medicine (1997a) has prepared a list of 31 items considered as potent herbs for public reference. The Central Health Education Unit of the Department of Health has also taken a more proactive role in promoting public education in Chinese Medicine by setting up a hot line and organising regular public exhibitions and seminars.

Health education on the use of Chinese medicine has long been a hot topic in the media. The associations of Chinese medicine practitioners also organise regular exhibitions and seminars to enhance public knowledge of Chinese medicine. By comparison, the government did very little in this area of public education in the past. This is indeed the first time for the pubic health care providers to include Chinese medicine in their formal health education. This implies that the official health care domain has at least implicitly recognised the role of Chinese medicine in health maintenance and medical treatment even though it has not been incorporated within the formal health care domain. Unlike Western medicine, Chinese medicine has not yet gained the status as part of formal medicine. As pointed out in Chapter 1, it is still a type of quasi-formal medicine, somewhere between formal medicine and informal health care.

In considering the function of public education, the Working Party emphasises that:

> [s]elf-prescription and self-medication of TCM are common practices. Public education on the safe and proper use of various traditional Chinese medicines is crucial to ensure consumer safety. (Working Party on Chinese Medicine, 1994:para.11.1)

Thus, the Working Party has regarded health education an appropriate measure in view of the prevalence of self-prescription and self-medication of Chinese medicine. Besides, it has also reaffirmed the practice of self-medication of Chinese medicine; or at least it does not regard it as an undesirable practice subjected to further control. A recent local study found that self-medication was a common and universal practice by Hong Kong Chinese with a prevalence of 32.5 per cent in 2 weeks. It was also found that Chinese medicine or Chinese tonics were the most frequently used self-medications. Very few who were not ill had used any medicine. However, Chinese tonics were used frequently by those with or without any illness. Among the respondents 14 per cent used Western medicine or western tonic, and 24.5 per cent used Chinese medicine or Chinese tonic. Whereas among those respondents who reported no illness, 13.5 per cent used Chinese tonic and 0.7 per cent used Chinese medicine, while only 4.3 per cent used Western tonic and 0.1 per cent used Western medicine (Lam et al., 1994). Hence, as far as self-medication is concerned, Chinese medicine and Chinese tonics have assumed much greater popularity than Western medicine and Western tonics.

Self medication may be viewed as an action taken by the user as being used for health related purposes that is not prescribed by a Western doctor or a Chinese medicine practitioner. Self medications may be used for the treatment of illness or the promotion of health. As the use of self-medications is a self-initiated behaviour, the users' subjective evaluation is the most important. The prevalence of traditional Chinese concepts on health maintenance and etiology of illness is therefore an important factor in explaining why Hong Kong Chinese people frequently use Chinese medicine and Chinese tonics. The publication of the list of potent Chinese medicinal materials, and public education on Chinese medicine could thus play a role to reaffirm and further encourage the self-prescription and self-medication behaviour of Hong Kong Chinese who constitute the majority of the population. Self-medication is an indication of self-care and health consciousness (Russell, 1986). The further promotion and use of Chinese medicine may therefore help to promote self-care and other health-conscious behaviour deemed important by the government in current health care reforms. (This point will be discussed in more detail in the section on the ideological and material implications for using Chinese medicine).

Recognising the Role of Chinese Medicine Dispensers   Most Chinese medicines are sold over the counter of retail herbal shops to customers with or without prescriptions. Chinese medicine dispensers play an important role in the delivery of Chinese medicines in that they are responsible for dispensing medicines to customers and patients. As they are allowed to dispense medicines without prescriptions, they may also advise customers on the use of Chinese medicines for treating simple illness or for health maintenance purpose according to the physical constitution of the customer. Therefore, dispensers can, to a certain extent, play a role as practitioners in prescribing Chinese medicines. Customers can also pass through Chinese medicine practitioners and go direct to dispensers for buying Chinese medicines. Since most families possess some knowledge of Chinese medicine, those who self-medicate, especially for health maintenance purpose or at the initial stage of illness, may not necessarily consult a Chinese medicine practitioner. They may instead consult family members, friends or dispensers for the regimen of a particular disease (Koo, 1987; Chi, 1994). So, dispensers can play an important role in assuring the proper and safe use of Chinese medicines. The Working Party recognises the role of dispensers in the delivery of Chinese medicine. Through such a recognition, the current practice of dispensers in dispensing and prescribing medicines for customers or patients is also reaffirmed.

Although the role of dispensers is recognised, the Working Party and the Preparatory Committee, probably for financial reasons, did not recommend on the government's subsidising the training of dispensers. Instead, they encourage schools in Chinese medicine, and Chinese medicine associations to provide training on Chinese medicine dispensing or refresher courses for current dispensers. Besides, tertiary education institutes in Hong Kong have either recently introduced or are planning to introduce dispensing courses on a self-financing basis (para.9.4). The Working Party recommended that the statutory body set up for governing the registration of Chinese medicine practitioners and development of Chinese medicine should consider registration of dispensers in due course (para.9.7). With the further promotion of the status of dispensers through their getting of formal qualifications and registration, the use of Chinese medicine would be further encouraged. The government wants to make the most of available community resources, and the academic interest in Chinese medicine, to enhance the training and knowledge of dispensers. Such an approach is consistent with that applied to the promotion of the status of Chinese medicine practitioners.

It appears that the incorporation of Chinese medicine into the formal health care system is still confronted with insurmountable difficulties. Firstly, the government limits itself to the promotion rather than subsidisation of Chinese medicine consumption. Being deprived of government's direct political and financial support, Chinese medicine will continue to be excluded from the official health care domain and the formal health care system as well. Secondly, the inequitable distribution of power between the providers of Western medicine and Chinese medicine is another major obstacle. Since the medical profession is vested with great power to control medical resources as well as health affairs in Hong Kong, a strong resistance from it is expected. Confronted with these two major obstacles, Chinese medicine is still consumed in the form of commodity, and remains subordinate to Western medicine as it was in the past.

Use of Chinese Medicine: Ideological and Material Implications for Informal Health Care

There has been a steady demand for Chinese medicine in Hong Kong despite the overwhelming majority of government medical resources allocated to Western medicine, and dominance of the medical profession in the government's organisation and policy-making of health care. The registration of Chinese medicine practitioners and public education on the proper and safe use of Chinese medicine would help to safeguard and promote quality of care on the one hand, and enhance public confidence on consulting Chinese medicine practitioners and on the use of Chinese medicine on the other hand. To the government itself, such a trend appears to agree with its cost containment objective in health care. The point to be made is that the increasing consumption of Chinese medicine will provide the ideological and material context for expanding informal health care financed and provided by individuals and families.

Health Maintenance and Self-responsibility

While informal health care refers also to the promotion of health of able-bodied persons, the community health care strategy has focused on the care of people who might otherwise require frequent hospitalisation and institutional care. The practice of Chinese medicine is, however, concerned with the maintenance of the natural balance of the human body and is considered relevant for the purposes of health maintenance and treatment of diseases, and for both able-bodied persons and dependants.

According to the philosophy of Chinese medicine, one has to pay attention to the natural balance of his or her own body in order to maintain health or prevent illness. In a study on contemporary Chinese concepts of health, three main sources of body energy were identified by Chinese informants in Taiwan and San Francisco: *jing* (sexual energy), *qi* (physical energy), and *sheng* (spiritual energy) (Koo, 1982). The key to good health was to accumulate as much of the three energies as possible, and to encourage their smooth flow in the body. To achieve such a purpose, one has to observe and practise various behavioural and dietary rules informed either by families, friends or Chinese medicine practitioners.

In her interview with some of the 20 Chinese medicine practitioners in Hong Kong during 1976-1978, McDermott (1986:192) found that not unlike their Western medicine counterparts, Chinese medicine practitioners often 'complained of their patients' bad living habits and the need for the patients to take more responsibility for their own health'. Thus, the focus of Chinese medicine practitioners is not only on medical treatment, but also on emphasising individual responsibility for health maintenance or illness prevention. In the eyes of Chinese medicine practitioners, patterns of living habit and nutrition become defined as health concerns and increasingly require individual efforts, or put in other words, informal health care in the form of self-care.

The emphasis of Chinese medicine on health maintenance and self responsibility constitutes the hallmark of the many 'holistic health' approaches. Lowenberg and Davis (1994) argue that these approaches move the locus of control for health back towards the self, and there is a tremendous emphasis placed on returning the responsibility for health, illness, and cure to the individual. Basically, the holistic model of health puts increasing emphasis on life-style modification. As Stone (1979:34) phrases it: 'Illness is seen here as an imbalance in the energy spheres of our emotional, rational, spiritual, physical and social selves. Healing is concerned with the individual balancing of these energies'.

For example, nutrition is of paramount importance in Chinese medicine. Lam et al. (1994) found that the commonest indication for self-medication was promotion of health (43.9%), and the majority of them used Chinese tonics for this purpose. Lee (1980) argues that it is a Chinese cultural belief that individuals need to take tonics regularly to maintain the body's equilibrium to prevent disease. In Chinese societies like Hong Kong, the division between food and medicine is not clear-cut. Chinese medicines are often cooked with other foods in the form of herbal soup or herbal tonic prepared by mother and taken by the whole family (Koo, 1982, 1989). Therefore, it is not surprising not to find any significant difference between the prevalence of self-medication in the different groups in the study of Lam et al. (1994).

The popularity of self-medication in the form of Chinese tonics is an indication of a sense of self-reliance and responsibility in the prevention of illness. However, this sense of self-responsibility for health maintenance has to be understood with particular reference to women's domestic health work in the family context. Topley (1976) emphasises that mothers play a key role in the health care of their families in Hong Kong. The mother is not only the first one to detect symptoms in her children, but she is the person who decides the course of treatment, either home-based treatment or the seeking of traditional or modern medical care, and also the one to take care of her sick family members. As discussed in Chapters 1 and 4, there is a stronger inclination of women than men towards a keen awareness of family health matters and in the pragmatic considerations in choosing traditional Chinese medicine or modern medicine. It is also found that in a modern Chinese society like Hong Kong, there still exists the tendency to blame women for certain diseases (Koo, 1987). Graham (1991) argues that women find themselves engaged in the care of family's health because they are engaged in the care of their family. In actual practice, family care or women's care has provided the context for realising the Chinese way of health maintenance emphasising so much the importance of self-responsibility or self-care.

The enhanced vitality of Chinese medicine consumption has major implications for providing the ideological and material context in expanding the role of self-care and family care in the area of health maintenance. If Chinese medicine practitioners can command more public confidence with the coming set-up of the registration system, their role in health maintenance or promotion would likely be enhanced. The moral overtones of living habits or life-style changes may place even wider areas of everyday life under the medical supervision and control of Chinese medicine practitioners. The relationship between the promotion of Chinese medicine and the promotion of self-care and healthy life-style is, however, subtle. It is because Chinese medicine is part of Hong Kong Chinese practice and part of the everyday life of Hong Kong people. As a result, with the increasing prevalence of Chinese medicine consumption, people may not be aware of the shift of responsibility more to individuals and families in taking care of their own health, or in strengthening the ideological orientation towards individual or family responsibility in maintaining healthy life-style or living habits.

Chinese Medicine and Medical Treatment The study of Lam et al. (1994) shows that Chinese medicines were used as often as Western medicines in the self-treatment of illnesses. The utilisation survey on Chinese medicine commissioned by the Working Party on Chinese Medicine (1991:para.4.7) showed that 73 per cent consulted a Western medicine doctor, 17 per cent resorted to self medication and 10 per cent consulted a Chinese medicine Practitioner. Thus, for most acute problems, there was no hesitation about consulting a Western medicine doctor for treatment if professional help rather than self-medication was deemed necessary. However, the utilisation survey showed a much higher proportion of respondents seeing a Chinese medicine practitioner as 'secondary action' if 'primary action' taken to seek professional help did not work: 47 per cent consulted a Western medicine doctor and 42 per cent consulted a Chinese medicine practitioner.

As far as medical help-seeking is concerned, Chinese medicine practitioners seem to fit into the same niche as chiropractors and homeopaths occupy in the West; they offer alternative professional services for those dissatisfied with Western medicine (Saks, 1994). However, Hong Kong people seem to adopt an eclectic approach in the use of Chinese and Western medicines for Chinese medicines prepared in the form of herbal soup or herbal tonics are used to complement Western medicine especially at the initial stage and the recuperation stage (Koo, 1987; 1989).

In a recent study on the pathway to health care for patients who had just finished consulting Chinese medicine practitioners at herbal shops, it was found that regarding the same sickness episode, nearly 30 per cent of respondents replied they had used a combination of both Chinese and Western medical services; and nearly 20 per cent of respondents had consulted Western medicine practitioners, then followed by Chinese medicine practitioners (Wong, 1998). In another study on the pathway to health care for orthopaedic inpatients in two regional hospitals in Hong Kong, it was found that more than half of the respondents (57.5%) had consulted bone-setting practice within the past six month prior to admission, which has a common concern with orthopaedics on health problems in connection with bones. Most respondents appeared to be assessing the degree of severity of bone problems and decided to go for bone-setting for some minor injuries. The study argued that bone-setting remains a popular quasi-formal treatment among other modes of health care for orthopaedic inpatients (Wong and Chiu, 1998). To the Hong Kong

Chinese, the use of Chinese medicine alone or in combination with Western medicine for dealing with health and illness is seemingly pragmatic in nature (Lee and Cheung, 1989; Koo, 1987). The two medical systems of Chinese medicine and Western medicine are not mutually exclusive; instead, they may perform complementary functions. Thus it appears more appropriate to describe Chinese medicine as complementary rather than alternative medicine in the context of Hong Kong.

As discussed before, the prevalence of chronic illnesses with which Western biomedicine has been largely ineffective in terms of treating or curing, has been viewed as a challenge to the official health care system nowadays. However, Chinese medicine is perceived by the public to have effectiveness in treating chronic illnesses (Lee, 1982; Koo, 1987). Moreover, Chinese medicine practitioners can explain in traditional etiological terms that patients can understand. Chinese medicine tends to adopt a multi-factorial approach in the understanding of etiological factors for disease. The focus is, however, more on life-style factors which are subjected to individual health actions in addition to the use of herbal medicine. As life-style becomes causative of illness, increasing emphasis is placed on life-style modifications, and individuals themselves are increasingly responsible for the treatment of chronic illness.

On the one hand, government's promotional measures applied to Chinese medicine play a role in recognising the role of Chinese medicine in treating diseases, in particular chronic illnesses. On the other hand, people's dissatisfaction with Western medicine in treating chronic illnesses may also encourage more and more people to seek Chinese medicine remedies in the health care market. Nowadays, more people will have experienced non-infectious health problems that linger on chronically, and which are usually not curable by Western medicine, will help to increase people's receptiveness to Chinese medicine both in terms of etiological explanations and methods of treatment. The implications of this trend of seeking Chinese medicine remedies may, in the long run, help to shift people's attention more to individual responsibility both in terms of financing the consumption of Chinese medicine, and in focusing on individual health actions. The increasing consumption of Chinese medicine for treating diseases, notably chronic illness, will enhance the role played by quasi-formal medicine not subsidised, though actively promoted, by the government. The increasing emphasis placed on modifying life-style patterns for the prevention and long-term treatment of chronic diseases will also increasingly enhance the individualistic orientation in health, and further expand the role of self-care or informal care as a consequence.

Chinese Medicine's Preparation: Labour-intensive and Time-consuming
In the survey commissioned by the Working Party on Chinese Medicine (1991:para.4.9), it is found that most herbalists (96%) prescribed herbal Chinese medicinal materials and only 11 per cent of them prescribed proprietary Chinese medicine which is now commonly available. An important factor for explaining this phenomenon is that the herbalists have to adjust the complex mix of different medicinal materials according to the particular physical constitution of the patient in order to produce the best effects. Because of this important factor, proprietary Chinese medicine, which can hardly be produced to suit every person's physical constitution, is rarely used alone. The domestic labour-intensive nature of the consumption of Chinese medicine incurs the (female) carers much physical energy and time in the preparation of Chinese medicine. Because of the inconvenience in relation to the use of herbal medicine, some herbal shops in Hong Kong also offer the service of medicine preparation. However, as the service is expensive, average patients could not afford to replace their own or family labour with this type of service. It is certain that herbal medicine will continue to be prepared and consumed within a family setting since it has not yet been recognised as part of formal medicine in Hong Kong. The increasing prevalence of Chinese medicine consumption will ultimately further increase the caring burden of women in taking care of their families' health.

The increasing receptiveness of Hong Kong people to Chinese medicine in health maintenance and medical treatment will further expand the role of informal care both in terms of care-for-self and care-for-others. The significance of informal care will be further reinforced not only by means of increasing the sphere of influence of Chinese medicine, but also by means of shifting more attention to individual responsibility and individual health actions. Alongside the expanding role of informal care with respect to the use of Chinese medicine, the consumption of Chinese medicine in the form of commodities may also shift the financial burden to individuals and families in health maintenance and medical treatment. It appears that the government has been actively encouraging the people of Hong Kong to resort to both Chinese and Western medicine, and 'integrate' the two approaches in one way or another by themselves, rather than to have both medical systems formally integrated by its active support. In other words, integration will continue to occur on 'users' level' rather than on 'institutional level' with individual preferences in medical care based mainly on a perception of the effectiveness of treatment and the nature and stage of illness and disease (Hyma and Ramesh, 1994). Precisely, the promotion of Chinese medicine is central to the state's re-shaping of the health care system in emphasising informal care and self-reliance both in terms of providing and financing health care.

'Family Care' Ideology and Informal Health Care

Domestication of Health Care

The government's emphasis placed on family responsibility in health care and Chinese medicine has signified the domestication of care in three interrelated areas: workplace for health work, labour functions and costs of health care.

Firstly, the site of health care or health work is much preferred to be the family - the only available 'community' to many elderly and chronically ill patients. The family as a domestic household can be represented as an informal workplace for health care in contrast with hospitals or clinics as formal ones providing 'professional' care. Feminists have already described the domestic household as a place where the majority of health care for both the dependent and able-bodied members is provided (Chapter 1). The shifting of health care from hospitals and infirmaries to families or patients' homes is conceived as a tactical move to cope with the long-term and non-acute health needs of patients. The family home 'should' be made available for not only as a place for residence but also a workplace catering for the health needs of the dependent members. As long as the trend is towards shifting the workplace to the home or domestic household, domestication of the health care workplace will take place irrespective of whether it is prompted by formal or informal providers. The domestication of the health care workplace does not necessarily require the dependent members to live with their family members. That is, domestication can be made possible as long as the workplace is a domestic household, and as long as informal or formal health care is provided within the living household of the care receiver.

In the use of Chinese medicine, the workplace for the preparation and final consumption of Chinese medicine is almost entirely confined to the home setting. Unlike the major concern of community health care strategy with respect to the dependent population, the promotion of Chinese medicine covers a wider scope to the extent of including the whole population for the purposes of both health maintenance and medical treatment. However, it is the government rather than the formal health care providers which appears to encourage the shifting of the health care workplace from the formal setting to the informal setting. Within the context of Hong Kong where there is a co-existence rather than an integration of Chinese medicine and Western medicine on the institutional level, it is very rare for Western medicine doctors to make patients referrals to Chinese medicine practitioners (Lee, 1980).

Secondly, another closely related process accompanied with the shifting from formal to household workplace is the transfer of labour functions from formal to family providers. It does not mean the provision of domiciliary health care with labour functions performed by paid labour. The labour functions performed by the family are involved in the production of informal health care which is used to supplement or enhance formal health care. The state has 'discovered' and expanded the family as a pool of valuable resources providing caring labour for its sick or dependent members. It has already been shown that priority is most often given to collective rather than domestic households as far as the provision of community health care services is concerned. Such a bias against domestic households has further perpetuated the domestication of labour functions for producing health care. The family is constructed not only as an 'ideal' place for health care, but also as potential resources for contributing caring labour. With regard to Chinese medicine, since it is not and will not be provided by formal health care providers, there will not be any shift of labour functions from the formal to family providers. Moreover, Chinese medicine practitioners and dispensers mainly provide consultation and dispensing services, while patients or their family members have to prepare the medicine or herbal soups by themselves. Thus, the use of Chinese medicine will still heavily rely on the labour functions performed by the individual or caregiver within a family context.

Thirdly, the domestication of health care also refers to the shifting of costs from the public sector to the family. It is within the context of cost containment that the informal sector, in particular the family, is implicitly viewed as a pool of unpaid caring labour that is not compensated by the state itself. That is, the shifting of labour functions from the formal sector to domestic households is not matched by the provision of adequate financial support. As discussed before, the social security system of Hong Kong is remedial in nature, and patients' needs, not to mention carers' needs, are not well addressed by the state. More often than not, families are left on their own to meet the needs of their chronically sick members. Moreover, costs are transferred to the family not only in terms of making use of its free caring labour, but also in terms of forcing it to be responsible for the extra medical expenditure incurred. The assumption is that the private wage earned by an individual family member can be and should be shared within the household. Such an assumption of putting an equal sign between private purse and family purse is similar to that held by neo-liberals (Chapter 1). As regards Chinese medicine, the case is simple. Users are totally responsible for financing the consumption of Chinese medicine, and the labour functions involved in the preparation of herbal medicine is taken for granted.

The domestication of health care is further reinforced by the policy and practice of regarding family care as the core of community care in the health and rehabilitation fields. The Working Group on Care for the Elderly (1994:para.71) re-affirms that people should be allowed to grow old in their home environment with minimal disruption. Although there is not the same explicit statement applied to the chronically ill or other dependants with a long-term need for help and support, policy and practice are similar since the goal is also aimed at keeping them out of institutional care and have them cared for in the domestic household.

The Working Group confirms that the premises of such a policy are consistent with community care policy applied to the care of old people proposed in 1973 and finally implemented ever since 1979. Firstly, it is assumed that old people would prefer to live in the familiar surroundings of their own home. Secondly, family members are believed to be capable of providing the best care for old people, and there is thus no exception to informal health care. The government asserts that informal care is superior since personal relationship involved in the caring process is irreplaceable. Thirdly, family members are expected to be most prepared than other community carers to care for their sick elderly members if they are provided with appropriate support or assistance from formal health care providers. Thus, the family has been viewed by the state as being central to the provision of both social and health care - a broad category of care and support provided by informal carers within the family context.

Community care can be the best form of care if it is properly resourced. However, in view of the inadequacy of community health care services in Hong Kong, the involvement of the informal sector in health care would largely mean the shifting of costs and work back to the family. The shifting of costs and work to the family is, to a great extent, obscured by the state's increasing emphasis placed on family responsibility or obligation in health care, and the paramount objective of cost containment in formal health care.

As regards the use of Chinese medicine, the government has made good use of the 'cultural' receptiveness of Hong Kong Chinese to Chinese medicine that will not be incorporated as part of the formal health care system. Because of the particular socio-cultural context of Hong Kong, it is not difficult to understand why the government can apply a 'cost-effective' approach to promoting the use of Chinese medicine. It should be emphasised that as death and pain are matters of great concern to patients, people are bound to be pragmatic and use whatever remedies which are believed to be effective. The prevalence of chronic illness may also be an important factor in boosting the demand for Chinese medicine, and thus further increase the domestication of health care in Hong Kong.

Family Care as Care by Women

The discourse of family responsibility for care of its members is implicitly built on the assumption that women are the most appropriate and available carers. In the Green and White Papers on Rehabilitation, it is stated that 'the responsibility for caring for disabled children, or other family members, usually lies with the wife or mother' (Hong Kong Government, 1992:para.2.18; 1995b:para.2.23). Thus women are most often under great psychological pressure induced by normative expectations to be responsible for their family's health as a whole. In a recent study on family care in a new town in Hong Kong, it was found that women (including daughter-in-law, wife, mother or daughter) are largely responsible for the care of the sick, elderly or disabled member(s) of the family (Chiu, Wong and Woo, 1993). The characteristic of the unequal gender division of informal care in the area of health is neither new nor exceptional (Stacey, 1988; Baldwin and Twigg, 1991). In Hong Kong today, this unequal gender division of labour in informal health care still remains very much the same despite the increase in female labour force participation, and the higher level of education of the female population.

The home or domestic household has traditionally been considered the 'women's natural domain' and caring is a 'natural female characteristic' (Sommers and Shields, 1987). Thus, the state takes for granted the health care work that women do in the domestic sphere, and sees it as an integral aspect of their caring role in the family. The practice of social policy continues to render the majority of women's health work invisible through lack of pay and lack of carers' benefits. This has well reflected the conception of women as occupying a family position primarily filling caring roles and only secondarily participating in the paid labour force (Estes and Swan, 1993). As a family's contribution in health care tends to be viewed as free and readily available resources, the magnitude of the sacrifices entailed by women's caregiving is obscured at best, and totally unrecognised at worst. Walker (1991:102) argues that there are three reasons for the state to reinforce the traditional division of caring labour along the line of gender. Firstly, the state has a direct financial interest in making use of the unpaid caring labour contributed by female carers. Secondly, the state avoids actions weakening family ties, and thus the gendered patterns of caring. (This point will be elaborated in more detail in the last sub-section). Thirdly, social policy is shaped by men and built upon a patriarchal society that is characterised by the dominant position of man and the subordinate one of women (Pascall, 1997). Through the implementation of the community health care strategy and the promotion of Chinese medicine, the traditional role of the family and thus the place for women has been further reproduced.

Since female carers predominantly perform the work of informal care, the economic and social costs of caring would be largely borne by them. The current provision of community health care and promotion of Chinese medicine continue to encourage the reproduction of 'double dependencies' in informal care. In such, family members have to depend on their families for the needs of care. At the same time, female informal carers have to be financially dependent on their husband because of the reduced opportunities in participating in the paid labour market as a result of performing caring work. In reality, current service provisions in health and rehabilitation fields depend on the uncompensated contribution of women's caring labour to maintain the provision. Their contribution is rendered invisible and is a 'socially constructed myth' to restrict their autonomy and confine them to the caring role. The normative expectation of family care as care by women is therefore reproduced.

Manthorple (1994:100) precisely summarises three levels of relationship between gender and informal health care that reinforce or perpetuate the gender division of labour in informal care. On a macro or policy level, the variable of gender is viewed as an available resource providing unpaid caring labour. On the mezzo or service delivery level, the presence of an available female member usually leads to a much lower priority for receiving formal support or service. In actual practice, the priority of service provision has long been given to those dependants without family (female carers') support in Hong Kong. Whereas in the case of Chinese medicine consumption, no formal support, except health education, is provided. Finally, on the micro-level women themselves may consider the tending of care as their duty or obligation, because they are normatively designated as carers. Walker (1991:106) argues that 'because family and other informal carers are constrained by normative obligations it is difficult for change to be achieved at an individual level'. Since the work of informal care is predominantly performed by female carers, the economic and social costs of caring would be disproportionately borne by them (Qureshi, 1990). The expanded role played by the family in informal health care will thus be largely operated on the basis of 'compulsory altruism' (Land and Rose, 1985) of the family and in particular, female kin.

Inadequacies and Limits of Informal Health Care

Within the context of Hong Kong, social policy in general and health care policy in particular have failed to examine in sufficient detail the dynamics and relations among the family, the community and the dependent themselves. The fact is that the government has not undertaken any study concerning the financial and caring burden that the family has to shoulder with respect to the likely increasing consumption of Chinese medicine. From the angle of the family, caring for their older or chronically ill members is an expensive one, physically, psychologically, emotionally and financially. Policy makers and health care providers are over-optimistic about the capacity of the family to provide continual and long-term care to look after its frail or chronically ill dependants. Because of the inadequate support given to the caring capacity of the family and the community, most of the caring load is passed back to the principal family caregivers who are mostly women themselves.

As informal care is largely provided through the bonds of kinship, those who are singletons or with fractured family networks can find themselves denied access to informal care. For example, the majority of older people in Hong Kong migrated into the territory after the end of the Second World War, and some of them have never succeeded in getting married (Ikels, 1983). Chu and Lo (1989) found that facing the 1997 issue, a substantial number of families, about 20,000 a year, had emigrated, very often leaving behind their elderly members. Besides, because women are more likely than men to live longer than their spouses, women are also more likely to be deprived of spousal care. In a study of the social support of cancer patients in Hong Kong, 16.7 per cent of respondents had no family members to look after them at all (Ma et al., 1990). Many elderly and chronically ill patients can therefore find themselves living alone on their own on the one hand, and on the other be excluded from both the formal and informal sectors of care.

In their study of disabled old people in two public housing estates in Hong Kong, Ngan and Kwok (1992) found that the size of the respondents' informal caring networks was negligible. The mean was 1.16 persons only, and over nine out of ten (91%) had a caring network size of not more than two persons. In fact, the availability of informal carers has been thrown in doubt with current ageing trend and increasing women's employment opportunities. For example, the White Paper on Rehabilitation states that 'the number of females in the labour force has increased by 15.6 per cent between 1983 and 1993, and the number of married females in the labour force increased by 20.8 per cent within the same period' (Hong Kong Government, 1995b:para.2.23). The notable growth in participation by women in paid work is partly accounted by the rising cost of living, and partly by the increasing emphases on owner occupation and consumption. As a result, many women have to work to cope with the pressures on household budgets. However, there is a contradiction between an economy that increasingly relies on women's labour and an increasing state's emphasis on expanding the role of the informal sector in the provision of both social and informal health care. Most women, especially those with dependent kin, are then torn between the formal and informal sectors as a result of the apparently contradictory demands upon their labour.

Female carers may be caught in a caring dilemma of either giving up a job to take care of their dependent members, or sorting out the problem by sending them to institutions against their own will. The former option is not without cost, both in terms of psychological stress and the opportunity cost of losing or quitting a job. The latter option may release the caring load but the carers may still feel obliged to provide informal care by themselves, and thus a strong feeling of guilt may result (Ngan and Kwok, 1994). Another possible option for female carers is to take up a full-time or part-time job, and continue to take care of their dependent members. Women carers of working class background may have no choice but to take up both sets of demand (Graham, 1991). It is apparent that the demand will be even heavier as these female carers have to play the dual role as care provider within the household and wage earner in the labour market.

Family Care and Self-reliance as Ideology

The discourse of informal health care or the call for increased family responsibility, whether made in an explicit or implicit way, has been central to the state mobilisation of uncompensated or unsubsidised resources for health care. However, the family and other informal carers, like friends and volunteers have already provided the bulk of long-term care. Thus, the re-emphasis put on family responsibility has to be understood with particular reference to the state's shaping of family care as ideology (Havas, 1995). Family care is portrayed by the state as the most appropriate form of care provided to dependants, both in terms of social organisation and preservation of Chinese culture (Chiu and Wong, 1998). The Social Welfare White Paper 1991 states that '[s]ocial networks are part of Chinese culture and tradition and have always existed in Hong Kong. They are most clearly demonstrated in the role of the family as the primary providers of care and welfare...' (Hong Kong Government, 1991:18).

The Working Group on Care for the Elderly (1994:para.74) also reveals a similar point of view as follows:

[t]he Chinese have traditionally relied on themselves and their families for assistance in times of need. Self-reliance, mutual support and a reluctance to be dependent on outside help are traditional Chinese values. These values are

still strong in Hong Kong, although there have been tremendous social and economic changes since the Pacific War.

As regards the promotion of Chinese medicine, the Working Party on Chinese medicine (1991:para.1.1) emphasises that '[Chinese medicine] is not just a traditional system of medical and health care but very much an integral part of Chinese culture'. The government's active promotion of Chinese medicine has indirectly strengthened Chinese culture in the sense of reinforcing the value of self-reliance and family care. It appears that the predominant role played by the family in the provision of care to its members is understood to be the reflection of the Chinese culture and tradition cherished by Hong Kong people. Most important of all, they are cherished and preserved by the state itself through social policies lest the ideological basis of family care should be undermined. While the increasing emphasis placed on informal health care, the policy of community health care and promotion of Chinese medicine appears to rest on a deeper ideological orientation about the role of families in providing care and welfare. In restructuring the health care organisation and delivery strategy, state policy emphasises continuity in 'family care' ideology upon which state intervention is based.

It also appears that the two respective strategies of promoting Chinese medicine and community health care also reflect the state's desire to further reinforce the prescriptive normative ideas and beliefs about the family which lie at the very foundation of the 'family care' or 'self-reliance' ideology. The importance and the needs of the carers have been identified in health field, but minimal aid is deemed by the state to be enough to strengthen the social organisation of care by the family. Whereas in the case of Chinese medicine, family care is entirely taken for granted. A proper and safe use of Chinese medicine has been officially emphasised, but no financial or tangible aid is given to individuals or families in the consumption of Chinese medicine. The family care ideology has played a role to legitimate the state's minimal support to the family. All this in turn perpetuates the ideological pressure upon families to take care of their dependants and family members.

Emphasis placed on the maintenance of Chinese culture in general and family responsibility and caregiving in particular diverts attention from broader structural problems of formal health care and the inadequacy of informal care, and consequently redirects attention toward the 'privatised' families. The discourse or social construction of informal health care and quasi-formal medicine is strongly reliant on self-responsibility and family responsibility. Such a conceptualisation tends to shift the responsibility of the state back to the family. This shift has given the state both political and economic advantages in assuming greater 'responsibilities' to enhance the integration of formal and informal health care and the promotion of Chinese medicine. In the health field, family care as ideology has adopted the notion of the family as source of health care support to its family members. Politically and economically, the family thus appears to be 'haven' to the state itself.

Conclusion

In an era emphasising cost containment in health care, the informal sector has been considered by the policy makers to be important in preventing institutionalisation and frequent hospitalisation of elderly and chronically ill patients. The role of the informal sector is set to be further expanded to cater for the long term needs of the dependent. The community health care strategy, which comprises a mix of social and health care services, is implemented to enhance informal health care and support to the carers so that the dependent can be kept at home as long as possible. Nevertheless, the discourse of informal health care largely features the contribution of the informal sector, and the family in particular, as free and available resource that should be further tapped by the health care providers. Moreover, in policy terms and in actual practice, the community health care strategy appears to marginalise those patients with family support.

The relationship between the promotion of Chinese medicine and the increasing emphasis placed on informal care is less explicit at first glance. With respect to the use of Chinese medicine, nothing has been mentioned about the needs of individuals or informal carers in official documents. However, the above discussion has shown that the use of Chinese medicine is strongly reliant on informal care, and is closely associated with individual or family health actions both for health maintenance and medical treatment purposes. As far as the use of Chinese medicine is concerned, self-care, family care or care by women is taken-for-granted. The further promotion of Chinese medicine and the more prevalent use of Chinese medicine will imply the expansion of informal care.

Social policy in general and health care policy in particular has reinforced the domestication of health care. The provision of informal health care within a domestic household is not a new phenomenon, but will be further expanded and exploited to tackle the problems of the formal health care system and the community-based long term care system in particular.

Already Hong Kong's major health care provider, the informal sector is expected to contribute more in the field of health and rehabilitation. Family-based care and quasi-formal or traditional Chinese medicine are seen as having a major role in tackling the problems in the public sector perpetuated by the high-tech orientation of Western medicine, the ageing trend and the prevalence of chronic illness. The 'family care' ideology, which is backed by the state's maintenance or preservation of Chinese cultural philosophy and practice, has played an important role in legitimating the increasing familial responsibility in health care, and in obscuring the heavy caring load of the informal (female) carers. The promotion of informal health care and quasi-formal medicine form the basis for shifting more caring responsibilities to the informal sector, with a less dominant role for the state in the financing or provision of health care and community-based long term care.

10 Conclusions

In this concluding chapter, I firstly aim to present a summary for the study. Then, I will propose major areas for further research or investigation, and make some speculations about the further development of health care in Hong Kong.

A Summary of the Theoretical Framework

Any picture of how the health care system develops and which direction health care reforms are heading towards in Hong Kong has to begin with a theoretical framework that can highlight the major elements or features shaping and reshaping health care policy. I suggest that the political economy perspective can provide a valuable framework for understanding how the polity, economy and society shape the field of health care within a capitalist society like Hong Kong. Precisely, the state has an important role in the formulation of health care policy and implementation of strategies and measures, but it has to consider the needs and context of capitalism, the political demand of its citizens on health care and the dominant power of the medical profession.

Informed by the political economy perspective, I suggest that the power of the state extends beyond the distribution of resources to the reproduction of social institutions, in particular the role of the family in formal and informal health care. Taking into specific consideration the local socio-cultural context, the role of Chinese medicine consumed in the form of quasi-formal medicine is included in examining the health care development and reforms in Hong Kong. The incorporation of the family and Chinese medicine in examining the political economy of health care development is considered essential - which is yet underdeveloped as an academic enquiry in Hong Kong.

Chapter 1 argues that the political economy of health care requires an expanded conceptualisation of resources for health consumption of which the private wage, the social wage and unpaid domestic labour are three major elements. This does not mean that they are the only resources for health consumption, but they provide the basis on which further analysis of state utilisation of societal resources can be made. Chapter 2 argues that focusing on the forms of state intervention in health care, rather than the entire health care systems, allows for a more in-depth analysis of the various changes with respect to the use of public medical services. A health care system is conceptualised as having three important interrelated constituent elements, namely access, financing and delivery, in influencing people's consumption or non-consumption of public sector health care. Chapter 3 is devoted to a critical examination of the clinical perspective of medicine, and the power, autonomy and dominance of the medical profession in the delivery and social organisation of health care. To illuminate the local context of Hong Kong, the professional dominance of the medical profession over Chinese medicine practitioners was also discussed.

A Summary of the Thesis

1) In spite of increasing state intervention in health care between 1945 and the mid-1980s, the period was also characterised by state utilisation of charity clinics, unregistered doctors and ex-subvented hospitals on the one hand, and the roles played by the family and Chinese medicine on the other. But the respective role of charity clinics, unregistered doctors and ex-subvented hospitals almost came to an end by the 1990s.

Between 1945 and 1950, state intervention in health care was minimal. Realising that immigrants were going to settle in the Colony, the state began to initiate planning for health care development in 1957, which finally led to the publication of the first Medical White Paper in 1964. This White Paper established the basis for the seemingly universalist practices of providing virtually free health care to the public for the next ten years until 1974. The second Medical White Paper published in 1974 further reaffirmed such practices even though citizens' right to health care was not mentioned at all. Within the constraints of maintaining a low-tax policy, the state gradually dominated in financing or providing expensive hospital care. As discussed in Chapters 4 and 5, in spite of its increasing intervention in health care before the health care reforms started, the state consistently highlighted the role played by the family in taking care of its sick and infirm members, and began to realise the importance of Chinese medicine in meeting part of the health care needs of the population since the mid-1960s.

Although the state had to play a very important role in subsidising hospital care provided by ex-subvented hospitals, it was initially able to capitalise the infrastructure set up by charitable organisations and to exploit the ongoing differences between ex-government and ex-subvented hospitals because health care practitioners or providers working in the latter type of hospitals were entitled to less attractive package of fringe benefits and promotion prospect than their counterparts employed within the civil service structure. However, the establishment of the Hospital Authority in the early 1990s finally brought an end to the government's exploitation of these differences.

As regards medical personnel, unregistered doctors played an important role in staffing the medical workforce of public hospitals and clinics especially from the end of the Second World War to the 1960s. Because of the availability of this type of doctor, charity clinics sponsored by different sorts of charitable organisations could run their services charging at low fees and with modest budgets. However, with the implementation of the revised Medical Ordinance 1963, the number of charity clinics employing unregistered doctor could no longer expand. Although there are still some one hundred charity clinics nowadays in Hong Kong, their role is undoubtedly insignificant. Moreover, the publication of the Report on Unregistrable Doctors in 1975 represented an end to the state's attempt to recruit unregistered doctors into its health services or to absorb these doctors into a proposed new roll of assistant medical practitioners.

2) *The health care reforms in Hong Kong since the mid-1980s have modified three important interrelated constituent elements of the health care system, namely access, financing and delivery, and such a modification has provided the state with the ideological and material context to expand the role of private spending in health care, including the cost recovery of public medical care, encouragement of private health insurance and market consumption of health care.*

Chapters 6 to 8 have shown that ever since the mid-1980s the three constituent elements of the public health care system, namely, access, financing and delivery, have gradually been reformed. The adoption of the safety-net approach is a strategy for the state to persuade the citizens to believe that to advocate for the universally free use of public medicine is beyond the original purposes of public health services. The pubic health care system is still open to universal use, but the state has used various justifications to legitimate its attempts to ask the patients and their families to contribute more towards their use of public medical services. Other more explicit criteria for rationing people's access to state-subsidised medicine have also increased, like itemised charges and means-testing on family rather than individual income. Some of the chronic patients' demands are also redirected to the market via the application of the shared care approach. In addition to expanding the role of out-of-pocket payment, the desire of the state to promote private health insurance via the regulation approach is also an attempt to contain the growth of the state's involvement in financing health services. As regards the element of delivery, the B-class product is an innovation which has greater potential for cost recovery. If the semi-private bed scheme can be widely introduced, it may have the effect of stimulating the growth of private health insurance and further blurring the boundaries of health care delivery between the public and private sectors. Confronting strong political pressures and opposition from some politicians and the public, the pricing structure of public sector health care cannot be completely reformed as the state would like to see, at least in the short run. Moreover, confronting the private health care providers' opposition to the implementation of the scheme of B-class bed at the moment, the promotion of private financing via the scheme and the state's approach to regulating private health insurance has become something uncertain. However, all the above changes have provided the state with an ideological context, and in some cases, a material context, which is amenable to expanding the role of private spending or financing in health care and redirecting of patients' demand for market consumption of health care.

3) *The health care reforms undertaken in Hong Kong have further expanded the roles of the informal sector and unsubsidised Chinese medicine in resourcing health care, and the family has been central to such a re-shaping of the health care system in Hong Kong.*

The health care reforms undertaken in Hong Kong have also placed increasing emphases on establishing a closer interface between the formal and informal health care system on the one hand; and on promoting the use of Chinese medicine in the form of quasi-formal medicine on the other hand. The re-organised community health care strategy is implemented to achieve the former objective; while the preparation for the registration of Chinese medicine practitioners and the promotion of the use of Chinese medicine are to achieve the latter objective. These two measures tend to further expand the roles of the informal sector and unsubsidised Chinese medicine in resourcing health care both in terms of unpaid caring labour and self-financing of health care. The expanding role played by the informal sector and Chinese medicine would reinforce the trend of the domestication of health care in three ways: gradual shifting of workplace, labour functions and cost of care from the formal sector back to the family that has been central to the reshaping of the health care system in Hong Kong. However, the state's making use of the 'cultural' receptiveness of Hong Kong people to Chinese medicine and the family care ideology obscures this process. In turn, the domestication of health care may further reinforce or strengthen the family care ideology in the context of Hong Kong.

Major Areas for Further Research

Based on the study, I propose two major areas for further research and investigation: firstly, the complexity of the relationship between formal, informal and quasi-formal health care, and secondly, the reshaping of the boundaries between public, market and informal sectors.

Redefine the Scope of Health Care

The complex relationship between formal and informal care has been well recognised especially in the study of the care of older people (Walker, 1991; Estes and Swan, 1993). The study of alternative medicine (quasi-formal medicine) and the response of the medical profession towards it has also begun to develop (Saks, 1995). However, the relationship between informal health care and quasi-formal medicine has not yet been explicitly identified as an important area for academic research and investigation. The study is so far the first one highlighting the complex relationship between informal health care and the use of Chinese medicine consumed in the form of quasi-formal medicine in the Hong Kong context.   In the Western world, alternative medicine has attracted increasing attention with respect to its effectiveness in handling certain diseases and its low-cost approach to health and illness.   While in China and some South-East Asian societies, like Singapore, Taiwan and Hong Kong, Chinese medicine plays a significant role despite the continuing dominance of Western medicine and the medical profession (Lee, 1982; Chi, 1994; Quah, 1989; Wong and Chiu, 1997).   Unlike alternative medicine in the West, Chinese medicine is viewed more as 'complementary' medicine and is part of the socio-cultural practices in these societies, and this may explain why people in these societies are more receptive to Chinese medicine mostly consumed in the form of quasi-formal medicine.   The inadequacy of Western medicine in explaining and curing many chronic illnesses is also identified as an important factor in boosting the demand for Chinese medicine in the local context.   The complex relationship and dynamics between these three forms of health care, and how they are perceived and reshaped by different parties, like the state, the medical profession, the family, Chinese medicine practitioners and patients themselves are certainly important and challenging areas for further academic research and investigation.

Reshaping and Blurring the Boundaries Between Public, Market and Informal Sectors

The health care reforms are important not just because of their material and ideological impact but because of the reshaping and blurring of the boundaries between public, market and informal sectors.   Private health insurance may be increasingly used to finance public health care, and further expand the private sub-system within the public health care system.   The state may also encourage the development of the public-private interface by means of applying regulatory change, contracting out, promoting managed competition or internal market, employing fiscal measures to stimulate the growth of private health insurance, etc. (Johnson, 1995).   In addition, the state may also further expand the role of the informal sector by shifting the workplace for health, labour functions and cost of care to the informal sector, in particular the family.   The trend of domestication discussed in the study has served to increasingly blur the boundaries between the public and informal sectors in the field of health. Formal market provision of domiciliary services is, in most countries, still relatively under-developed.   At present, the most extensive development appears to have been in the US (Twigg, 1994). In an era of health care reforms, these three sectors no longer exist side-by-side as separate or independent entities but are closely interrelated and have their boundaries further blurred. All this is worth researching in depth.

The Future: Some Speculations

Further Development of the Six Strategies

Health care reforms are very unlikely to be reversed and will therefore be further extended into the next century. Health care problems and health care reforms would still capture increasing attention from policy makers, politicians, the mass media and the public. Dominated by the objective of cost-containment, it is likely that the six strategies identified, namely, the safety-net approach, the shared care approach, introduction of B-class beds, promotion of private health insurance, adoption of a community health care strategy, and promotion of Chinese medicine will continue to be experimented or implemented. The pace of each strategy will not be the same, and the government will still be 'politically sensitive' to the reactions of the public, politicians and the medical profession.

However, changes will gradually take place and the role of private spending and informal health care will be further expanded. It is estimated that the increase of fees and charges for public medicine will induce most public criticism. The trends of the domestication of health care and increasing stress put on female caregivers will most likely continue, and the state will still manoeuvre the family care or self reliance ideology to obscure all these processes.

Further Development of Chinese Medicine

So far, Mainland China is the only Chinese society to fully and formally integrate Western medicine and Chinese medicine. With the change of sovereignty in Hong Kong after June 30, 1997, Chinese medicine may therefore get a better chance for further development. China has rich experience in the use and development of Chinese medicine, and lots of academic and experienced personnel involved in the research and delivery of Chinese medicine. Moreover, alongside the coming registration of Chinese medicine practitioners, the training and education of Chinese medicine practitioners is now formally incorporated into the tertiary education system of Hong Kong. This indeed will help promote the status of Chinese medicine and that of its practitioners as well. Academics may have more research interest in Chinese medicine and its relationship with social policy. The medical profession in Hong Kong may also show increasing interest in Chinese medicine, and in the future, there may have some co-operation between the medical profession and Chinese medicine practitioners both in the areas of research and practice.

However, in the foreseeable future at least, the status of Chinese medicine would not be changed from quasi-formal medicine to formal medicine. There are two reasons for this. First, the Government of the Hong Kong Special Administrative Region would not risk subsidising people's self-initiated demand for Chinese medicine so as to prevent itself from allocating extra public health care resources. Second, the medical profession in Hong Kong is still very critical of the seemingly unscientific basis of Chinese medicine, and is determined to protect its economic and social interests from being undermined by alternative health care providers. The fact is that even though Mainland China has incorporated Chinese medicine into the formal health care system, the medical profession of Western medicine still holds the dominant power in the distribution of resources and delivery of health care. Therefore Chinese medicine will continue to prosper in the market, but its status as a quasi-formal medicine being kept out of the formal health care system, in particular hospital medicine, is likely to continue for a long period.

Concluding Remarks

The political economy perspective is suggested in this book as a sound theoretical framework for critically examining health care development and reforms in Hong Kong. The study has also highlighted the respective role of informal health care and Chinese medicine consumed in the form of quasi-formal health care and their complex relationship with formal health care in the local context. I shall be more than satisfied if this piece of study can contribute towards further academic inquiries in the fields of health policy and health care.

Bibliography

Aaron, H.J. and Schwartz, W.B. (1984), *The Painful Prescription - Rationing Hospital Care*, The Brookings Institution, Washington.

Abbott, A. (1988), *The System of Professions: An Essay on the Division of Expert Labour*, University of Chicago Press, Chicago.

Abel, E.K. (1993), 'Negotiating Dignity: Family Caregivers and Formal Health Care Providers', *Research in the Sociology of Health Care*, vol. 10, pp. 177-191.

Abel-Smith, B. (1976), *Value for Money in Health Services*, Heinemann, London.

Abel-Smith, B. (1992), *Cost Containment and New Priorities in Health Care: A Study of the European Community*, Avebury, Aldershot.

Abel-Smith, B. (1994), *An Introduction to Health: Policy, Planning and Financing*, Longman, London.

Aday, L.A. (1994), 'Equity, Accessibility, and Ethical Issues: Is the US Health Care Reform Asking the Right Question?', in P.V. Rosenau (ed) *Health Care Reform in the Nineties*, Sage, California.

Advisory Committee on Clinics, Hong Kong Government (1966), *Report of Advisory Committee on Clinics*, Government Printer, Hong Kong.

Advisory Committee on Reviewing the Doctor Problem in the Hong Kong Government Service, Hong Kong Government (1969), *Report of the Committee Appointed to Review the Doctor Problem in the Hong Kong*

Alford, R. (1972), 'The Political Economy of Health Care: Dynamics without Change', *Politics and Society*, vol. 2, pp. 127-64.

Allen, I. (ed) (1993), *Rationing of Health and Social Care*, PSI, London.

Anderson, E.N. and Anderson, M.L. (1975), 'Folk Dietetics in Two Chinese Communities, and its Implications for the Study of Chinese Medicine', in A. Kleinman, P. Kunstadter, E.R. Alexander, and J.L. Gale (eds) *Medicine in Chinese Cultures: Comparative Studies of Health Care in Chinese and other Societies*, US Department of Health, Education and Welfare and National Institution of Health, New York.

Appleby, J. (1992), *Financing Health Care in the 1990s*, OUP, London.

Armstrong, D. (1987), 'Bodies of Knowledge: Foucault and the Problem of Human Anatomy', in G. Scambler (ed) *Sociological Theory and Medical Sociology*, Tavistock Publications, London.

Arrow, K.J. (1963), 'Uncertainty and the Welfare Economics of Medical Care', *American Economic Review*, vol. Liii, Dec, 1993, pp. 941-73.

Atkinson, A.B. and Stiglitz, J.E. (1980), *Lectures on Public Economics*, McGraw-Hill, Maidenhead.

Atkinson, P. (1988), 'Discourse, Descriptions and Diagnoses: Reproducing Normal Medicine', in M. Lock and D. Gordon (eds) *Biomedicine Examined*, Kleuwer Academic Publishers, London.

Baer, H.A., Singer, M. and Johnsen, J.H. (1986), 'Toward a Critical Medical Anthropology', *Social Science and Medicine*, vol. 23, no. 2, pp. 95-8.

Bailey, S.J. and Bruce, A. (1994), 'Funding the National Health Service: the Continuing Search for Alternatives', *Journal of Social Policy*, vol. 23, no. 4, pp. 489-516.

Ball, J. (1993), 'First the Baby, Now the Nuptials: An Interview with Elizabeth Wong, Secretary for Health and Welfare', *Hong Kong Accountant*, Sept/Oct, 1993.

Bamford, T. (1993), 'Rationing: A Philosophy of Care', in I. Allen (ed) *Rationing of Health and Social Care*, Policy Studies Institute, London.

Barber, B. (1963), 'Some Problems in the Sociology of Professions'. *Daedalus*, vol. 92, pp. 669-88.

Barry, J. and Jones, C. (eds) (1991) *Medicine and Charity before the Welfare State*, Routledge, London.

Bauman, S. (1988), *Freedom*, Open University Press, Milton Keynes.

Bennett, L., May, C. and Wolfson, D.J. (1994) 'Sharing Care between Hospital and the Community: A Critical Review of Developments in the UK', *Health and Social Care*, vol. 2, no. 2, pp. 105-112.

Bennholdt-Thomsen, V. (1981), 'Subsistence Production and Extended Reproduction', in K. Young, C. Wolkowitz and R. McCullagh (eds) *Of Marriage and the Market*, CSE Books, London.

Berlant, J.L. (1975), *Profession and Monopoly: A Study of Medicine in the United States and Great Britain*, University of California Press, Berkeley.

Binney, E.A. and Swan, J.H. (1990), 'The Political Economy of Mental Health Care for the Elderly', in M. Minkler, and C.L. Estes (eds) *Critical Perspectives on Aging: The Political and Moral Economy of Growing Old*, Baywood, New York.

Birdsall, N. (1994), 'Pragmatism, Robin Hood, and Other Themes: Good Government and Social Well-being in Developing Countries', in L.C. Chen, A. Kleinman and N.C. Ware (eds) *Health and Social Change in International Perspective*, Havard University Press, Boston.

Black, D. (1993), 'Inequalities in Health', in D.E. Rogers and E. Ginzberg (eds) *Medical Care and the Health of the Poor*, Westview Press, Boulder.

Bond, J. (1992), 'The Politics of Caregiving: The Professionalisation of Informal Care', *Aging and Society*, vol. 12, pp. 5-21.

Boorse, C. (1975), 'On the Distinction Between Disease and Illness'. *Philosophy and Public Affairs*, vol. 5, pp. 49-68.

Brody, E.M. and Brody, S.J. (1989), 'The Informal System of Health Care', in C. Eisdorfer, D.A. Kessler and A.N. Spector (eds) *Caring for the Elderly: Reshaping Health Policy*, The Johns Hopkins University Press, Baltimore.

Brody, S., Poulshock, S. and Masciocchi, C. (1978), 'The Family Caring Unit: A Major Consideration in the Long-term Care Support System', *The Gerontologist*, vol. 18, pp. 555-561.

Brown, E.H.P. (1971), 'The Hong Kong Economy: Achievements and Prospects', in K. Hopkins (ed) *Hong Kong, The Industrial Colony: A Political, Social and Economic Survey*, Oxford University Press, Hong Kong.

Burrows, R. and Marsh, C. (eds) (1992), *Consumption and Class: Divisions and Change*, St. Martin's Press, New York.

Busfield, J. (1990), 'Sectoral Divisions in Consumption: The Case of Medical Care', *Sociology*, vol. 24, no. 1, pp. 77-96.

Busfield, J. (1992), 'Medicine and Markets: Power, Choice and the Consumption of Private Medical Care', In R. Burrows and C. Marsh (eds) *Consumption and Class: Divisions and Change*, St. Martin's Press, New York.

Business and Professionals Federation of Hong Kong (1991), *A Review of Benefits for the Elderly and a Policy for the Provisions of Social Security and Retirement Benefits in Hong Kong*, BPF, Hong Kong.

Calnan, M., Cant, S. and Gabe, J. (1993), *Going Private: Why People Pay for Their Health Care*, Open University Press, Buckingham.

Caplan, R.L. (1989), 'The Commodification of American Health Care', *Social Science and Medicine*, vol. 3, no. 1, pp. 104-13.

Castells, M. (1973), 'Advanced Capitalism, Collective Consumption and Urban Contradictions', in L.N. Lindberg et al. (eds) *Stress and Contradiction in Modern Capitalism*, Lexington D.C.Heath.

Castells, M. (1978), *City, Class and Power*, MacMillan, London.

Census and Statistics Department, Hong Kong Government (1961), *Hong Kong Census, 1961: Population Projections 1961-1971*, Government Printer, Hong Kong.

Census and Statistics Department, Hong Kong Government (1969), *Hong Kong Statistics 1947-1967*, Government Printer, Hong Kong.

Census and Statistics Department, Hong Kong Government (1972), *Annaul Digest of Statistics 1971*, Government Printer, Hong Kong.

Census and Statistics Department, Hong Kong Government (1986), *Report on the Household Expenditure Survey 1984-85*, Government Printer, Hong Kong.

Census and Statistics Department, Hong Kong Government (1990), *Annual Digest of Statistics 1989*, Government Printer, Hong Kong.

Census and Statistics Department, Hong Kong Government (1991), *Report on the Household Expenditure Survey 1989-90,* Government Printer, Hong Kong.

Census and Statistics Department, Hong Kong Government (1992), *Monthly Statistics 1992*, Government Printer, Hong Kong.

Census and Statistics Department, Hong Kong Government (1993), 'Medical Benefits Provided by Employer/Company and Medical Insurance', *Social Data Collected by the General Household Survey: Special Topics Report No. VIII*, Government Printer, Hong Kong.

Census and Statistics Department, Hong Kong Government (1995), *Annual Digest of Statistics 1994*, Government Printer, Hong Kong.

Central Policy Unit, Hong Kong Government (1993), 'Background Information', Paper Presented at Seminar *After Retirement: Income Support in an Aging Population* organised CPU of Hong Kong Government, Hong Kong.

Chan, C. et al. (1992), *Report of a Survey of the Members of Self-Help Groups for Persons with Chronic Illness in Hong Kong*, Department of Social Work and Social Administration, University of Hong Kong, Hong Kong.

Chan, C.M.A. et al. (1993), *Comparative Experience of Psychological Symptoms of Frail Elderly People in Need of Residential Care*, Department of Applied Social Studies, City Polytechnic of Hong Kong, Hong Kong.

Cheal, D. (1990), 'Social Construction of Consumption', *International Sociology*, vol. 5, no. 3, pp. 299-317.

Cheng, D.W.L. (1986), 'The Aspect of International Commercial Relations', in A.Y.H. Kwan and D.K.K. Chan (eds) *Hong Kong Society: A Reader*, Writers' and Publishers' Cooperative, Hong Kong.

Cheung, A.B.L. (1994), 'Medical and Health', in D.H. McMillen and S.W. Man (eds) *The Other Hong Kong Report 1994*, The Chinese University Press, Hong Kong.

Chi, C.H. (1994), 'Integrating Traditional Medicine into Modern Health Care Systems: Examining the Role of Chinese Medicine in Taiwan', *Social Science and Medicine*, vol. 39, no. 3, pp. 307-321.

Chi, I. and Lee, J.J. (1989), *A Health Survey of the Elderly in Hong Kong*, Department of Social Work and Social Administration, the University of Hong Kong, Hong Kong.

Childress, J. (1987), 'Sociocultural Metaphors', in H. Schwartz (ed) *Dominant Issues in Medical Sociology* (2nd ed.), Random House, New York.

Ching, F. (1993), 'Politics, Politicians and Political Parties', in P.K. Choi and L.S. Ho (eds) *The Other Hong Kong Report 1993*, The Chinese University Press, Hong Kong.

Chiu, S.W.S. and Wong, V.C.W. (1998), 'Social Policy in Hong Kong: from British Colony to Special Administrative Region of China', *European Journal of Social Work*, vol. 1, no. 2, pp. 231-242.

Chiu, S.W.S., and Yu, S.W.K. (1992), 'The Paradox of Social Service Privatization in Hong Kong', *Hong Kong Journal of Social Work*, vol. 26, no.1, pp. 13-20.

Chiu, S.W.S., Wong, V.C.W. and Woo, J. M.L. (1993), *An Exploratory Study of Family Needs and Family Support in Yuen Long District*, Yuen Long District Board, Hong Kong (in Chinese).

Choa, G.H. (1967), 'Chinese Traditional Medicine and Contemporary Hong Kong', in M. Topley (ed) *Some Traditional Chinese Ideas and Conceptions in Hong Kong Social Life Today*, The Hong Kong Branch of the Royal Asiatic Society, Hong Kong.

Choa, G.H. (1981), *The Life and Times of Sir Kai Ho Kai - A Prominent Figure in Nineteenth-Century Hong Kong*, The Chinese University Press, Hong Kong.

Chow, C. (1956), *The Honorary Secretary's Annual Report, Hong Kong Chinese Medical Association, 1955-56*, Hong Kong Chinese Medical Association, Hong Kong.

Chow, N.W.S. (1982), 'Development and Functions of Social Services in Hong Kong', in J.Y.S. Cheng (ed) *Hong Kong in the 1980s*, Summerson Eastern Publishers, Hong Kong.

Chow, N.W.S. (1986a), 'The Image of the Elderly and Their Need for Community Support Services', in T.P. Khoo (ed) *Mental Health in Hong Kong 1986*, Mental Health Association of Hong Kong, Hong Kong.

Chow, N.W.S. (1986b), 'A Review of Social Policies in Hong Kong', in A.Y.H. Kwan and D.K.K. Chan (eds) *Hong Kong Society: A Reader*, Writers' and Publishers' Cooperative, Hong Kong.

Chow, N.W.S. (1987), 'Factors Influencing the Support of the Elderly by their Families', *Hong Kong Journal of Gerontology*, vol. 1, no. 1, pp. 4-9.

Chow, N.W.S. (1988), *Caregiving for the Elderly Awaiting Admissions into Care and Attention Homes*, Department of Social Work and Social Administration, The University of Hong Kong, Hong Kong.

Chow, N.W.S. (1992), 'Hong Kong: Community Care for Elderly People', in P.R. Phillips (ed) *Ageing in East and South East Asia*, Edward Arnold, London.

Chow, N.W.S. (1994), 'Social Welfare Development in Hong Kong - An Ideological Apprisal', in B.K.P. Leung and T.Y.C. Wong (eds) *25 Years of Social and Economic Development in Hong Kong*, Centre of Asian Studies, The University of Hong Kong, Hong Kong.

Chu, D.K.W. (1988), *Cost-effectiveness of General Hospitals under Two Different Hospital Reimbursement Systems: An International Study of Hong Kong and Indiana*, Unpublished PhD thesis, University of Indiana, Indiana.

Chu, D.K.W. (1992), 'Global Budgeting of Hospitals in Hong Kong', *Social Science and Medicine*, vol. 35, no. 7, pp. 857-868.

Chu, I.P.L. and Lo, K.Y. (1989), 'An Exploratory Study on Adjustment of the Elderly Separated from Family Members Who Had Emigrated to Overseas Countries', *Hong Kong Journal of Gerontology*, vol. 3, no. 2, pp. 34-36.

Churchill, L.R. (1987), *Rationing Health Care in America: Perceptions and Principles of Justice*, University of Notre Dame Press, Nortre Dame, Indiana.

Coburn, D., Torrance, G. and Kaufert, J. (1983), 'Medical Dominance in Canada in Historical Perspective', *International Journal of Health Services*, vol. 13, pp. 407-432.

Commission of Inquiry, Hong Kong Government (1966), *Report on Kowloon Disturbances 1966*, Government Printer, Hong Kong.

Committee on Community Nursing Service, The (1973), *Bridging the Gaps: A Report on Community Nursing in Hong Kong*, The Committee on Community Nursing Service, Hong Kong.

Conrad, P. (1989), 'The Experience of Illness: Recent and New Directions', *Research in the Sociology of Health Care*, vol. 6, pp. 53-69.

Conrad, P. and Brown, P. (1993), 'Rationing Medical Care: A Sociological Reflection', *Research in the Sociology of Health Care*, vol. 10, pp. 3-22.

Contandriopoulos, A-P., Lesemann, F. and Lemay, A. (1995) 'Canada', in N. Johnson (ed) *Private Markets in Health and Welfare: An International Perspective*, Berg, Oxford.

Corbin, J.M., and Strauss, A. (1988), *Unending Work and Care: Managing in the Home*, Jossey-bass, San Francisco.

Culyer, A.J. (1971), 'The Nature of the Commodity Health Care and Its Efficient Allocation', *Oxford Economic Papers*, vol. 5, pp. 293-313.

Culyer, A.J., Maynard, A. and Posnett, J. (eds) (1990), *Competition in Health Care: Reforming the NHS*, MacMillan, Oxford.

Davies, D.P. (1989), 'Doctors at Large - So Much to Learn, But Too Little Time: An Educational Challenge to Clinical Teaching in the Undergraduate years', *Hong Kong Practitioner*, vol. 11, no. 10, pp. 490-499.

Davies, S.N.G. (1977), 'One Band of Politics Rekindled', *Hong Kong Law Journal*, vol. 7, pp. 44-80.

De Kadt, E. (1982), 'Ideology, Social Policy, Health and Health Services: A Field of Complex Interactions', *Social Science and Medicine*, vol. 16, pp. 741-752.

Dickinson, J. and Russell, B. (eds) (1986), *Family, Economy and Society: The Social Reproduction Process under Capitalism*, Croom Helm, London.

Donaldson, C. and Gerard, K. (1993), *Economics of Health Care Financing: The Visible Hand*, Macmillan, London.

Doorslaer, E.V., Wagstaff, A. and Rutten, F. (eds) (1993), *Equity in the Finance and Delivery of Health Care: An International Perspective*, Oxford University Press, Oxford.

Doty, P. (1986), 'Family Care of the Elderly: The Role of Public Policy', *The Milbank Quarterly*, vol. 64, no. 1, pp. 34-75.

Downey, M.J. (ed) (1993), *Hong Kong Staff Employment Manual*, Asia Law and Practice Ltd, Hong Kong.

Doyal, L. (1979), *The Political Economy of Health*, Pluto Press, London.

Eastern Express, 1 June 1995.

Economist, 2 November 1968.

Education Department, Hong Kong Government (1971), 'Hong Kong', in UNESCO (ed) *World Survey of Education*, UNESCO, Paris.

Edwards, M. (1981), 'Financial Arrangements within Families', *Social Security Journal*, vol. 7, pp. 1-16.

Ellencweig, A.Y. (1992), *Analysing Health Systems: A Modular Approach*, Oxford University Press, Oxford.

Elling, R.H. (1994), 'Theory and Method for the Cross-National Study of Health Systems', *International Journal of Health Services*, vol. 24, no. 2, pp. 285-309.

Elston, M.A. (1991), 'The Politics of Professional Power: Medicine in a Changing Health Service', in J. Gabe, M. Calnan and M. Bury (eds) *The Sociology of the Health Service*, Routledge, London.

Endacott, G.B. (1958), *A History of Hong Kong*, Oxford University Press, Hong Kong.

Endacott, G.B. (1964), *Government and People in Hong Kong 1841-1962: A Constitutional History*, Hong Kong University Press, Hong Kong.

Endacott, G.B. and Hinton, A. (1962), *Fragrant Harbour: A Short History of Hong Kong*, Greenwood Press, Connecticut.

England, J. and Rear, J. (1981), *Industrial Relations and Law in Hong Kong*, Oxford University Press, Hong Kong.

Enthoven, A.C. (1988), *Theory and Practice of Managed Competition in Health Care Finance*, Elsevier Science Publishers, Amsterdam.

Estes, C.L. and Swan, J.H. and Associates (1993), *The Long Term Care Crisis - Elders Trapped in the No-Care Zone*, Sage, Newsbury Park.

Evans, D.E. (1987), *Constancy of Purposes: An Account of the Foundation and History of the Hong Kong College of Medicine and the Faculty of Medicine of the University of Hong Kong 1887-1987*, Hong Kong University Press, Hong Kong.

Evans, R.G. (1984), *Strained Mercy: the Economics of Canadian Medical Care*, Butterworths, Toronto.

Evans, R.G. (1989), 'The Canadian Health Care System: The Other Part of North America is Rather Different', Paper presented at *International Symposium on Health Care Systems*, December 18-19, 1989, Taipei, Taiwan.

Fein, R. (1989), *Medical Care, Medical Costs: The Search for a Health Insurance Policy*, Harvard University Press, Massachusetts.

Field, M.G. (1989), 'Introduction', in M.G. Field (ed) *Success and Crisis in National Health Systems: A Comparative Approach*, Routledge, London.

Folland, S., Goodman, A.C. and Stano, M. (1993), *The Economics of Health and Health Care*, MacMillan, New York.

Foucault, M. (1973), *The Birth of the Clinic: An Archaeology of Medical Perception*, Translated by S. Smith, Pantheon, New York.

Freidson, E. (1970), *Profession of Medicine*, Dodd, Mead, New York.

Freidson, E. (1983), 'The Theory of Professions - State of the Art', in R. Dingwall and P. Lewis (eds) *The Sociology of the Professions*, MacMillan, London.

Freidson, E. (1985), 'The Reorganisation of the Medical Profession', *Medical Care Review*, vol. 42, pp. 11-35.

Frenk, J. (1993), 'The Public/Private Mix and Human Resources for Health', *Health Policy and Planning*, vol. 8, no. 4, pp. 315-326.

Frenk, J. and Donabedian, A. (1987), 'State Intervention in Medical Care: Types, Trends and Variables', *Health Policy and Planning*, vol. 2, pp. 17-31.

Friedland, R. and Sanders, J. (1986), 'Private and Social Wage Expansion in the Advanced Market Economies', *Theory and Society*, vol. 15, pp. 193-222.

Fuchs, V. (1974), *Who Shall Live? Health, Economics and Social Choice*, Basic Books, New York.

Fuchs, V. (1986), *The Health Economy*, Harvard University Press, Massachusetts.

Fulcher, D. (1974), *Medical Care Systems: Public and Private Health Coverage in Selected Industrialized Countries*, International Labour Organisation, Geneva.

Fung, H.L. (1992), 'Privatising the Medical Service: The Call for a Comprehensive Medical Insurance Scheme for Hong Kong', *Hong Kong Journal of Social Work*, vol. XXVI, no. 1, pp. 28-34.

Fung, W.Y.L. (1991), 'Proposed Framework for the Better Delivery of Contract Medicine', in Hong Kong Medical Association *Discussion Paper on Contract Medicine for Another Open Forum on 24 July 1991*, HKMA, Hong Kong.

Gabe, J., Kelleher, D. and Williams, G. (eds) (1994), *Challenging Medicine*, Routledge, London.

George, V. and Wilding, P. (1984), *The Impact of Social Policy*, RKP, London.

Gerhardt, U. (1989), *Ideas about Illness: An Intellectual and Political History of Medical Sociology*, New York University Press, New York.

Gerhardt, U. (1990), 'Patient Careers in End Stage Renal Failure', *Social Science and Medicine*, vol. 30, no. 11, pp. 1211-1224.

Gershuny, J. (1982), 'Household Tasks and the Use of Time', in S. Wallman (ed) *Living in South London*, Gower, Aldershot.

Giddens, A. (1984), *The Constitution of Society*, Polity Press, Cambridge.

Gill, D. (1980), *The British National Health Service*, Department of Health and Human Services, New York.

Ginzberg, E. (1990), *The Medical Triangle: Physicians, Politicians and the Public*, Harvard University Press, Cambridge, Mass.

Glaser, W.A. (1991), *Health Insurance in Practice: International Variations in Financing, Benefits, and Problems*, Jossey-Bass Publishers, San Francisco.

Glendinning, C. (1992), *The Costs of Informal Care: Looking Inside the Household*, HMSO, London.

Glennerster, H. (1992), *Paying for Welfare: The 1990s*, Harvester Wheatsheaf, London.

Goldberg, D. and Jackson, G. (1992), 'Interface between Primary Care and Specialist Mental Health Care', *British Journal of General Practice*, vol. 42, pp. 267-269.

Gough, I. (1979), *The Political Economy of the Welfare State*, MacMillan, London.

Government Secretariat, Hong Kong Government (1987), *Report on the Delivery of Medical Services in Hospital - A Summary of Public Opinion*, Government Printer, Hong Kong.

Government Secretariat, Hong Kong Government (1992), *Consultation Paper: A Community-wide Retirement Protection System*, Government Printer, Hong Kong.

Government Secretariat, Hong Kong Government (1994), *A Consultation Paper on the Government's Proposals for an Old Age Pension Scheme*, Government Printer, Hong Kong.

Graham, H. (1984), *Women, Health and the Family*, Wheatsheaf, Brighton.

Graham, H. (1985), 'Providers, Negotiators, and Mediators: Women as the Hidden Carers', in E. Lewin and V. Olesen (eds) *Women, Health, and Healing: Toward a New Prspective*, Tavistock Publication, London.

Graham, H. (1987), 'Women's Poverty and Caring', in C. Glendinning and J. Millar (eds) *Women and Poverty in Britain*, Wheatsheaf, Bridgton.

Graham, H. (1991), 'The Informal Sector of Welfare: A Crisis in Caring?', *Social Science and Medicine*, vol. 32, no. 4, pp. 507-515.

Grantham, Sir Alexander (1965), *Via Ports: From Hong Kong to Hong Kong*, Hong Kong University Press, Hong Kong.

Green, D. (1986), *Which Doctor?*, Institute of Economic Affairs, London.

Griffin, C.C. (1992), *Health Care in Asia: A Comparative Study of Cost and Financing*, Regional and Sectoral Studies, World Bank, Malaysia.

Habermas, J. (1984), *The Theory of Communicative Action, Volume I: Reason and Rationalisation in Society*, Translated by T. McCarthy, Heinemann, London.

Hadden-Cave, P. (1980), 'Introduction: The Making of Some Aspects of Public Policy in Hong Kong', in D.G. Lethbridge (ed) *The Business Environment in Hong Kong*, Oxford University Press, Hong Kong.

Ham, C.J. (1985), *Health Policy in Britain: The Politics and Organisation of the National Health Service* (2nd ed), MacMillan, London.

Hambro, E. (1955), *Hong Kong Refugee Survey Mission, The Problem of Chinese Refugees in Hong Kong: Report Submitted to the United Nations High Commissioner for Refugees*, United Nations, Leyden.

Harris, C. (1983), *The Family and Industrial Society*, Allen and Unwin, London.

Harris, P. (1978), *Hong Kong: A Study in Bureaucratic Politics*, Heinemann Asia, Hong Kong.

Harris, R. (1969), *A Sacred Trust*, Penguin Books, Baltimore.

Harrison, S. (1991), 'Working the Markets: Purchaser/Provider Separation in English Health Care', *International Journal of Health Services*, vol. 21, no. 4, pp. 625-635.

Harrison, S., Hunter, D.J. and Pollitt, C. (1990), *The Dynamics of British Health Policy*, Routledge, London.

Haug, M. (1981), 'The Erosion of Professional Authority: A Cross-Cultural Inquiry in the Case of the Physician', in J. McKinlay (ed) *Health Care Consumers, Professionals, and Organizations*, MIT Press, Cambridge.

Haug, M.R. (1990), 'The Interplay of Formal and Informal Health Care: Theoretical Issues and Research Needs', *Advances in Medical Sociology*, vol. 1, pp. 207-231.

Havas, E. (1995), 'The Family as Ideology', *Social Policy and Administration*, vol. 29, no. 1, pp. 1-9.

Hay, J.W. (1992), *Health Care in Hong Kong: An Economic Policy Assessment*, The Chinese University Press, Hong Kong.

Hedley, A.J. et al. (1990), *Surveys on Health and Medical Care in Hong Kong*, Department of Community Medicine, the University of Hong Kong and Department of Health, Hong Kong Government, Hong Kong.

Helms, R.B. (ed) (1993), *Health Care Policy and Politics: Lessons from Four Countries*, The AEI Press, Washington, D.C.

Henke, K-D. (1992), 'Cost Containment in Health Care: Justification and Consequences', in P. Zweifel and H.E. Frech, III (eds) *Health Economics Worldwide*, Kluwer Academic Publishers, Boston.

Heung, S.K. (1990), *Towards Building a Theoretical Model of Welfare Policy Development: The Case of Health Care Policy in Advanced Capitalist Countries*, Unpublished PhD thesis, University of Illinois, Illinois.

Hewitt, M. (1992), *Welfare, Ideology and Need: Developing Perspectives on the Welfare State*, Harvester Wheatsheaf, Hertfordshire.

Higgins, J. (1988), *The Business of Medicine: Private Health Care in Britain*, Macmillan Education, London.

Hodge, P. (1976), 'The Poor and the People of Quality: Social Policy in Hong Kong', *Hong Kong Journal of Social Work*, vol. X, no. 2, pp. 2-17.

Hodge, P. (1981), 'The Politics of Welfare', in J.F. Jones (ed) *The Common Welfare: Hong Kong's Social Services*, Chinese University Press, Hong Kong.

Holliday, I. (1992), *The NHS Transformed*, Baseline Books, Manchester.

Hollinsworth, J.R., Hage, J. and Hanneman, R.A. (1990), *State Intervention in Medical Care: Consequences for Britain, France, Sweden, and the United States, 1890-1970*, Cornell University Press, Ithaca.

Holton, R.J. and Turner, B.S. (1986), *Talcott Parsons on Economy and Society*, Routledge, London.

Hong Kong Council of Social Service (1995), *Submission for the Governor's 1995 Policy Address*, HKCSS, Hong Kong.

Hong Kong Government (1949), *Hong Kong Annual Report 1948*, Government Printer, Hong Kong.

Hong Kong Government (1950), *Hong Kong Annual Report 1949*, Government Printer, Hong Kong.

Hong Kong Government (1960), *Hong Kong Annual Report 1959*, Government Printer, Hong Kong.

Hong Kong Government (1961), *Hong Kong Annual Report 1960*, Government Printer, Hong Kong.

Hong Kong Government (1963), *Hong Kong Annual Report 1962*, Government Printer, Hong Kong.

Hong Kong Government (1964), *Development of Medical Services in Hong Kong*, Government Printer, Hong Kong.

Hong Kong Government (1965), *Aims and Policy for Social Welfare in Hong Kong: A White Paper*, Government Printer, Hong Kong.

Hong Kong Government (1967), *A Report by the Inter-Departmental Working Party to Consider Certain Aspects of Social Security*. Hong Kong: Government Printer.

Hong Kong Government (1973), *Social Welfare in Hong Kong: The Way Ahead*, Government Printer, Hong Kong.

Hong Kong Government (1974), *The Further Development of Medical and Health Services in Hong Kong*, Government Printer, Hong Kong.

Hong Kong Government (1977a), *Help for Those Least Able to Help Themselves: A Programme of Social Security Development*, Government Printer, Hong Kong.

Hong Kong Government (1977b), *Hong Kong Hansard 1976-7*, pp. 827-30, Government Printer, Hong Kong.

Hong Kong Government (1977c), *Green Paper: Service for the Elderly*, Government Printer, Hong Kong.

Hong Kong Government (1979), *Social Welfare into the 1980's*, Government Printer, Hong Kong.

Hong Kong Government (1982), *Hong Kong Hansard 1982*, Government Printer, Hong Kong.

Hong Kong Government (1991), *Social Welfare into the 1990s and Beyond*, Government Printer, Hong Kong.

Hong Kong Government (1992), *Equal Opportunities and Full Participation: A Better Tomorrow For All*, Government Printer, Hong Kong.

Hong Kong Government (1993a), *Towards Better Health*, Government Printer, Hong Kong.

Hong Kong Government (1993b), *Hong Kong Hansard 1993*, Government Printer, Hong Kong.

Hong Kong Government (1995a), *Government Gazette*, GN(S) 66 of 1995, Government Printer, Hong Kong.

Hong Kong Government (1995b), *White Paper on Rehabilitation: Equal Opportunities and Full Participation: A Better Tomorrow for All*, Government Printer, Hong Kong.

Hong Kong Legislative Council (1993), *Hong Kong Legislative Council Paper* No. 4260/92-93, Government Printer, Hong Kong.

Hong Kong Medical Association (1991), *Discussion Paper on Contract Medicine for Another Open Forum on 24 July 1991*, HKMA, Hong Kong.

Hong Kong Medical Association (1992), *Opinion Survey on Health Care Financing*, HKMA, Hong Kong.

Hong Kong Medical Association (1993), *Medical and Dental Directory of Hong Kong*, HKMA, Hong Kong.

Hong Kong National Committee, International Conference of Social Work (1966), *Urban Development, Implications for Social Welfare: The Hong Kong Report*, A Report submitted to the The Thirteenth International Conference of Social Work, September, 1966, Washington D.C.

Hong Kong Special Administrative Region Government (1997), *The 1997 Policy Address: Progress Report*, Government Printer, Hong Kong.

Hong Kong Standard, 1 June 1995; 2 November 1995; 29 November, 1995.

Hong Kong Workers' Health Centre (1993), *Report of a Survey of the Needs of Pneumoconiotics*, HKWHC, Hong Kong (in Chinese).

Hospital Authority (1993), *Answers to Questions raised by Hon Mr. Li Wah-ming on 6 November, 1993*, Unpublished materials, Hospital Authority, Hong Kong.

Hospital Authority (1994), *Hospital Authority Business Plan 1994-1995*, Hospital Authority, Hong Kong.

Hospital Authority (1995), *Annual Plan 1995-1996*, Hospital Authority, Hong Kong.

Hospital Authority (1998), *Hospital Authority Annual Plan 1998-1999*, Hospital Authority, Hong Kong.

Huang, C.Y. (1991), 'Medical and Health', in Sung, Y.W. and Lee M.K. (eds) *The Other Hong Kong Report 1991*, The Chinese University Press, Hong Kong.

Hyma, B. and Ramesh, A,. (1994), 'Traditional Medicine: Its Extent and Potential for Incorporation into Modern National Health Systems', in D.R. Phillips and Y. Verhasselt (eds) *Health and Development*, Routledge, London.

Ikels, C. (1983), *Aging and Adaptation: Chinese in Hong Kong and the United States*, Archon, Connecticut.

Illich, I. (1975), *Medical Nemesis*, Calder & Boyars, London.

James, J.H. (1993), 'Health Care Rationing: Lessons from a District Health Authority', in Allen, I. (ed) *Rationing of Health and Social Care*, Policy Studies Institute, London.

Johnson, N. (ed) (1995), *Private Markets in Health and Welfare: An International Perspective*, Berg, Oxford.

Johnson, T. (1972), *Professions and Power*, MacMillan, London.

Jones, L.J. (1994), *The Social Context of Health and Health Work*, MacMillan, London.

Joseph, M. (1994), *Sociology for Nursing and Health Care*, Polity Press, Cambridge.

Judge, K. (1980), *Pricing the Social Service*, MacMillan, London.

Judge, K. and Methews, J. (1980), *Charging for Social Care*, George Allen and Unwin, London.

Kelman, S. (1971), 'Towards a Political Economy of Health Care', *Inquiry*, vol. 8, pp. 30-8.

Kelman, S. (ed) (1975), 'Special Section on Political Economy of Health', *International Journal of Health Service*, vol. 5, pp. 535-642.

Kennedy, I. (1981), *The Unmasking of Medicine*, Allen & Unwin, London.

Kerr, M. and Charles, N. (1986), 'Servers and Providers', *Sociological Review*, vol. 34, pp. 115-57.

Klein, R. (1983), *The Politics of the National Health Service*, Longman, London.

Klein, R. (1989), *The Politics of the NHS*, Longman, London.

Knapp, M. (1984), *The Economics of Social Care*, MacMillan, London.

Kohn, R. and White, K.L. (1976), *Health Care: An International Study*, Oxford University Press, Oxford.

Konner, M. (1993), *The Trouble with Medicine*, BBC Books, London.

Koo, L.C. (1987), 'Concepts of Disease Causation, Treatment and Prevention among Hong Kong Chinese: Diversity and Eclecticism', *Social Science and Medicine*, vol. 25, no. 4, pp. 405-417.

Koo, L.C. (1982), *Nourishment of Life*, Hong Kong Commerical Press, Hong Kong.

Koo, L.C. (1989), 'Ethnomedicine in Hong Kong: Local Concepts of Disease Causation, Treatment and Prevention', *Hong Kong Practitioner*, vol. 11, no. 4, pp. 178-183.

Kuan, C.H. (1958), *Report of the Honorary Secretary of Hong Kong Chinese Medical Association for the Year 1957/58*, Hong Kong Chinese Medical Association, Hong Kong.

Kwok, J. and Yueng, T.W. (1993), 'Income Allowance and Rehabilitation: Hong Kong's Challenges into the 21st Century', in Hong Kong Council of Social Services (ed) *Asia Regional Conference on Social Security - A Conference Proceeding*, HKCSS, Hong Kong.

Labour Department, Hong Kong Government (1960), *Annual Departmental Report 1959*, Government Printer, Hong Kong.

Lam, C.L.K. et al. (1994), 'Self-Medication Among Hong Kong Chinese', *Social Science and Medicine*, vol. 39, no. 12, pp. 1641-1647.

Land, H. and Rose, H. (1985), 'Compulsory Altruism or an Altruistic Society for All?', in Bean, P. et al., *In Defence of Welfare*, Tavistock, London.

Larkin, G.V. (1988), 'Dominance in Britain: Image and Historical Reality', *The Milbank Quarterly*, vol. 66, suppl. 2, pp. 117-32.

Larson, M. (1978), *The Rise of Professionalism*, Universitty of California Press, Berkeley.

Law, R.C.L. (1993), 'The Integration of Private and Public Specialist Medical Services in Hong Kong - A Necessary Evil?', in Hong Kong Medical Association (ed) *Medical and Dental Directory of Hong Kong*, Hong Kong Medical Association, Hong Kong.

Le Grand, J. (1982), *The Strategy of Equality*, Allen & Unwin, London.

Le Grand, J. and Estrin, S. (eds) (1989), *Market Socialism*, Oxford University Press, Oxford.

Le Grand, J. and Robinson, R. (1984), 'Privatisation and the Welfare State: An Introduction', in J. Le Grand and R. Robinson (eds) *Privatisation and the Welfare State*, George Allen & Unwin, London, pp.1-18.

Lee, C.Y. (1990), *Statement by the Joint Committee on Medical Services*, Hong Kong Confederation of Trade Unions, Hong Kong.

Lee, R.P.L. (1975), 'Health Services System in Hong Kong: Professional Stratification in a Modernizing Society', *Inquiry*, vol. 12, pp. 51-62.

Lee, R.P.L. (1980), 'Perceptions and Uses of Chinese Medicine among the Chinese in Hong Kong', *Culture, Medicine and Psychiatry*, vol. 4, pp. 345-75.

Lee, R.P.L. (1981), 'Chinese and Western Health Care Systems: Professional Stratification in a Modernizing Society', in A.Y.C. King and R.P.L. Lee (eds) *Social Life and Development in Hong Kong*, Chinese University Press, Hong Kong.

Lee, R.P.L. (1982), 'Comparative Studies of Health Care Systems', *Social Science and Medicine*, vol. 16, pp. 629-642.

Lee, R.P.L. and Chueng, Y.W. (1989), 'Receptivity to Traditional Chinese and Modern Medicine among Chinese Adolescents in Hong Kong', in S.R. Quah (ed) *The Triumph of Practicality: Tradition and Modernity in Health Care Utilization in Selected Asian Countries*, Institute of Southeast Asian Studies, Singapore.

Leichter, H. (1979), *A Comparative Approach to Policy Analysis: Health Care Policy in Four Nations*, Cambridge University Press, Cambridge.

Leong, C.H. (1987), 'The Medical Profession at Its Crossroad', in Hong Kong Medical Association (ed) *Medical Directory of Hong Kong* (1987 ed), Hong Kong Medical Association, Hong Kong.

Leung, B.K.P. (1990), 'Power and Politics: A Critical Analysis', in Leung, B.K.P. (ed), *Social Issues in Hong Kong*, Oxford University Press, Hong Kong.

Leung, J.C.B. (1994), 'Comunity Participation: Past, Present, and Future', in B.K.P. Leung and T.Y.C. Wong (eds) *25 Years of Social and Economic Development in Hong Kong*, Hong Kong University Press, Hong Kong.

Lewis, C.E. and Lewis, M.A. (1977), 'The Potential Impact of Sexual Equality on Health', *The New England Journal of Medicine*, no. 297, p. 863.

Lichtig, L.K. (1986), *Hospital Information Systems for Case Mix Management*, John Wiley & Sons, New York.

Lichtman, R. (1971), 'The Political Economy of Medical Care', in H. Dreitzel (ed) *The Social Organisation of Health*, Macmillan, New York.

Light, D. (1995), 'Countervailing Powers: A Framework for Professions in Transition', in T. Johnson, G. Larkin and M. Saks (eds) *Health Professions and the State in Europe*, Routledge, London.

Light, D.W. and Schuller, A. (1986), *Political Values and Health Care: The German Experience*, MIT Press, Cambridge.

Little, V.C. (1979), 'Planning and Delivering Elderly Services: The Hong Kong Experience', *Hong Kong Journal of Social Work*, vol. XII, no. 1.

Liu, E. and Wong, E. (1997), *Health Care for Elderly People*, Research and Library Services Division, Provisional Legislative Council Secretariat, Hong Kong.

Lo, S.H. (1988), 'Decolonization and Political Development in Hong Kong: Citizen Participation', *Asian Survey*, vol. 28, pp. 613-29.

Lo-Cheng, S.S. (1990), *Public Budgeting in Hong Kong: An Incremental Decision-Making Approach*, Writers' & Publishers' Cooperative, Hong Kong.

Lock, S. (1986), 'Self Help Groups - the Fourth Estate in Medicine', *British Medical Journal*, vol. 293, pp. 159-160.

Lopez-Casasnovas, G. (ed) (1989), *Incentives in Health Systems*, Springer-Verlag, Berlin.

Lowenberg, J.S. and Davis, F. (1994), 'Beyond Medicalisation-Demedicalisation: the Case of Holistic Health', *Sociology of Health and Illness*, vol. 16, no. 5, pp. 579-599.

Luft, H. and Miller, R.H. (1988), 'Patient Selection in a Competitive Health System', *Health Affairs*, vol. 7, no. 3, pp. 97-119.

Lupton, D. (1994), *Medicine as Culture: Illness, Disease and the Body in Western Societies*, Sage, London.

Ma J.L.C. et al. (1990), *A Study of the Social Support of Cancer Patients Receiving Chemotherapy in Hong Kong*, Department of Social Work and Social Adminsitration, the University of Hong Kong, Hong Kong.

Mackenzie, D.J.M. (1961), *Report on the Outbreak of Cholera in Hong Kong Covering the Period 11th August to 12th October, 1961*, Government Printer, Hong Kong.

MacLehose, Sir Murray (1973), *Governor Speech at the 1973/74 Opening Session of the Legislative Council*, Government Printer, Hong Kong.

Macleod, Sir Hamish (1994), *Managing Prosperity: 1994-95 Budget*, Government Printer, Hong Kong.

Malcolm, L. (1994), 'Primary Health Care and the Hospital: Incompatible Organisational Concepts?', *Social Science and Medicine*, vol. 39, no. 4, pp. 455-458.

Manthorple, J. (1994), 'Family and Informal Care', in N. Malin (ed) *Implementing Community Care*, Open University Press, Buckingham.

Marmor, T.R. (1995), 'Patterns of Fact and Fiction in the Use of Canadian Experience', in D. Seedhouse (ed) *Reforming Health Care: The Philosophy and Practice of International Health Reform*, Wiley, Chichester.

Martin, C.J. (1994), 'Managing National Health Reform: Business and the Politics of Policy Innovation', in P.V. Rosenaur (ed) *Health Care Reform in the Nineties*, Sage, California.

Marx, K. (1970), *A Contribution to the Critique of Political Economy*, International Publishers, New York.

Maxwell, R. (1974), *Health Care, The Growing Dilemma: Needs Versus Resources in Western Europe, the U.S., and the U.S.S.R.*, McKinsey and Co., New York.

McDermott, K. (1986), 'Community Health and Reform in Hong Kong', *Social Science and Medicine*, vol. 23, no. 2, pp. 191-199.

McDouall, J.C. and Keen, K. (1955), 'The Kaifong Welfare Association', *Community Development Bulletin*, vol. 7, no. 1.

McGhee, S. (1995), 'Shared Care: From Theory to Practice', in Hospital Authority (ed) *Proceedings of the Hospital Authority Convention '95*, Hospital Authority, Hong Kong.

McIntosh, M. (1979), 'The Welfare State and the Needs of the Dependent Family', in Burman, S. (ed) *Fit Work for Women*, Croom Helm, London.

McKee, J. (1988), 'Holistic Health and the Critique of Western Medicine', *Social Science and Medicine*, vol. 26, no. 8, pp. 775-784.

McKeown, T. (1971), 'A Historical Appraisal of the Medical Task', in G. McLachlan and T. McKeown (eds) *Medical History and Medical Care*, Oxford University Press, London.

McKeown, T. and Record, A. (1963), 'Reasons for the Decline of Mortality in England and Wales during the Nineteenth Century', *Population Studies*, vol. 16, pp. 94-122.

McKeown, T., Brown, R. and Record, R. (1972), 'An Interpretation of the Modern Rise of Population in Europe', *Population Studies*, vol. 26, pp. 345-82.

McKinlay, J. et al. (1989), 'A Review of the Evidence Concerning the Impact of Medical Measures on Recent Mortality and Morbidty in the United States', *International Journal of Health Services*, vol. 19, no. 2, pp. 181-208.

Medical and Health Department, Hong Kong Government (1949), *Annual Departmental Report for 1948/49*, Government Printer, Hong Kong.

Medical and Health Department, Hong Kong Government (1951), *Annaul Departmental Report for 1950/51*, Government Printer, Hong Kong.

Medical and Health Department, Hong Kong Government (1957), *Annual Departmental Report for 1956/57*, Government Printer, Hong Kong.

Medical Development Advisory Committee (1979), *The 1979 Review of the Medical Development Programme*, Government Printer, Hong Kong.

Miliband, R. (1977), *Marxism and Politics*, Oxford University Press, Blackwell.

Miller, D. (1990), *Market, State and Community: Theoretical Foundations of Market Socialism*, Clarendon Paperbacks, Oxford.

Miners, N. (1989), 'Constitutional Reform in Hong Kong, 1945-1952 and 1984-1989', *Asian Journal of Public Administration*, vol. 11, no. 1, pp. 92-103.

Miners, N. (1991), *The Government and Politics of Hong Kong* (5th ed), Oxford University Press, Hong Kong.

Miners, N. (1994), 'The Transformation of the Hong Kong Legislative Council 1970-1994: From Consensus to Confrontation', *Asian Journal of Public Administration*, vol. 16, no. 2, pp. 224-248.

Ming Pao, 16 May 1994; 18 July 1994; 31 October 1994.

Mishler, E.G. et al. (1981), *Social Contexts of Health, Illness, and Patient Care*, Cambridge University Press, Cambridge.

Mishra, R. (1984), *The Welfare State in Crisis: Social Thought and Social Change*, Wheatsheaf Books, Sussex.

Mishra, R. (1990), *The Welfare State in Capitalist Society: Policies of Retrenchment and Maintenance in Europe, North America and Australia*, Harvester Wheatsheaf, New York.

Mok, H.T.K. (1994), 'Elderly in Need of Care and Financial Support', in D.H. McMillen and S.W. Man (eds) *The Other Hong Kong Report 1994*, The Chinese University Press, Hong Kong.

Morgan, M., Calnan, M. and Manning, N. (1985), *Sociological Approaches to Health and Medicine*, Croom Helm, London.

Moroney, R.M. (1980), *Families, Social Services and Social Policy*, Department of Health and Human Services, US.

Mullen, P.M. (1990), 'Which Internal Market? The NHS White Paper and Internal Markets', *Financial Accountability and Management*, vol. 6, no. 1, pp. 33-50.

Murphy, H. (1994), 'Making the Patient Pay: Are Hong Kong's Doctors Getting Away with Financial Murder?', *Window*, September 2, 1994, pp. 33-37.

Mushkat, M. (1982), *The Making of the Hong Kong Adminsitrative Class*, Centre of Asian Studies, University of Hong Kong, Hong Kong.

Myles, J. (1991), 'Editorial: Women, the Welfare State and Care-giving', *Canadian Journal on Aging*, vol. 10, no. 2, pp. 82-85.

Navarro, V. (1975), 'The Political Economy of Medical Care', *International Journal of Health Service*, vol. 5, no. 1, pp. 65-94.

Navarro, V. (1976), *Medicine Under Capitalism*, Prodist, New York.

Nettleton, S. (1992), *Power, Pain and Dentistry*, Open University Press, Buckingham.

Nettleton, S. (1995), *The Sociology of Health and Illness*, Polity Press, Cambridge.

Ng, A. (1990), 'Medical and Health', in R.Y.C. Wong and J.Y.S. Cheng (eds) *The Other Hong Kong Report 1990*, The Chinese University Press, Hong Kong.

Ngan, R.M.H. (1990), 'The Availability of Informal Support Networks to the Chinese Elderly in Hong Kong and Its Implications for Practice', *Hong Kong Journal of Gerontology*, vol. 4, no.2, pp. 19-25.

Ngan, R.M.H. and Kwok, J. (1992), 'Informal Caring Network among Chinese Elderly with Disabilities in Hong Kong', *International Journal of Rehabilitation Research*, vol. 15, pp. 199-207.

Ngan, R.M.H. and Kwok, J. (1993), 'Assisting Disabled Chinese Old People through Informal Caring Network', *Asia Pacific Journal of Social Work*, vol. 3, no. 2, pp. 21-29.

Ngan, R.M.H. and Kwok, J. (1994), 'The Politics of Community Care: From Rhetoric to Reality', in Hong Kong Council of Social Service (ed) *International Conference on Family and Community Care - Conference Proceedings*, HKCSS, Hong Kong.

Northcott, H.C. (1983), 'Who Stays Home? Working Parents and Sick Children', *International Journal of Women's Studies*, vol. 6, pp. 387-394.

O'Connor, J. (1973), *The Fiscal Crisis of the State*, St. Martin's, New York.

OECD (1992), *The Reform of Health Care: A Comparative Analysis of Seven OECD Countries*, OECD, Paris.

OECD (1996), *Health Care Reform: The Will to Change*, OECD, Paris.

Offe, C. (1984), *Contradictions* of the Welfare State, Hutchinson, London.

Offe, C. and Ronge, V. (1982), 'Thesis on the Theory of the State', in Giddens, A. and Held, D. (eds) *Classes, Poser and Conflict*, University of California Press, Berkeley.

Open University (1985a), *Care for Health: History and Diversity*, Open University Press, London.

Open University (1985b), *Medical Knowledge: Doubt and Certainty*, Open University Press, London.

Orme, M. (1991), 'How to Pay for Expensive Drugs', *British Medical Journal*, vol. 303, pp. 593-594.

Øvretveit, J. (1995), *Purchasing for Health*, Open University Press, London.

Owen, N.C. (1971), 'Economic Policy', in Hopkins, K. (ed) *Hong Kong, The Industrial Colony: A Political, Social and Economic Survey*, Oxford University Press, Hong Kong.

Pahl, J. (1988), 'Earning, Sharing, Spending', in R. Walker and G. Parker (eds) *Money Matters*, Sage, London.

Parsons, T. (1937), *The Structure of Social Action*, McGraw-Hill, New York.

Parsons, T. (1951), *The Social System*, RKP, London.

Parsons, T. and Smelser, N.J. (1956), *Economy and Society*, RKP, London.

Pascall, G. (1997), *Social Policy: A Feminist Analysis*, Routledge, London.

Patten, C. (1993), *Governor Speech at the 1992/93 Opening Session of the Legislative Council*, Government Printer, Hong Kong.

Pepper Commission (1990), *A Call for Action, US Bipartisan Commission on Comprehensive Health Care*, US Government Printing Office, Washington DC.

Pierson, C. (1991), *Beyond the Welfare State? The New Political Economy of Welfare*, Polity Press, Cambridge.

Pirie, M. and Butler, E. (1988), *The Health Alternatives*, Adam Smith Institute, London.

Pneumoconiosis Mutual Aid Association (1994), *Report of a Survey of the Opinion of the Members of Pneumoconiosis Mutual Aid Society on the Compensation Ordinance*, PMAC, Hong Kong (in Chinese).

Portes, A., Castells, M. and Benton, L. (1989), *The Informal Economy*, Johns Hopkins University Press, Baltimore.

Pratt, L. (1976), *Family Structure and Effective Health Behaviour: The Energized Family*, Houghton Mifflin Co, Boston.

Preparatory Committee on Chinese Medicine (1997a), *Report of the Preparatory Committee on Chinese Medicine*, Government Printer, Hong Kong.

Preparatory Committee on Chinese Medicine (1997b), *Consultation on the Development of Traditional Chinese Medicine*, Government Printer, Hong Kong.

Preteceille, E. and Terrail, J-P. (1985), *Capitalism, Consumption and Needs*, Translated by S. Matthews, Basil Blackwell, Oxford.

Provisional Hospital Authority (1989), *Provisional Hospital Authority Report*, Government Printer, Hong Kong.

Quah, S.R. (ed) (1989), *The Triumph of Practicality: Tradition and Modernity in Health Care Utilization in Selected Asian Countries*, Institute of Southeast Asian Studies, Singapore.

Qureshi, H. (1990), 'Boundaries Between Formal and Informal Caregiving Work', in C. Ungerson (ed) *Gender and Caring*, Harvester Wheatsheaf, London.

Qureshi, H. and Walker, A. (1986), 'Caring for Elderly People: the Family and the State', in C. Phillipson and A. Walker (eds) *Ageing and Social Policy: A Critical Assessment*, Gower, England.

Qureshi, H. and Walker, A. (1989), *The Caring Relationship: Elderly People and Their Families*, Temple University Press, Philadelphia.

Rabushka, A. (1976), *Value for Money: The Hong Kong Budgetary Process*, Hoover Institution Press, Standford.

Radley, A. (1994), *Making Sense of Illness: The Social Psychology of Health and Disease*, Sage, London.

Raffel, M.W. (ed) (1984), *Comparative Health Systems: Descriptive Analyses of Fourteen National Health Systems*, Pennsylvania State University Press, Pennsylvania.

Rayack, E. (1967), *Professional Power and American Medicine: The Economics of the American Medical Association*, The World Publishing Company, New York.

Rear, J. (1971), 'The Law of the Constitution', in Hopkins, K. (ed) *Hong Kong: The Industrial Colony*, Oxford University Press, Hong Kong.

Reisman, D. (1993), *The Political Economy of Health Care*, St Martin's Press, New York.

Renaud, M. (1975), 'On the Structural Constraints to State Intervention in Health', *International Journal of Health Services*, vol. 5, no. 4, pp. 559-72.

Renaud, M. (ed) (1977), 'Special Issue on the Political Economy of Health', *Review of Radical Political Economy*, vol. 9, Spring.

Renshaw, J. et al. (1988), *Care in the Community: the First Steps*, Gower, Aldershot.

Rhodes, D. (1985), *An Outline of History of Medicine*, Butterworth, London.

Rodrigues, A. et al. (1966), *Special Committee on Higher Education Interim Report 1966*, Government Printer, Hong Kong.

Roemer, M.I. (1991), *National Health Systems of the World* (two volumes), Oxford University Press, New York.

Roemer, M.I. (1993), 'National Health Systems Throughout the World', *Annual Review of Public Health*, vol. 14, pp. 335-53.

Roth, J. and Ruzek, S. (eds) (1986), *Research in the Sociology of Health Care, Vol 4: The Adoption and Social Consequences of Medical Technologies*, JAI Press, Connecticut.

Russell, E. (1986), 'Self-care - Opting out or Opting in?', *Journal of Royal College of General Practitioner*, vol. 36, pp. 538-542.

Saks, M. (1994), 'The Alternatives to Medicine', in J. Gabe, D. Kelleher and G. Williams (eds) *Challenging Medicine*, Routledge, London.

Saks, M. (1995), 'The Changing Response of the Medical Profession to Alternative Medicine in Britain: A Case of Altruism or Self-interest?', in T. Johnson, G. Larkin and M. Saks (eds) *Health Professions and the State in Europe*, Routledge, London.

Saltman, R.B. and Von Otter, C. (1992), *Planned Markets and Public Competition: Strategic Reform in Northern Enuropean Health Systems*, Open University Press, Buckingham.

Saunders, P. (1985), *Social Theory and the Urban Question* (2nd ed), Hutchison, London.

Schiffer, J.R. (1991), 'State Policy and Economic Growth: A Note on the Hong Kong Model', *International Journal of Urban and Regional Research*, vol. 115, no. 2, pp. 180-196.

Schneider, S. (1982), 'The Sequential Development of Social Programs in Eighteen Welfare States', *Comparative Social Research*, vol. 5, pp. 195-219.

Schulz, R. and Harrison, S. (1986), 'Physician Autonomy in the Federal Republic of Germany, Great Britain and the United States', *International Journal of Health Planning and Management*, vol. 2, pp. 335-55.

Schwartz, H. (1987), 'Irrationality as a Feature of Health Care in the United States', in H. Schwartz (ed) *Dominant Issues in Medical Sociology* (2nd ed), Random House, New York.

Scott, I. (1995), 'Political Transformation in Hong Kong: From Colony to Colony', in R.Y.W. Kwok and A.Y. So (eds) *The Hong Kong-Guangdong Link: Partnership in Flux*, Hong Kong University Press, Hong Kong.

Scott, I. and Cheek-Milby, K. (1986), 'An Overview of Hong Kong's Social Policy-making Process', *The Asian Journal of Public Administration*, vol. 8, pp. 166-176.

Scott, W.D. (1985), *The Delivery of Medical Services in Hospitals*, Government Printer, Hong Kong.

Secretary for Chinese Affairs, Hong Kong Government (1952), *Annual Departmental Report 1951-52*, Government Printer, Hong Kong.

Shultz, S. (1991), 'Health Insurance: A Comparison of Medical Benefits in the United States and Hong Kong', *AmCham*, vol. 23, no. 5, pp. 37-40.

Sidell, M. (1995), *Health in Old Age: Myth, Mystery and Management*, Open University Press, Buckingham.

Sing Tao Daily, 22 April 1996 (in Chinese).

Sinn, E. (1989), *Power and Charity: The Early History of the Tung Wah Hospital, Hong Kong*, Oxford University Press, Hong Kong.

Smith, A. (1985), *An Inquiry into the Nature and Causes of the Wealth of Nations* (5th ed), Modern Library, New York.

Smith, M.J. (1993), *Pressure, Power and Policy: State Autonomy and Policy Networks in Britain and the United States*, Harvester Wheatsheaf, London.

So, K.M. (1991), 'A Proposal for Contract Medicine', in Hong Kong Medical Association (ed) *Discussion Paper on Contract Medicine for Another Open Forum on 24 July 1991*, HKMA, Hong Kong.

Social Welfare Department, Hong Kong Government (1960), *Annual Departmental Report 1959/60*, Government Printer, Hong Kong.

Social Welfare Department, Hong Kong Government (1993), *Five Year Plan Review 1993*, Government Printer, Hong Kong.

Sommers, T. and Shields, L. (1987), *Women Take Care: The Consequences of Caregiving in Today's Society*, Triad, Gainesville.

Sorell, T. (1991), *Scientism: Philosophy and the Infatuation with Science*, Routledge, London.

South China Morning Post, 4 June 1991; 21 April, 1994.

Squires, P. (1990), *Anti-Social Policy: Welfare, Ideology and the Disciplinary State*, Harvester Wheatsheaf, London.

Stacey, M. (1976), 'The Health Service Consumer: A Sociological Misconception', in M. Stacey (ed) *The Sociology of the National Health Service*, University of Keele, Keele.

Stacey, M. (1988), *The Sociology of Health and Healing: A Textbook*, Unwin Hyman, London.

Staples, C. (1989), 'The Politics of Employment-Based Insurance in the US', *International Journal of Health Services*, vol. 19, no. 3, pp. 414-31.

Starr, P. (1993), 'The Politics of Health Care Inequalities', in D.E. Rogers and E. Ginzberg (eds) *Medical Care and the Health of the Poor*, Westview Press, Boulder.

Starr, P. and Immergut, E. (1987), 'Health Care and the Boundaries of Politics', in C.S. Maier (ed) *Changing Boundaries of the Political*, Cambridge University Press, Cambridge.

Stone, H. (1979), 'Wholistic Healing: Historic Base and Short History', in H.A. Otto and J.W. Knight (eds) *Dimensions in Wholistic Healing*, Nelson-Hall, Chicago.

Sub-Committee of Task Force on Community Health, United Christian Service (1970), *Survey of Kwun Tong Medical and Health Services*, United Christian Service, Hong Kong.

Sung, Y.W. (1986), 'Fiscal and Economic Policies in Hong Kong', in J.Y.S. Cheng (ed) *Hong Kong in Transition*, Oxford University Press, Hong Kong.

Swedberg, R. (1986), 'The Critique of the "Economy and Society" Perspective During the Paradigm Crisis', *Acta Sociologica*, vol. 29, pp. 91-112.

Swedberg, R. (1987), 'Economic Sociology', *Current Sociology*, vol. 35, pp. 1-215.

Tai Kun Pao, 24 October 1993 (in Chinese).

Tang, D. (1978), 'Regionalisation of the Medical and Health Services', *Society of Community Medicine Hong Kong Bulletin*, vol. 9, pp. 101-104.

Tang, J.T.H. and Ching, F. (1994), 'The MacLehose-Youde Years: Balancing the "Three-Legged Stool", 1971-1986', in M.K. Chan and J.D. Young (eds) *Precarious Balance: Hong Kong between China and Britain, 1842-1992*, Hong Kong University Press, Hong Kong.

Taylor, S.E. et al. (1988) 'Sources of Satisfaction and Dissatisfaction among Members of Cancer Support Groups', in B.H. Gottlieb (eds) *Marshalling Social Support*, Sage, New York.

Ten Have, H.A.M.J. (1995), 'Choosing Core Health Services in the Netherlands', in D. Seedhouse (ed) *Reforming Health Care: The Philosophy and Practice of International Health Reform*, Wiley, Chichester.

Terris, M. (1978), 'The Three World Systems of Medical Care: Trends and Prospects', *American Journal of Public Health*, vol. 68, pp. 1125-1131.

Titmuss, R.M. (1974), *Social Policy: An Introduction*, Allen and Unwin, London.

Titmuss, R.M. (1976), *Essays on 'The Welfare State'* (3rd ed), George Allen and Unwin, London.

Topley, M. (1969), 'The Role of Savings and Wealth Among Hong Kong Chinese', in I.C. Jarvie (ed) *Hong Kong: A Society in Transition*, RKP, London.

Topley, M. (1976), 'Chinese Traditional Etiology and Methods of Cure in Hong Kong', in C. Leslie (ed) *Asian Medical Systems: A Comparative Study*, University of California Press, Berkeley.

Topley, M. (1978), 'Chinese and Western Medicine in Hong Kong: Some Social and Cultural Determinants of Variation, Interaction and Change', in Klienman, et al. (ed) *Culture and Healing in Asian Societies: Anthropological, Psychiatric and Public Health Studies*, Shenkman Publishing Co, Massachusettes.

Townsend, P. and Davidson, N (1982), *The Black Report*, Penguin, London.

Tsang, S.Y.S. (1988), *Democracy Shelved: Great Britain, China and Attempts at Constitutional Reform in Hong Kong, 1945-1952*, Oxford University Press, Hong Kong.

Tung Wah Group of Hospitals (1961), *Development of the Tung Wah Hospital, 1870-1960*, Tung Wah Group of Hospitals, Hong Kong.

Tung Wah Group of Hospitals (1971), *One Hundred Years of the Tung Wah Group of Hospitals, 1870-1970*, Tung Wah Group of Hospitals, Hong Kong.

Tung Wah Group of Hospitals (1990), *Tung Wah Group of Hospitals: Annual Report 1989*, Tung Wah Group of Hospitals, Hong Kong.

Turner, B.S. (1988), *Medical Power and Social Knowledge*, Sage London.

Turshen, M. (1975), *The Political Economy of Health with a Case Study of Tanzania*, Unpublished Ph.D thesis, University of Sussex, Sussex.

Turshen, M. (1977), 'The Political Ecology of Disease', *Review of Radical Political Economics*, vol. 9, pp. 45-60.

Turshen, M. (1989), *The Politics of Public Health*, Rutgers University Press, New Jersey.

Twigg, J. (1993), 'Integrating Carers into the Service System: Six Strategic Responses', *Ageing and Society*, vol. 13, pp. 141-170.

Twigg, J. (1994), 'Community Care', *Ageing and Society*, vol. 14, pp. 619-22.

Twigg, J. and Atkin, K. (1994), *Carers Perceived: Policy and Practice in Informal Care*, Open University Press, Buckingham.

United Democrats of Hong Kong (1990), 'Provisional Hospital Authority Report Policy Document', *UDHK Policy Documents* No. EC/39/90, UDHK, Hong Kong.

Urry, J. (1981), *The Anatomy of Capitalist Societies: The Economy, Civil Society and the State*, MacMillan, London.

Waddington, I. (1973), 'The Role of the Hospital in the Development of Modern Medicine: A Sociological Analysis', *Sociology*, vol. 7, pp. 211-24.

Wagstaff, A. and Doorslaer, E.V. (1993), 'Equity in the Finance and Delivery of Health Care: Concepts and Definitions', in E.V. Doorslaer, A. Wagstaff and F. Rutten (eds) *Equity in the Finance and Delivery of Health Care: An International Perspective*, Oxford University Press, Oxford.

Waitzkin, H. (1983), 'A Marxist View of Health and Health Care', in D. Mechanic (ed) *Handbook of Health, Health Care, and the Health Professions*, Free Press, New York.

Waldron, S. (1980), *Fire on the Rim: A Study in Contradictions in the Left-wing Political Mobilization in Hong Kong, 1967*, Unpublished PhD thesis, University Microfilms International, Ann Arbor, Michigan.

Walker, A. (1981), 'Towards a Political Economy of Old Age', *Ageing and Society*, vol. 1, no. 1, pp. 73-94.

Walker, A. (1984a), 'The Political Economy of Privatisation', in J. Le Grand and R. Robinson (eds) *Privatisation and the Welfare State*, George Allen & Unwin, London.

Walker, A. (1984b), *Social Planning: A Strategy for Socialist Welfare*, Basil Blackwell, Oxford.

Walker, A. (1988), *Social Policy Versus Economic Policy: The Future of Social Planning*, Department of Social Work, University of Hong Kong, Hong Kong.

Walker, A. (1991), 'The Relationship Between the Family and the State in the Care of Older People', *Canadian Journal on Aging*, vol. 10, no. 2, pp. 94-112.

Walker, A. (ed) (1982), *Community Care: The Family, the State and Social Policy*, Blackwell, Oxford.

Walton, J. (1979), 'Urban Political Economy', *Comp. Urban Res.*, vol. 7, no. 1, pp. 5-17.

Warde, A. (1990), 'Sociology of Consumption', *Sociology*, vol. 24, no. 1, pp. 1-5.

Warde, A. (1992), 'Notes on the Relationship between Production and Consumption', in R. Burrows and C. Marsh (eds) *Consumption and Class: Divisions and Change*, St. Martin's Press, New York.

Weisbrod, B.A. et al. (1973), *Disease and Economic Development*, The University of Wisconsin Press, Wisconsin.

Weller, G.R. and Manga, P. (1983), 'The Push for Reprivatization of Health Care Services in Canada, Britain and the United States', *Journal of Health Politics, Policy and Law*, vol. 8, no. 3, pp. 495-518.

WHO (1985), *Targets for Health for All*, Regional Office for Europe, Copenhagen.

WHO (1987), *Hospitals and Health for All*, WHO, Geneva.

Wildavsky, A. (1977), 'Doing Better and Feeling Worse: The Political Pathology of Health Policy', in J. Knowles (ed) *Doing Better and Feeling Worse*, W.W. Norton, New York.

Wilk, R. (ed) (1989), *The Household Economy*, Westview Press, Boulder.

Wilkin, D. and Hughes, B. (1986), 'The Elderly and the Health Services', in C. Phillipson and A. Walker (eds) *Ageing and Social Policy: A Critical Assessment*, Gower, Hants.

Willcocks, A. (1967), *The Creation of the National Health Service: A Study of Pressure Groups and a Major Policy Decision*, RKP, London.

Williams, E.L. and Fritton, F. (1988), 'Factors Affecting Early Unplanned Readmission of Elderly Patients to Hospital', *British Medical Journal*, vol. 297, pp. 784-787.

Williams, S.J. (1995), *Essentials of Health Services*, Delmar Publishers, New York.

Wilson, E. (1982), 'Women, the "Community" and the "Family"', in A. Walker(ed) *Community Care: The Family, the State and Social Policy*, Blackwell, Oxford.

Wilson, Sir David (1989), *Governor Speech at the 1988/89 Opening Session of the Legislative Council*, Government Printer, Hong Kong.

Wilson, Sir David. (1990), *Governor Speech at the 1990/91 Opening Session of the Legislative Council*, Government Printer, Hong Kong.

Wistow, G., Knapp, M., Hardy, B. and Allen, C. (1994), *Social Care in a Mixed Economy*, Open University Press, Buckingham.

Wolfe, J.R. (1993), *The Coming Health Crisis: Who will Pay for Care for the Aged in the Twenty-first Century?*, The University of Chicago Press, Chicago.

Wolfe, P.R. and Moran, D.W. (1993), 'Global Budgeting in the OECD Countries', *Health Care Financing Review*, vol. 14, no. 3, pp. 55-76.

Wong, A.K. (1972), *The Kaifong Associations and the Society of Hong Kong*, University of Singapore, Singapore.

Wong, E. (1990), 'Elizabeth Wong's Address to the Legislative Council on April 4, 1990', *Hong Kong Hansard 1989/90*, pp. 1165-69, Government Printer, Hong Kong.

Wong, E. (1994), *More Choice to the Public: Press Release by Mrs. Elizabeth Wong on 18 January 1994*, Government Information Service, Hong Kong.

Wong et al. (1993a), 'Traditional Chinese Medicine and Western Medicine in Hong Kong: A Comparison of the Consultation Process and side effects', *Journal of Hong Kong Medical Association*, vol. 45, no. 4, pp. 278-284.

Wong et al. (1993b), 'A Study of Traditional Chinese Medicine Practitioners in Hong Kong', *Journal of Hong Kong Medical Association*, vol. 45, no. 4, pp. 285-290.

Wong, V.C.W. (1992), 'Towards a Recommodification of Medical Care: The Case of Hong Kong'. *Occassional Paper Series, Department of Social Work*, no. 6, Hong Kong Baptist College, Hong Kong.

Wong, V.C.W. (1996), 'Medical and Health', in Nyaw, M.K. and Li, S.M. (eds), *The Other Hong Kong Report 1996*, The Chinese University Press, Hong Kong, pp. 449-468.

Wong, V.C.W. (1998), *The Pathway to Health Care for Patients of Traditional Chinese Medicine Practitioners*, Hong Kong Council of Social Service, Hong Kong.

Wong, V.C.W. (1999), 'Medical and Heath Care Policy in Hong Kong: A Critical Examination', in J.K.C. Lee, S.W.S. Chiu, L.C. Leung and K.W. Chan (eds), *New Social Policy*, The Chinese University Press, Hong Kong, pp. 195-212 (in Chinese).

Wong, V.C.W. and Chiu, M.Y.L. (1998), 'The Pathway to Health Care for Orthopaedic Inpatients', *Health Information*, no. 193, pp. 32-33 (in Chinese).

Wong, V.C.W. and Chiu, S.W.S. (1997), 'Health-Care Reforms in the People's Republic of China: Strategies and Social Implications', *The International Journal of Public Sector Management*, vol. 10, nos. 1&2, pp. 76-92.

Woo, J. (1994), 'A Survey of Elderly People Discharged from Hospital', in Hong Kong Council of Social Service (ed) *International Conference on Family and Community Care Conference Proceedings*, Hong Kong Council of Social Service, Hong Kong.

Working Group on Care for the Elderly (1994), *Report of the Working Group on Care for the Elderly*, Government Printer, Hong Kong.

Working Group on Research for International Year of the Family (1994), *Role of the Family in Community Care*, Hong Kong Council of Social Service, Hong Kong.

Working Party on Chinese Medicine (1991), *Working Party on Chinese Medicine, Interim Report*, Government Printer, Hong Kong.

Working Party on Chinese Medicine (1994), *Report of the Working Party on Chinese Medicine*, Government Printer, Hong Kong.

Working Party on Primary Health Care (1990), *Health for All: The Way Ahead: Report of the Working Party on Primary Health Care*, Government Printer, Hong Kong.

Working Party on the Future Needs of the Elderly (1973), *Services for the Elderly*, Government Printer, Hong Kong.

Working Party on Unregistrable Doctors (1975), *Report of the Working Party on Unregistrable Doctors*, Government Printer, Hong Kong.

Woronoff, J. (1980), *Hong Kong: Capitalist Paradise*, Heinemann Asia, Hong Kong.

Youngson, A.J. (1982), *Hong Kong Economic Growth and Policy*, Oxford University Press, Hong Kong.

Yuen, P.P. (1994), 'The Corporatisation of Public Hospital Services in Hong Kong: A Possible Public Choice Explanation', *Asian Journal of Public Administration*, vol. 16, no. 2, pp. 165-181.

Yuen, P.P. (1988a), 'The Characteristics of Private Hospital Patients in Hong Kong: A Discriminant Analysis Approach', *Proceedings of the 1988 Pan-Pacific Conference V*, Singapore.

Yuen, P.P. (1988b), 'The Private Medical Insurance Market in Hong Kong: Implications for the Privatization of Health Services', *Proceedings of the 1988 Annual Conference of the Academy of International Business* (South East Asia Region), Bangkok.

Yuen, P.P. (1992), *Cost Containment Strategies and Fee Policies for Public Hospitals*. Paper No. FWC 5/92, Health and Welfare Branch, Hong Kong Government.

Yuen, P.P. (1994), 'Health-Care Systems and Demands', in J. Fry and N. Yuen (eds) *Principles and Practice of Primary Care and Family Medicine: Asia-Pacific Perspective*, Radcliffe Medical Press Ltd, Oxford.

Index